Surgical Management of Endometriosis

Surgical Management of Endometriosis

Edited by

David B Redwine MD
Endometriosis Institute of Oregon
Bend, Oregon
USA

© 2004 Martin Dunitz, an imprint of the Taylor & Francis Group plc

First published in 2004

Published in the USA and Canada by
Martin Dunitz, Taylor & Francis Group
29 West 35th Street, New York, NY 10001
and in the UK by
Martin Dunitz, Taylor & Francis Group
11 New Fetter Lane, London EC4P 4EE
Tel.:   +44 (0) 20 7583 9855
Fax.:   +44 (0) 20 7842 2298
E-mail: info@dunitz.co.uk
Website: http://www.dunitz.co.uk

All rights reserved. No part of this publication may be reproduced, stored in a retrieval system, or transmitted, in any form or by any means, electronic, mechanical, photocopying, recording, or otherwise, without the prior permission of the publisher or in accordance with the provisions of the Copyright, Designs and Patents Act 1988 or under the terms of any licence permitting limited copying issued by the Copyright Licensing Agency, 90 Tottenham Court Road, London W1P 0LP.

Although every effort has been made to ensure that all owners of copyright material have been acknowledged in this publication, we would be glad to acknowledge in subsequent reprints or editions any omissions brought to our attention.

A CIP record for this book is available from the British Library.
ISBN 1 84184 248 6
Distributed in the USA by
Fulfilment Center
Taylor & Francis
10650 Toebben Drive
Independence, KY 41051, USA
Toll Free Tel.: +1 800 634 7064
E-mail: taylorandfrancis@thomsonlearning.com

Distributed in Canada by
Taylor & Francis
74 Rolark Drive
Scarborough, Ontario M1R 4G2, Canada
Toll Free Tel.: +1 877 226 2237
E-mail: tal_fran@istar.ca

Distributed in the rest of the world by
Thomson Publishing Services
Cheriton House
North Way
Andover, Hampshire SP10 5BE, UK
Tel.: +44 (0)1264 332424
E-mail: salesorder.tandf@thomsonpublishingservices.co.uk

Composition by J&L Composition, Filey, North Yorkshire, UK

Printed and bound in Spain by Grafos S.A. Arte Sobre Papel

Table of contents

List of contributors	vii
Preface	ix
1. Was Sampson wrong? *David B Redwine*	1
2. Berkson's fallacy and endometriosis *David B Redwine*	13
3. Modern medical therapy of endometriosis *David L Olive*	25
4. Patient preparation *David B Redwine*	47
5. Principles of monopolar electrosurgery *David B Redwine*	61
6. Electrosurgical resection of endometriosis *Ray Garry*	71
7. Laser vaporization and electrocoagulation of endometriosis *Chrisopher Sutton*	87
8. Excision of endometriosis with the carbon dioxide laser *Robert Albee*	109
9. Fiber laser excision of endometriosis *Thomas L Lyons*	127
10. Harmonic scalpel excision of endometriosis *Martin Robbins*	137
11. Ovarian endometriosis *David B Redwine*	149

12. Intestinal endometriosis 157
    David B Redwine

13. Rectovaginal endometriosis 175
    Jeremy Wright

14. Endometriosis of the urinary tract 191
    David B Redwine

15. Diaphragmatic endometriosis 205
    David B Redwine

16. Conservative excision of endometriosis at laparotomy 211
    David B Redwine

17. Endometriosis in distant sites 223
    David B Redwine

    Index 235

Contributors

Robert B. Albee Jr. MD
Medical Director
Center for Endometriosis Care
Atlanta, Georgia
USA

Ray Garry MD FRCOG FRNCOG
Professor of Clinical Gynaecology
University of Western Australia
School of Women's and Infant's Health
King Edward Memorial Hospital
374 Bagot Rd
Subiaco Perth
WA 6008
Australia

Thomas L Lyons MD
Director
Center for Women's Care and
Reproductive Surgery
Suite 6230
1140 Hammond Drive
Atlanta, Georgia GA 30328
USA

David Olive MD
Professor of Obstetrics and Gynecology
University of Wisconsin Medical School
600 Highland Avenue
Madison, Wisconsin 53792
USA

David B. Redwine MD
Endometriosis Institute of Oregon
2190 NE Professional Court
Bend, Oregon
OR 97701
USA

Martin L. Robbins MD
New England Center for Endometriosis
148 State Street
Portland, Maine 04101
USA

Christopher Sutton MD
Honorary Consultant Gynaecologist
Royal Surry County Hospital, Guildford;
Emeritus Consultant
Chelsea and Westminster Hospital
Imperial College School of Medicine
London;
Professor of Gynaecological Surgery
University of Guildford,
UK

Jeremy Wright FRCOG
Centre for Endometriosis and Pelvic Pain
Woking Nuffield Hospital
Shores Road, Woking GU21 4BY;
Consultant Gynaecologist and
Minimal Access Surgeon
Ashford & St. Peters NHS Trust,
Guildford Road
Chertsey KT16 0PZ
UK

Preface

If you are a gynecologist dealing with endometriosis, you know the trite drill dictated by conventional wisdom: in the office diagnose pelvic pain as a sexually transmitted pelvic inflammatory disease (PID) and treat with antibiotics; diagnose recurrent pelvic pain as recurrent PID in a woman with loose morals and treat again with antibiotics; when the patient (sometimes virginal) re-presents with pain thought to be due to yet another recurrent sexually transmitted disease, perform a laparoscopy and finally diagnose endometriosis; shine a coherent beam of light at the disease or put a metal electrode on the various spots and step on a foot pedal to unleash unseen electrons and pronounce that the disease is treated; after surgery administer powerful and expensive medical agents with multiple side-effects and reassure the patient that this combination of treatment will be the best treatment for her disease since this is what most clinicians use; shuffle the suffering patient to various other practitioners, including psychiatrists and pain clinics; question her about childhood sexual abuse when her pain does not respond well; repeat a laparoscopy; repeat the same therapies which did not seem to work the first time; repeat these a third time to be certain they did not work the second time; perform a total abdominal hysterectomy and bilateral salpingo-oophorectomy; rush off to perform a routine vaginal delivery when the patient returns to the office complaining of pain and vasomotor menopausal symptoms. What is wrong with this picture? Modern therapy of endometriosis has become unimaginative, rigid and dogmatic.

It is universally acknowledged that endometriosis is a confusing, enigmatic, mysterious disease, but this need not be so. Confusion is an opportunity for change if this confusion is recognized for what it is: lack of accurate information. Whereas the debate about the origin of the disease rages confusingly, the debate on treatment has become quite distilled. The word 'treatment' is used here in the same manner as when one talks about treatment of a urinary tract infection: the disease is gone when treatment is concluded, and symptoms once caused by the disease are gone as well. This use of the word 'treatment' is familiar and comforting to patients and physicians and can be used to summarize modern therapy of endometriosis accurately in one sentence – Since no available medicine eradicates endometriosis, surgery is its only treatment. It thus becomes a question simply of which type of surgical treatment most effectively eradicates the disease. This book will help the reader answer that question.

The introductory chapters written by me present my thoughts on various topics related to the history and treatment of endometriosis which I think are important in understanding the confusion accompanying the disease. These chapters are based on a deep and broad familiarity of the literature as well as a quarter century of personal and professional interest in the disease.

Most of the confusion regarding endometriosis stems from long-held biases that are rooted in misinformation. Our profession must grapple with the probability that Sampson's theory of origin is incorrect because the facts upon which it was based were incorrect. Sampson did not have all the facts we have today when he devised this theory. It seems unlikely that he would have supported reflux menstruation as the origin of endometriosis if he had been aware of the information in Chapter 1. Continuing support for his theory of origin is not just an intellectual question, because this theory directly affects the treatment of most women today. If the theory is wrong, then it is probable that most women with the disease are being poorly treated.

Misunderstanding about endometriosis is due to a predictable phenomenon which has a name: Berkson's fallacy. This fallacy has operated from the very beginning of our understanding of the disease and its effects are discussed in Chapter 2. Because Berkson's fallacy has operated unidentified and uncorrected for many decades, its deleterious effects on our understanding have been magnified over time and have become huge. This has led to enormous inertia in understanding, treatment and research because we have been unwilling to give up the past, partly because of the fear that we have been so wrong for so long. Things can be made right by leaving our minds open to new thoughts regarding the disease, with the possibility that we must reject much of what we think we know. Understanding clearly the origins of our current confusion will make it easier to face a future which contains the real truth about the disease.

The practice of medicine is sublimely simple because there are only three choices available for almost any ailment: (1) Do nothing. (2) Treat with medicine. (3) Treat with surgery. The patient with endometriosis will already have tried doing nothing, and that did not work because she is now in your office. This simplifies greatly the care of patients with endometriosis, because once the diagnosis is made surgically, there are only two treatment options: medicine or surgery. (Observation of a treatable disease which has led to surgery is not rational by anyone's judgment. If observation seems rational, then surgery should not have been done.) To decide between these two modalities, more information is needed, and this book provides that information. The history of development of medical therapy is outlined in Chapter 3, and modern medical therapy and possibilities for the future are discussed in Chapter 4. It should be apparent after reading these chapters that endometriosis is a disease which requires surgery for diagnosis and treatment, and this should be a part of the process of informed consent with the patient.

The remainder of the book is its *raison d'être*: how to treat virtually any manifestation of endometriosis surgically using any one of a number of surgical energy systems. Since surgery is a visual as well as a tactile and judgmental art, an effort has been made to provide illustrations of surgical strategies with the hope that if a surgeon sees what is supposed to happen, it can be made to happen in that surgeon's hands. The chapters by experts in surgical treatment of endometriosis will allow readers to compare surgical energy systems and perhaps choose one that is most adaptable to their surgical style. There is admittedly a heavy emphasis on excision, which alone is able to treat both superficial and invasive endometriosis completely anywhere in the body.

Many of the chapters and accompanying illustrations were produced by myself. These images were selected to illustrate what I consider to be important points gained through the surgical treatment of over 2500 patients with endometriosis from around the world. Most of these patients have had multiple surgeries and several rounds of medical therapy. One common thread clearly stands out: their disease has never been completely eradicated. They are dealing not with recurrent disease, but with persistent disease. Everything possible has been done to them and to their disease except one thing: the disease has never been removed from their bodies.

This book will help surgeons to eradicate endometriosis from any location in the body. Endometriosis surgery is rightfully considered the most difficult surgery to be done in gynecology, and some cases will seem to be the most difficult surgery possible anywhere in the human body, maximally taxing the mental and physical strength of the surgeon. For those surgeons who relish challenge, endometriosis is the perfect disease.

David B Redwine

1

Was Sampson wrong?

David B Redwine

Endometriosis is the presence outside the uterus of tissue which somewhat resembles endometrium from the uterine lining. It affects approximately 10% of the female population in their reproductive years and may cause non-menstrual or menstrual pain as well as infertility. The most widely held theory of origin is Sampson's theory of reflux menstruation. Sampson's final version of his theory[1] proposed that endometriosis occurs as a result of the reflux of menstrual blood out through the end of the fallopian tubes, this blood carrying with it viable cells from the endometrial lining which could attach to peritoneal surfaces, proliferate, invade, and become the disease known as endometriosis.

This theory has undergone successive mutations by Sampson and others to accommodate new information. It is helpful to read Sampson's earlier papers with one of his last papers as a guide to understand fully the thought processes which resulted in this theory.[2]

Sampson burst on the endometriosis scene in 1921,[3] with a study of 23 cases of ovarian chocolate cysts, although endometriosis was confirmed histologically in only 9 cases. This focus on the ovaries convinced him that the ovaries were the most common site of disease and he proposed that endometriosis appeared on or within the ovaries as a result of metaplasia or embryonic rests. He noted that ovaries involved by endometriosis were frequently adherent to the pelvic sidewall or uterus, in which locations endometriosis could also be found. He surmised that the endometriosis on these contiguous pelvic surfaces was the result of direct extension or seeding from menstrual bleeding from ovarian endometriotic cysts or from superficial disease of the ovarian cortex. Like Cullen,[4-7] Stevens,[8] and Lockyer[9] before him, he described thick adhesions in the cul de sac between the rectum and uterus which could accompany ovarian endometriomas and proposed that such adhesions were the result of repeated irritation of the peritoneum by monthly leakage of blood from the ovarian cysts. Although he recognized that endometriosis could be present in an 'adenomyomatous' form beneath the visible adhesions with involvement of both the rectal wall and the cervical stroma, his focus on this morphologic feature (which now is commonly referred to as obliteration of the cul de sac) revolved around an adhesive process rather than an endometriotic process. Observing that only 9 of 16 married women had been pregnant in an era when the normal pregnancy rate was thought to approach 100%, Sampson introduced the notion that pregnancy protected against endometriosis or that infertility promoted it. This was before tubal, ovulatory or male factors were commonly recognized as possible contributors to infertility, and certainly well before the current knowledge that pain (not infertility) is the most common and most specific symptom of the disease. In that day, the term 'adenomyoma' was used to reflect the histologic appearance of what is now commonly called invasive or deep endometriosis, where glands and stroma of endometriosis are surrounded by dense fibromuscular metaplasia somewhat resembling tissue which can be seen in a uterine leiomyoma.

With increasing experience and reading of the older literature, Sampson shifted his thoughts by 1922, although not necessarily toward greater clarity.[10] He noted that Russel in 1899 had referred to earlier works by Nagel and Waldeyer who had found that the germinal epithelium of the posterior fetal pelvis was the origin of all Müllerian structures. In fact, evidence existed that the germinal epithelium of the mature ovary itself could give rise to endometriosis since germinal epithelium could be traced in serial sections of ovarian cortex and seen to transform into tubular structures containing glandular structures resembling endometrium. While this seemed to solidify the concept of an embryonic origin of endometriosis, Sampson headed in another direction based on speculation and specious concepts which must have seemed correct to him at the time:

- He observed that the surface of the ovary could contain ciliated epithelium resembling the epithelial lining of the Fallopian tube, bringing to mind the possibility that Müllerian epithelium of the Fallopian tube could slough and shed out of the end of the tube and attach and implant on the ovary.
- He concluded that the ovarian tubules of Nagel and Waldeyer must be the result of implantation of epithelium from the Fallopian tube or endometrium on the ovary with secondary formation of tubules.
- He concluded that these tubules were the origin of ovarian endometriosis and that the ovaries are the most common site of disease in part because they are so near the ostia of the Fallopian tubes.
- He concluded that endometriosis formed later in life, usually after the age of 30, because he had only seen two patients younger than 30, so endometriosis could not possibly be a congenital or developmental process, otherwise it could be seen shortly after menarche.
- By a method of study which is unclear, he noted that ovarian and peritoneal endometriosis appeared to be of the same chronological age, so they must have a common source and time of origin such as retrograde menstruation.
- Observing obliteration of the cul de sac, uterine leiomyomas and endometrial polyps in some, but not all patients, he concluded that these pathologies might result in retrograde passage of menstrual blood out of the Fallopian tubes, which always appeared to be open, thus facilitating development of endometriosis.
- He noted that the ovarian adhesions associated with endometriosis were similar in location to adhesion resulting from salpingitis spreading out from the end of the tubes so they must have a similar transtubal origin, such as reflux menstruation.
- He noted that some patients could have adenomyomatous endometriosis without coexisting ovarian endometrioma cysts, indicating that infrequently peritoneal endometriosis might exist without ovarian disease.

In his final version[1] of the theory of reflux menstruation, he had concluded that the ovaries are not as commonly involved by endometriosis as he had once thought. Peritoneal disease could occur in the absence of ovarian disease and actually seemed more common and clinically more important than ovarian disease, a position he later affirmed.[2] Since he had seen menstrual blood exiting the tubal ostia during surgery performed during menses, and since some Fallopian tubes removed at hysterectomy had endometrial fragments within them, he concluded that refluxed endometrium was likely the source of ovarian and pelvic endometriosis, and that rupture or bleeding of ovarian endometrioma cysts could result in peritoneal disease by secondary implantation. It is clear in his writings that the mode of spread of ovarian cancer weighed heavily in his conclusions about the spread of endometriosis. It is also clear that he considered endometriosis to be identical to endometrium and that the tubes were usually open. Among 293 cases of endometriosis surgically diagnosed by that time in his career, six had bilateral tubal blockage and he concluded that reflux menstruation must have occurred before blockage of the tubes. Much of the rest of his career was spent defending his theory against attacks by Emil Novak, one of the pre-eminent gynecologists of the first half of the 20th century. Dr Novak was highly skeptical of the evidence supporting reflux menstruation as the origin of endometriosis and favored coelomic metaplasia instead.[11]

Where to begin? How could an initial study with such small numbers in which most patients did not have histologic confirmation of ovarian endometrioma cysts be accepted as a seminal paper on the disease? Sampson's intimation of a cause and effect between endometriosis and infertility seems unsupportable since other fertility factors were not considered, and the notion that normal fertility approaches 100% seems unreasonable today. Sampson could have easily argued that since most of his married patients with endometriosis had been pregnant, that pregnancy or fertility causes endometriosis. There was no evidence whatsoever that tubal epithelium sloughs, attaches to the ovary and grows into the ovarian tubules of Nagel and Waldeyer. Sampson also took evidence which had previously been interpreted by those who developed it as showing development of ovarian cortical epithelium into glandular tissue (from the 'inside out') and turned it on its head, now introducing an interpretation whereby glandular elements alight upon the ovary and begin to penetrate it (from the 'outside in'). Again, there was no real evidence to support this usurpation of intellectual primacy. The youngest patient with endometriosis was noted to be 10.5 years,[12] and an entire literature on the visual appearance of endometriosis shows that teenagers can, indeed, have endometriosis which is often not identified because it is so subtle. Sampson's incorrect conclusion that endometriosis forms only in later years was clearly the result of selection bias since he was concentrating on disease which was apparently easily and more frequently diagnosed because of the presence of ovarian endometrioma cysts, which occur more commonly in older age groups. His conclusion that endometriosis could not be congenital was unsustainable since it arose from incorrect data, so another of the initial pillars supporting his belief in his theory topples. Regarding the notion that uterine structural or positional abnormalities might encourage reflux menstruation and development of endometriosis, he apparently did not consider the likelihood that endometriosis might have been present before the development of fibroids or uterine retroversion related to obliteration of the cul de sac, thus rendering moot the notion of facilitation of menstrual reflux by these conditions. The conclusion that adhesions of endometriosis must have a tubal origin since they are similar to adhesions resulting from salpingitis is obviously comparing apples to oranges. The most common site of involvement by disease began to shift in Sampson's mind from the ovaries to the peritoneum, especially the cul de sac, a process thought to be facilitated by the effects of gravity, although a plausible alternate explanation based on fetal pelvic organogenesis across the posterior coelomic cavity exists.[13] The notion that endometriosis is identical to endometrium has been thoroughly dispelled by modern data.[14]

Most of Sampson's theory was promulgated on the basis of speculation, errors of interpretation or leaps of faith, aided and abetted by Berkson's fallacy (discussed in Chapter 2) and skewed by the very small number of cases seen in his career. Additionally, Sampson obviously had a personal bias toward supporting this theory and was its greatest champion for over two decades. If his theory is misleading and incorrect, he can be forgiven since he was doing the best with the evidence at hand. But what of modern support for this theory? We have much more evidence than did Sampson. How have we used it? Sadly, not well. In Sampson's absence, generations of authors have become apologists for this theory. What has been written in the distant past has often been repeated without thought or consideration of more recent available evidence. Circumstantial evidence is sometimes grotesquely twisted in an effort to support the theory. There are several examples of this which are readily identifiable to modern clinicians.

Continuing errors of interpretation

It is still possible to read that the ovaries are the most common site of disease. This notion was on its way out in 1927 by Sampson's own evidence and has no place in rational discussion of endometriosis. Modern studies of endometriosis in all its morphologic forms clearly indicate that the cul de sac is the most common area of pelvic involvement.[15] Even if the frequency of involvement of the right ovary were added to that of the left and the total taken as one area, the frequency of involvement of the ovaries would still trail the cul de sac, left broad ligament, left uterosacral ligament, right broad ligament and right uterosacral ligament.

One of the consequences predicted by Sampson's theory is that more of the pelvis should be involved by endometriosis with the passing of time. If monthly seedings of menstrual endometrium were occurring, the pelvis should fill up with endometriosis like a pasture filling up with dandelions. Older age groups should have more disease than younger age groups, and most untreated patients should develop more extensive disease over time. Such a progressively spreading character of endometriosis is a widely held belief among clinicians. But what is the evidence that this occurs? Actually none at all. Older age groups do not have more disease than younger age groups regardless of whether disease extent is measured by the number of pelvic areas involved,[16] the revised American Fertility Society (rAFS) classification system,[17] or by the square centimeters of peritoneum involved by disease.[18] Most untreated patients do not have disease progression between surgical investigations.[19-22]

Another of the consequences predicted by Sampson's theory is that it should be impossible to cure endometriosis since the pelvis will only be re-seeded by monthly reflux menstruation. Actually, it has been known for over half a century that endometriosis can be cured by conservative surgery,[23] and recurrence rates following conservative surgery are surprisingly low.[24-31] And cure rates of over 50% following one conservative surgery in 'resistant' or difficult cases have been confirmed by modern studies at laparoscopy[32] or laparotomy.[33]

The mysterious circulation within the peritoneal cavity

A slight increased frequency of involvement of the left side of the pelvis has been explained by an especially strained mutation of Sampson's theory. An alleged intraperitoneal circulation of fluid from the left upper quadrant down across the cul de sac and ascending to the right upper quadrant is thought by some to alter the pelvic microenvironment. Thus, eddies of this circulation caused by the protective effect of the sigmoid colon's physiologic attachment to the left pelvic brim supposedly predispose to the deposition of regurgitant cells in the left side of the pelvis which is more protected by the sigmoid. The 'proof' of existence of such a circulation is dubious. In one experiment on stillborn infants, artificial perforations were created in intestines, and barium was injected continuously over 3 hours and x-rays were taken to follow the course of the barium.[34] Depending on where the perforation was created, barium could literally disperse in any direction. In one stillborn female infant, the uterus was perforated and barium was injected at a pressure of 100 mmHg and was seen to travel into the right upper quadrant! In another study,[35] a catheter was passed through the right subcostal margin of the abdominal wall of rhesus monkeys and led down to the right iliac fossa. Another catheter was placed into the left upper quadrant of the peritoneal cavity and not advanced. Radioactive albumen was injected through the second catheter and was found to eventually track up the path of the first catheter, which is unsurprising. It is astounding that such evidence is offered to support the theory of reflux menstruation.

The immune system arm of Sampson's theory

One persistent question about reflux menstruation is why all women do not develop endometriosis. It has been found that between 80%[36] and 90%[37] of women with patent Fallopian tubes have bloody peritoneal fluid during menses, while only 15% of women with tubal blockage have bloody fluid during menses.[37] This suggests that the actual rate of bloody peritoneal fluid due to reflux menstruation may be about 75–80% of women rather than 100% as is often stated. In any event, it seems safe to say that a great majority of women have reflux menstruation but most do not develop endometriosis. While one possible conclusion that comes quickly to mind would be that reflux menstruation has nothing to do with development of endometriosis, supporters of Sampson's theory have provided yet another mutation to explain this on an immune basis.

The immune arm of Sampson's theory alleges that women with endometriosis have decrepit immune systems which cannot identify and destroy refluxed menstrual endometrium and so these cells are allowed to attach to peritoneal surfaces and to proliferate and invade to become the disease known as endometriosis. In women with normal immune systems, the refluxed cells are supposedly attacked and digested before attachment can occur. Since the immune system functions in part to identify 'non-self', one immediate objection to this notion is that the immune system should not be expected to attack refluxed endometrial cells in the first place since they are 'self'.

If all women destined to develop endometriosis have decrepit immune systems, then there should be an extraordinarily high rate of immune system diseases, cancers, and opportunistic infections perhaps approaching 100% in women with endometriosis. However, a large questionnaire survey of women with surgically proved endometriosis found that most women with endometriosis did not have endocrinological disease, autoimmune inflammatory diseases, or chronic pain and fatigue, with the prevalence of these conditions ranging between 0.5% and 9.6%. Nonetheless, these prevalence rates were increased by between 0.9 times and 180.5 times over the prevalence of historical population controls.[38] A population-based study in Sweden found a slight increase of ovarian, breast and hematopoietic cancers among patients with endometriosis, but it was clear that most women with endometriosis will not develop cancer,[39] and no one has documented a high rate of opportunistic infections in women with endometriosis. Another problem with this concept is that no one has produced evidence of the immunological warfare which is alleged to occur in the pelvis of women with normal immune systems who do not develop endometriosis. Presumably, there should be easily obtained photomicrographic evidence of macrophage destruction of refluxed endometrium since this must be occurring in billions of instances.

Decreased natural killer (NK) cell activity against autologous endometrium has been identified as due to both a defect in NK activity as well as resistance of the endometrium to NK activity,[40] and this defect is more pronounced with increasing stage of disease.[41] This defect persists after excision of endometriosis, indicating that it apparently is not a result of the effect of endometriosis but a primary defect originating elsewhere in the body.[42] The NK defect may be secondary to an unknown effect of the uterus or ovarian endometriomas since removal of these organs results in an improvement of NK activity.[43] Thus, the evidence suggests that NK activity is not directly related to endometriosis and seems unlikely related to its origin in the manner postulated.

The immune system can be activated in patients with endometriosis, with increased macrophage activity found both within the peritoneal fluid itself,[44] as well as within the endometriotic lesion itself.[45]

It is clear that most women with endometriosis do not have immune system problems but that their immune systems are dynamic and active, producing an appropriate inflammatory response to the effects of the disease. Some, but not all, may have accompanying abnormalities of the immune system but it would be incorrect to conclude that these abnormalities have anything at all to do with facilitating attachment of refluxed endometrial cells.

Where is the evidence?

Despite almost 100 years of research, Sampson's theory remains a theory supported only by circumstantial evidence. The simplest evidence to prove Sampson's theory would be to display photomicrographs of the steps that are missing: (1) Initial attachment of endometrial fragments to peritoneal surfaces. (2) Secondary proliferation and invasion of the attached cells. These two steps occur by the billions during the course of any year so it would be simple to photograph one or both of these steps and our textbooks should be filled with clear photographic evidence of hundreds or thousands of examples of initial attachment. Despite the ease of such proof, no convincing photomicrographs exist as such proof. Researchers examining the concept of microscopic endometriosis found no evidence of initial attachment in hundreds of biopsies of normal peritoneum in patients with endometriosis.[46–51]

The dangers of Sampson's theory

While it is difficult to say anything positive about the theory of reflux menstruation as the origin of endometriosis, the story worsens. Sampson's theory of reflux menstruation is stifling progress in research and treatment of endometriosis. Because all treatment failures can be explained away by this theory, a clinician does not have to worry about whether the treatment used has efficacy since 'everybody knows that the disease comes back because of reflux menstruation'. Thus, medical therapists may beat their chests and exult that pain is decreased during ovarian suppression with the thought that the disease might be eradicated or 'dried up'. When pain returns after the return of ovarian function, the patient can be told that the reason was not failure of the medicine to eradicate the disease, but because it is the nature of the disease to recur. Similarly, when endometriosis is treated by shining a light at it or by spraying electrons at its surface, Sampson's theory can be used to explain any treatment failures. Endometriosis is thought to be an incurable, chronic, enigmatic, recurrent, progressively spreading disease which can only be treated by removal of the uterus, tubes and ovaries (which are uncommonly involved by endometriosis) with retention of the disease. This pessimistic view seems to be the result of several generations of clinicians observing the results of ineffective medical therapy or less effective surgical therapy, blaming treatment failures on Sampson's theory and ignoring the possibility of cure by removal of all disease from the body.

Research on endometriosis is hampered by Sampson's theory because so many dollars and minds are devoted to chasing this theory and various intellectual spinoffs which have led nowhere. It would be much cheaper and more productive for effort to be spent in trying to obtain photomicrographs of initial attachment. If initial attachment does not occur, then it would be unnecessary to waste more time on the theory of reflux menstruation and real progress could then be made.

The new endometriosis paradigm: what is old is new again

In the vacuum left by revocation of the reflux menstruation theory of origin of endometriosis, coelomic metaplasia as championed by Novak,[11] Moench,[52] and Gruenwald[53] rises to the top of the short list of possible causes of the disease, with certain modern alterations and insights: polygenic and/or environmental factors present at the moment of conception result in estrogen-responsive target mesenchymal substrate being laid down during embryogenesis in tracts or fields which roughly follow the pathways of fetal pelvic organogenesis caudally across the posterior coelomic epithelium. The distribution of these tracts may vary from female to female, and the inherent potential biologic activity of these tracts may also vary even at different sites in the same pelvis. For example, tracts laid down in parenchymal structures, such as the uterosacral ligaments, or within the muscularis of bowel or bladder have the potential of undergoing fibromuscular metaplasia which is not seen with simple peritoneal or ovarian endometriosis. Undifferentiated substrate tracts in girls or young women have no distinctive morphology that would allow them to be identified at surgery. During puberty, rising estrogen production by the ovaries causes these tracts to begin to undergo metaplasia into various preordained forms of endometriosis or endosalpingiosis with the many possible differences in histology, morphology and function that have been observed. In a metaplastic process similar in timing to squamous metaplasia of the cervix, by their mid-twenties women have developed essentially all of the sites of endometriosis they will have. Those sites destined to develop fibromuscular hyperplasia or adenomyotic changes may continue to do so until the mid-thirties. This model of embryologically patterned metaplasia, a derivation of the concept of Mülleriosis,[13] predicts the surgical results that have been observed following conservative excisional surgery.[32,33] If surgery is performed and if all endometriosis and all underlying substrate which is destined to form endometriosis are removed, then endometriosis can be cured by a single conservative surgery. If all existing endometriosis is removed but not all underlying or adjacent undifferentiated estrogen-targeted substrate is removed, then recurrence of new disease is possible. However, such recurrent disease will almost always be much less than the initial amount of disease,[32] since the majority of substrate will have already changed into endometriosis. If the uterus, tubes and ovaries are removed but endometriosis is left untreated, patients are at risk for continuing symptoms, especially if they have deep disease or intestinal involvement.[54] Local growth factors associated with the metaplasia of healing can induce formation of only small amounts of superficial endometriosis within or at the margin of the surgical site. Some patients can have endometriosis-associated Müllerian disorders of the uterus, such as adenomyosis or fibroids, which may necessitate surgery later. Gruenwald pointed out that this model can explain the occurrence of endometriosis anywhere in the body or in males,[55-57] since between 6 and 8 weeks of fetal development, all fetuses contain both Müllerian and Wolffian tracts.

The high probability that reflux menstruation is not the origin of any form of endometriosis is one of the main reasons to learn about aggressive excision of the disease, for cure of endometriosis is within the grasp of gifted surgeons around the world. The other reason to learn about excision is that patients are truly helped by the process and excision of endometriosis becomes a life-changing experience for both patient and surgeon.

References

1. Sampson JA. Peritoneal endometriosis due to the menstrual dissemination of endometrial tissue into the peritoneal cavity. Am J Obstet Gynecol 1927;14:422–69.
2. Sampson JA. The development of the implantation theory for the origin of peritoneal endometriosis. Am J Obstet Gynecol 1940;40:549–57.
3. Sampson JA. Perforating hemorrhagic (chocolate) cysts of the ovary. Arch Surg 1921;3:245–323.
4. Cullen TS. Adenomyoma of the rectovaginal septum. JAMA 1914;62:835–9.
5. Cullen TS. Adenomyoma of the rectovaginal septum. JAMA 1916;67:401–6.
6. Cullen TS. Adenomyoma of the recto-vaginal septum. Johns Hopkins Hosp Bull 1917;321:343–8 (plus plates).
7. Cullen TS. The distribution of adenomyomas containing uterine mucosa. Arch Surg 1920;1:215–83.
8. Stevens TG. Adenomyoma of the recto-vaginal septum. Proc Roy Soc Med 1916;9 (Obtstet Gynaecol section):1–17.
9. Lockyer C. Adenomyoma in the recto-uterine and recto-vaginal septa. Proc Roy Soc Med 1913;4:112–6 (plus Discussion).
10. Sampson JA. Ovarian hematomas of endometrial type (perforating hemorrhagic cysts of the ovary) and implantation adenomas of the endometrial type. Bost Med Surg J 1922;186:445–56.
11. Novak E. The significance of uterine mucosa in the fallopian tube, with a discussion of the origin of aberrant endometrium. Am J Obstet Gynecol 1926;12:484–526.
12. Goldstein DP, DeCholnoky C, Emans SJ. Adolescent endometriosis. J Adolesc Health Care 1980;1:37–41.
13. Redwine DB. Mulleriosis: the single best fit model of origin of endometriosis. J Reprod Med 1988;33:915–920.
14. Redwine DB. Was Sampson wrong? Fertil Steril 2002;78:686–93.
15. Redwine DB. Ovarian endometriosis: A marker for more severe pelvic and intestinal disease. Fertil Steril 1999;73:310–5.
16. Redwine DB. The distribution of endometriosis in the pelvis by age groups and fertility. Fertil Steril 1987;47:173–5.
17. Marana R, Muzii L, Caruana P, Dell'Acqua S, Mancuso S. Evaluation of the correlation between endometriosis extent, age of the patients and associated symptomatology. Acta Europaea Fertilitatis 1991;22:209–12.
18. Koninckx PR, Meuleman C, Demeyere S, Lesaffre E, Cornillie FJ. Suggestive evidence that pelvic endometriosis is a progressive disease, whereas deeply infiltrating endometriosis is associated with pelvic pain. Fertil Steril 1991;55:759–65.
19. Mahmood TA, Templeton A. The impact of treatment on the natural history of endometriosis. Hum Reprod 1990;5:965–70.
20. Thomas EJ, Cooke ID. Impact of gestrinone on the course of asymptomatic endometriosis. Brit Med J 1987;294:272–4.
21. Telimaa S, Ronnberg L, Kauppila A. Placebo-controlled comparison of danazol and high-dose medroxyprogesterone acetate in the treatment of endometriosis after conservative surgery. Gynecol Endocrinol 1987:1;363–71.
22. Harrison RF, Barry-Kinsella C. Efficacy of medroxyprogesterone treatment in infertile women with endometriosis: a prospective, randomized, placebo-controlled study. Fertil Steril 2000;74:24–30.
23. Meigs JV. Endometriosis. Etiologic role of marriage age and parity. Obstet Gynecol 1953;2:46–53.
24. Bacon WB. Results in 138 cases of endometriosis treated by conservative surgery. Am J Obstet Gynecol 1949;57:953–8.
25. McCoy JG, Bradford WZ. Surgical treatment of endometriosis with conservation of reproductive potential. Am J Obstet Gynecol 1963;87:394–8.
26. Green TH. Conservative surgical treatment of endometriosis. Clin Obstet Gynecol 1966;9:293–308.

27. Ranney B. Endometriosis: I. Conservative operations. Am J Obstet Gynecol 1970; 107: 743–50.
28. Punnonen R, Klemi P, Nikkanen V. Recurrent endometriosis. Gynecol Obstet Invest 1980;11: 307–12.
29. Wheeler JM, Malinak LR. Recurrent endometriosis. Contrib Gynecol Obstet 1987;16: 13–21.
30. Fayez JA, Collazo LM, Vernon C. Comparison of different modalities of treatment for minimal and mild endometriosis. Am J Obstet Gynecol 1988;159:927–32.
31. Ahmed MS, Barbieri RL. Reoperation rates for recurrent ovarian endometriomas after surgical excision. Gynecol Obstet Invest 1997;43: 53–4.
32. Redwine DB. Conservative laparoscopic excision of endometriosis by sharp dissection: life table analysis of reoperation and persistent or recurrent disease. Fertil Steril 1991;56:628–34.
33. Wheeler JM, Malinak LR. Recurrent endometriosis. Contrib Gynecol Obstet 1987;16: 13–21.
34. Mitchell GAG. The spread of acute intraperitoneal effusions. Br J Surg 1941;28: 291–313.
35. Rosenshein N, Blake D, McIntyre PA, Parmley T, Natarajan TK, Dvornicky J, Nickoloff E. The effect of volume on the distribution of substances instilled into the peritoneal cavity. Gynecol Oncol 1978;6:106–10.
36. Blumenkrantz MJ, Gallagher N, Bashore RA, Tenckhoff H. Retrograde menstruation in women undergoing chronic peritoneal dialysis. Obstet Gynecol 1981;57:667–70.
37. Halme J, Hammond MG, Hulka JF, Raj SG, Talbert LM. Retrograde menstruation in healthy women and in patients with endometriosis. Obstet Gynecol 1984; 64:151–4.
38. Sinaii N, Cleary SD, Ballweg ML, Nieman LK, Stratton P. High rates of autoimmune and endocrine disorders, fibromyalgia, chronic fatigue syndrome and atopic diseases among women with endometriosis: a survey analysis. Hum Reprod 2002;17:2715–24.
39. Brinton L, Gridley G, Persson I et al. Cancer risk after a hospital discharge diagnosis of endometriosis. Am J Obstet Gynecol 1997;176: 572–9.
40. Oosterlynck DJ, Cornillie FJ, Waer M, Vandeputte M, Koninckx PR. Women with endometriosis show a defect in natural killer activity resulting in a decreased cytotoxicity to autologous endometrium. Fertil Steril 1991;56: 45–51.
41. Oosterlynk DJ, Meuleman C, Waer M, Vandeputte M, Koninckx PR. The natural killer activity of peritoneal fluid lymphocytes is decreased in women with endometriosis. Fertil Steril 1992;58:290–5.
42. Oosterlynck DJ, Meuleman C, Waer M, Koninckx PR. CO_2-laser excision of endometriosis does not improve the decreased natural killer activity. Acta Obstet Gynecol Scand 1994;73: 333–7.
43. Kikuchi Y, Ishikawa N, Hirata J, Imaizumi E, Sasa H, Nagata I. Changes of peripheral blood lymphocyte subsets before and after operation of patients with endometriosis. Acta Obstet Gynecol Scand 1993;72:157–61.
44. Halme J, Becker S, Hammond MG, Raj MHG, Raj S. Increased activation of pelvic macrophages in infertile women with mild endometriosis. Am J Obstet Gynecol 1983;145:333–7.
45. Cirkel U, Ochs H, Mues B, Zwadlo G, Sorg C, Schneider HPG. Inflammatory reaction in endometriotic tissue: an immunohistochemical study. Eur J Obstet Gynecol Reprod Biol 1993;48:43–50.
46. Murphy et al. Unsuspected endometriosis documented by scanning electron microscopy in visually normal peritoneum. Fertil Steril 1986; 46:522–4.
47. Jansen RPS, Russell P. Nonpigmented endometriosis: Clinical, laparoscopic, and pathologic definition. Am J Obstet Gynecol 1986;155:1154–9.
48. Redwine DB. Is 'microscopic' peritoneal endometriosis invisible? Fertil Steril, 1988;50: 665–6.
49. Redwine DB, Yocom L. A serial section study of visually normal peritoneum in patients with endometriosis. Fertil Steril 1990;54:648–51.
50. Nezhat F, Allan CJ, Nezhat C, Martin DC. Nonvisualized endometriosis at laparoscopy. Int J Fertil 1991;36:340–3.
51. Balasch J, Creu M, Fabregues, Carmona F, Ordi J, Martinez-Roman S, Vanrell JA. Visible and non-visible endometriosis at laparoscopy in

fertile and infertile women and in patients with chronic pelvic pain: a prospective study. Hum Reprod 1996;11:387–91.
52. Moench GL. The histogenesis of adenomyositis. Surg Gynecol Obstet 1929;49:332–45.
53. Gruenwald P. Origin of endometriosis from the mesenchyme of the coelomic walls. Am J Obstet Gynecol 1942;44:470–4.
54. Redwine DB. Endometriosis persisting after castration: Clinical characteristics and results of surgical management. Obstet Gynecol 1994;83:405–13.
55. Oliker AJ, Harris AE. Endometriosis of the bladder in a male patient. J Urol 1971:106:858–9.
56. Pinkert TC, Catlow CE, Straus R. Endometriosis of the urinary bladder in a man with prostatic carcinoma. Cancer 1979;43:1562–7.
57. Beckman EN, Pintado SO, Leonard GL, Sternberg WH. Endometriosis of the prostate. Am J Surg Path 1985;9:374–9.

2

Berkson's fallacy and endometriosis

David B Redwine

When a disease is studied only in patients in a hospital, the symptomatic and morphologic features seen in those hospitalized patients may not accurately reflect the wild type disease which is prevalent in the population as a whole. This may result in an inaccurate picture of the disease. This is called 'Berkson's fallacy' (he described it but did not commit it),[1,2] and it may result in an increased chance of a positive or negative correlation being found where no or weak correlation actually exists. Since a description by Rokitansky in 1869,[3] endometriosis has usually required surgery in a hospital or other health care facility for diagnosis. Thus, the risk has always silently existed that endometriosis could be spuriously linked to symptoms or other disease states due to the effects of Berkson's fallacy acting unrecognized in hospitalized patients. Modern hindsight suggests that the decades-old effects of Berkson's fallacy have led to misinterpretation of the symptoms of infertility and pain associated with endometriosis. This in turn has led to confusion and ineffective treatment which are the unfortunate modern hallmarks of the disease.

Pregnancy as prophylaxis

The historical origin of the notion that endometriosis is positively associated with infertility began in an earlier, simpler time when it was thought that the pregnancy rate in married women should approach 100%. Early studies[4-6] of surgically diagnosed patients with obliteration of the cul-de-sac, large ovarian chocolate cysts (most of which were non-endometriotic), and pelvic adhesions found a pregnancy rate of only 40% in married women[5] without accounting for other important fertility factors, such as the male factor, age, and duration of conception attempts. Such patients today would be classified as Stage III or IV by the revised American Fertility Society (rAFS) classification system for endometriosis.[7] However, even in a modern large referral practice devoted almost exclusively to patients with endometriosis, rAFS Stage III and IV patients constitute only about 18% of surgically diagnosed patients.[8] Therefore, these early studies inaccurately characterized the morphological spectrum of endometriosis toward the severe end. Then, as now, the true prevalence of endometriosis and the symptom of pregnancy among the general population of women was unknown. Without these important prevalence figures, the observation of a 60% rate of infertility[5] among patients with chocolate cysts of the ovary has no relevance.

Observing this fertility rate of about 40%, Meigs[6] postulated that repeated pregnancies delayed the appearance of endometriomata of the ovaries, thus introducing the concept of pregnancy as prophylaxis or therapy which was later repeated by others.[9] He did not pause to wonder why parous women in his own study were not protected against the disease. So convinced was Meigs that early and frequent childbearing would help prevent endometriosis, that in later years he urged parents to support their newly married children so the young couples could reproduce early without economic pressures.[10] He was especially interested in educated couples having children and his views generated a storm of controversy at the time.[11]

In the modern era, we can easily identify the causes and effects of Berkson's fallacy on such early mischaracterization of disease. For example, the actual visual spectrum of disease is far greater than that found by Sampson and Meigs, and we now realize that most women do not have Stage III or IV disease. Also, the ovaries are not as commonly involved by endometriosis as suggested by these earlier studies. Unfortunately, the history of study of endometriosis is marked by authors simply repeating what has been published in the past, even if their own findings are contradictory.

Haydon also favored the concept that endometriosis is more common in infertile women.[12] Support for his conclusion came from his retrospective study of 569 cases. He found that 262 patients were parous, whereas 302 were not. He concluded that the incidence of relative infertility was therefore 53%. However, his numbers were not corrected for patients not attempting pregnancy. When 122 of his unmarried patients are eliminated from consideration, the birth rate in his population was actually 58%. However, follow-up was available in only 291 of his patients, so the actual eventual birth rate may have been higher. This important distinction regarding his work has been overlooked to this day.[13]

Counsellor and Crenshaw found in a retrospective study of patients with endometriosis that 56.2% of married couples were sterile.[14] They acknowledged the possibility that patients presenting for surgery for infertility constituted a biased population.

Pregnancy as 'treatment'

From observations of decreased fertility in patients with endometriosis, authors began to make unsupported leaps of faith. Beecham believed pregnancy to be a cure for endometriosis and dogmatically stated: 'Nature (since the beginning of time) has employed an efficient prophylactic and curative measure for endometriosis, i.e. pregnancy.' No reference or evidence was offered to support this speculation.[15]

Modern studies have found infertile patients to be more likely to have disease than fertile controls undergoing laparoscopic tubal ligation.[16–18] This would seem to support the notion that pregnancy is a good treatment for endometriosis. However, fertile patients undergoing tubal ligation could be a 'super fertile' and therefore an unrepresentative subset of the total population of women. The notion of pregnancy as treatment seems to be a charade resulting from misinterpreting the reduced fecundity of women with the disease as positive evidence of a beneficial effect of pregnancy in those without the disease, compounded by the observation of symptom reduction during pregnancy in women with the disease.

No one has ever done the simple study which would have proven whether pregnancy eradicates endometriosis. This would require making a surgical diagnosis of endometriosis in a woman and not treating the disease. After an intervening pregnancy, the pelvis could be checked by reoperation to see if the disease were gone.

Does endometriosis cause fertility? Does pregnancy cause endometriosis?

Not all authors, however, have found a high rate of infertility among patients with endometriosis. At odds with his later published work,[14] Counseller[19] observed a 61.3% crude birth rate and a 71.5% crude pregnancy rate among 737 married patients with endometriosis. Bennet found a corrected birth rate of 88% in patients with only endometriosis.[20] Dougherty and Anderson found that 87% of their patients with endometriosis had previously been pregnant and wondered whether pregnancy caused endometriosis.[21] Andrews and Larsen found that 72% of their married patients with endometriosis had been pregnant prior to their diagnosis.[22] One modern longitudinal cross-section study of largely untreated patients with endometriosis found no clearly consistent protective effect of parity against extent of disease as measured by number of pelvic areas involved and found that most patients had previously conceived, even though this study population included women never attempting pregnancy.[23] Although it might be tempting, as Dougherty and Anderson did, to conclude from observations such as these that pregnancy causes endometriosis or that fertility is caused by endometriosis, this would be as outrageous as observing a higher rate of infertility associated with endometriosis and concluding, as did Meigs and several generations of gynecologists, either that lack of childbearing causes endometriosis or that infertility is caused by endometriosis.

Pregnancy effects on endometriosis

The notion that pregnancy has a cytotoxic effect on endometriosis has been refuted by several authors. MacArthur and Ulfelder reviewed the behavior of 24 cases of endometriosis during pregnancy in a literature review.[24] They were unable to verify that pregnancy had a beneficial effect on endometriosis. They concluded that its behavior in pregnancy is highly variable, that permanent regression after pregnancy is the exception and may never truly occur, and that regression of endometriosis in the rare instances in which it occurred during pregnancy appeared to be ascribable to diminished tissue responsiveness to hormonal stimulation postpartum, rather than to necrosis and actual disappearance of endometriosis.

Further evidence that pregnancy is not toxic to endometriosis has been reported. Hanton et al described two cases of symptomatic ovarian endometrioma, one during pregnancy, the other immediately postpartum.[25] Norenberg et al reported a case of diaphragmatic pregnancy adjacent to endometriosis.[26]

It was clearly a leap of faith to observe a slightly higher percentage of nulligravidas than gravidas with endometriomas and then conclude that endometriosis is a cause of sterility or caused by delayed childbearing when parous women in the same study also suffered from it.[5,6,27] Still lacking is a simple prospective study with accurate antenatal and postpartum laparoscopic control proving histologically that untreated endometriosis is improved or absent after pregnancy.

Although the scientific evidence supporting pregnancy as prophylaxis or treatment of endometriosis seems unconvincing, this did not stop efforts to mimic its presumed beneficial state as suggested by Berkson's fallacy.

Pseudopregnancy treatment of endometriosis

Kistner initiated the concept of pseudopregnancy as treatment for endometriosis.[28] Pseudopregnancy was based on the unproven 'fact' that pregnancy improves existing endometriosis or prevents its development. There was no proof of this 'fact' at that time.[28] The anecdotal impetus for pseudopregnancy came from observations on a 25-year-old patient without a proven diagnosis of endometriosis. A dark brown, collapsed cystic structure on her right ovary was removed at Cesarean section and submitted for microscopy. Although no glandular element was found, it was claimed that microscopic evidence of endometrial stroma was found in a field of decidual change and occasional necrosis. The term 'necrobiosis' was coined to describe this histologic finding, and because endometriosis was not found, it was concluded that pregnancy had cured her disease. It was postulated that eventually all of the endometriotic stroma might have undergone complete necrosis and resorption if exposed to the hormonal effects of pregnancy long enough. Beyond the scientifically objectionable assumption of 'fact' and the obvious observation that if nine months of pregnancy had not resulted in complete necrosis of endometriosis then pregnancy is incomplete therapy for the disease, it is risky to base an entire ethos of treatment on a single patient who did not have proven endometriosis. This study was small (12 patients) and loose: it did not require biopsy proof of disease, used several dose regimens, assessed endometrial but not endometriotic response to therapy, did not attempt to quantify extent of disease, and did not mention length of follow-up.

A second loosely designed study of 58 patients, 30 of whom had previous conservative surgery, treated with several medicines in several dose regimens for varying lengths of time found a 'satisfactory' response in 93.3% of surgical-medical patients but in only 75% of medically treated patients.[29] Six of 24 medical patients had subsequent surgery and all had endometriosis. Two of 30 surgical-medical patients had subsequent surgery and one had endometriosis. Four patients with vaginal endometriosis were treated medically, but one had repeated biopsies to assess treatment. Disease was eventually absent in that patient, who was judged a medical cure despite the obvious possibility that the disease was surgically removed by repeated biopsies. This surgically treated patient has been referred to by other authors as an example of successful medical therapy.[18] Beyond the complexity of again using multiple dose regimens of multiple medications, with or without surgery, in patients whose extent of disease is not known, the apparent superior results obtained with surgery were not emphasized. It was concluded that medical therapy with norethynodrel was optimal.

Other reports on pseudopregnancy followed,[30–32] mentioning endometrial biopsy as a way to assess response of endometriosis to therapy since it was assumed that endometriosis was simply misplaced normal endometrial tissue. It is now realized that endometriosis has low and varying populations of hormone receptors,[33–35] as compared with native endometrium, so a difference in response would be expected. Therefore, the response of the endometrium is not pertinent to the treatment of endometriosis.

It is actually impossible to assess the response of endometriosis to medical treatment, since it is impossible to obtain biopsies before and after treatment from the same group of cells. An assumption must be made that any biopsy taken either before or after treatment will be an accurate representation of all other disease in the pelvis. Considering the protean visual, histologic, biochemical and hormonal characteristics of endometriosis, this assumption may not be valid.

Although some patients with endometriosis may have diminution of symptoms while on therapy or successful conception following therapy, these observations by themselves do not prove eradication of disease by pseudopregnancy therapy. Considering the historical context in which it was developed, it came as no surprise that rates of persistence of disease of 90–100% were reported after pseudopregnancy therapy.[22,36]

The effect of the menopause on endometriosis

It has been observed for many years that endometriosis is primarily a disease of the menstrual years. Goldstein et al.[37] reported the youngest patient with the disease, 10.5 years old, while the oldest patient, mentioned by Haydon, was 78.[12] It has long been held that the hypoestrogenic state accompanying menopause improves or cures endometriosis, while estrogen stimulates or perhaps causes it.

Sampson observed the relative rarity of postmenopausal endometriosis and made the optimistic and highly qualified conclusions that: 'I hope and expect that the cessation of ovarian function will cause any adenomatous tissue which was left in the pelvis to atrophy',[5] and that: '. . . the implantations will usually, possibly always, atrophy after all ovarian tissue is removed . . . . All of them probably cease to grow and actually atrophy after the menopause'.[38]

Meigs reinforced the concept of the importance of the cyclic action of estrogen and progesterone on the maintenance of endometriosis.[6] Although two of his 16 patients with ovarian endometriomas were menopausal, he nonetheless believed that without the estrogenic stimulus provided by the ovaries, endometriosis shrinks and atrophies. In addition, he proposed bilateral oophorectomy as treatment which would make the catamenial activity of the ovarian endometrioma cysts stop. He reasoned that removal of the ovaries would make the cysts within the ovaries stop growing and slowly atrophy (sic). He referred to 'case number 8946' as an example of shrinkage of residual endometriosis after castration. There is no case number 8946 in the paper, but there is a case number 8496. This patient had a lime-sized mass which persisted on the left side of the pelvis for 25 months postoperatively, it then disappeared within 2 months. Although both ovaries had been removed, it was assumed that this was a remnant of the left ovary. Beyond the obvious observations that Meigs did not really know what the mass was and therefore made unjustified conclusions and that parts of his paper may have been poorly worded at best, if 25 months of castration did not make endometriosis go away, then castration is not an efficient treatment of the disease.

Although the notion that lack of cyclic estrogenic activity will result in physical eradication of endometriosis may not have been specifically stated by early authors, many authors up to the present have mentioned castration with retention of disease as satisfactory treatment of endometriosis.

In 1936, Cattell and Swinton[39] stated that castration 'will cause the lesion to recede and usually relieve symptoms'. No supporting references were offered.

Cattell,[40] later noting that 6 of 11 patients with significant bowel disease continued to have symptoms or abnormal x-rays after removal of the ovaries and retention of disease, stated: 'It seems safe to remove the ovaries without resecting the bowel if the diagnosis of endometriosis is confirmed by frozen section'. The rationale for favoring a treatment that usually left pathology behind was not explained.

Fallon et al.[41] stated that: '. . . all endometriosis . . . regresses after removal of the ovaries . . . Following ovarian deactivation, endometriosis gradually regresses, with insignificant residua'. Partial oophorectomy was mentioned as a means of slightly reducing estrogen production, possibly with diminution of symptoms. No references were offered in support of these opinions.

Counseller and Crenshaw[14] noted the difficulty sometimes encountered in attempting conservative surgery in extensive disease, and left ovarian tissue in only 38.5% of their patients. They stated that: 'Obviously, the quickest and most certain way for the relief of pain is the destruction of the ovarian function . . .' Counseller[19] had stated this earlier. No references were offered in support of their opinions.

None of the above studies showed actual destruction of endometriosis resulting from decreased estrogen effect, but relied on symptomatology to gauge success of treatment. As with pregnancy, absence or diminution of symptoms does not prove elimination of disease.

Probably because endometriosis is less symptomatic after the menopause, and because fewer menopausal patients seek treatment for it, not as much is known about the disease in postmenopausal patients as following pregnancy. However, it is clear from published reports that older women can have problems due to endometriosis.

In two studies of large numbers of patients with endometriosis, 2.5% and 3.7% of the patients were postmenopausal.[42,43]

In another study of postmenopausal endometriosis by Kempers et al.[44] 138 patients 45 years of age or older who were menopausal for at least two years were compiled. Only one patient had been on estrogen replacement therapy. Forty-one had clinically significant disease including intestinal disease, widespread pelvic involvement or endometriomas over 3 centimeters in diameter (61% of these patients were fertile, another indication of the baseline fertility potential among these patients). Among eight patients with intestinal endometriosis, the disease was classified histologically as atrophic in all, including two with small bowel obstruction. In 26 patients with histologic proof of disease, 20% had histologic evidence of cellular activity of their disease, but none of these was symptomatic. The conclusions were that: symptomatic postmenopausal endometriosis occurs, albeit less prevalent than symptomatic premenopausal disease, postmenopausal disease can be independent of estrogen support, and the histologic appearance of the disease is not helpful in predicting whether it is symptomatic.

Although some reports of postmenopausal endometriosis have detailed patients who have not been exposed to endogenous or exogenous estrogen, one patient with postmenopausal endometriosis associated with ovarian hyperthecosis has been reported.[45]

Although there is no question that the disease usually appears visually to be quiescent post menopause, and microscopically the glands may appear atrophic, scientific evidence of an actual toxic effect of the menopause on endometriosis is lacking. Nonetheless, menopause has frequently been proposed as treatment of endometriosis, and many physicians believe that this will cure a patient in the absolute sense of the word: that the disease will ultimately be gone as a result of anticellular toxicity of low estrogen levels. In a reprise of the developments preceding initiation of pseudopregnancy therapy, the fact that postmenopausal patients are less commonly afflicted with symptomatic disease has led to the conclusion that endometriosis is cured by the hypoestrogenic states of natural or surgical menopause.[46] Castration or medical suppression of ovarian function is a natural suggestion for treatment of endometriosis if it is believed that women do not need estrogen and that endometriosis is cured by some type of anticellular activity resulting from the lack of estrogen characterizing menopause. Ovarian suppression, therefore, is the goal of pseudomenopausal treatments of endometriosis.

Pseudomenopausal treatments of endometriosis

Danazol was the first medicine introduced for the treatment of endometriosis by pseudomenopause. Gonadotropin-releasing hormone (GnRH) agonists were the second.

One of the first studies on danazol was illustrated by many 'before and after' photographs of the female pelvis purporting to show resolution of endometriosis after danazol therapy.[47] This led immediately to great hopes that endometriosis could be cured by medical therapy which mimicked nature. However, not all the patients had biopsies taken after therapy, and the notion of consistent, profound antigonadotropin suppression by danazol was later found to be erroneous.[46,48] It is now realized that danazol does not eradicate endometriosis of any stage or location,[49–53] and the hopes dashed by danazol seem to be a combined result of historically misplaced expectations, errors of visual identification and of not confirming clinical observations by biopsy.[50,54] Recent reports on the use of danazol for endometriosis have shown an actual decrease in fertility in treated women with minimal or mild disease compared to operative laparoscopy[52] or observation only,[55–57] while the improved pregnancy rate following surgical therapy for disease associated with pelvic adhesions has long been recognized. Since there is a surprisingly high background pregnancy rate in untreated disease in infertile patients,[55,56,58] the true effect of medical or surgical therapy on fertility is difficult to determine, since it may be small. It seems most likely that much of the 'improved' fertility after treatment is due to the natural history of endometriosis, not to the treatment itself.

Urologists have questioned the use of danazol for endometriosis involving the urinary tract, noting it to be ineffective for relief of obstructive ureteral endometriosis.[59] Since danazol does not eradicate endometriosis, it is not surprising that it is ineffective in long-term relief of pain.[60–63] Danazol has been found to reduce high density lipoprotein (HDL) cholesterol.[64]

GnRH agonists seek to mimic the hypoestrogenic menopausal state by inducing a profound suppression of pituitary gonadotropins. However, since this approach shares danazol's historical basis of origin, one would naturally predict that GnRH agonists would replicate danazol's shortcomings, although with different side-effects.

An early report[65] on the efficacy of GnRH agonists assessed response of the endometrium rather than endometriosis, assessed the visual appearance of endometriosis at the conclusion of therapy when errors of visual identification are common,[50] and spoke of disappearance and resorption of lesions without biopsy proof. The definite impression was left that GnRH agonist therapy resulted in physical eradication of disease.

A large multicenter randomized, double-blind, study of 213 treated patients was based on the undefined and unreferenced statement that: 'endometriosis resolves after ovariectomy and menopause,'[66] and went on to find that treatment with a GnRH agonist, nasal nafarelin, was as effective as danazol in reduction of symptoms and severity of disease while on treatment. A post-treatment pregnancy rate of 39% was reported for all stages of disease. Treatment response was evaluated by laparoscopy done at the end of the treatment period, presence or absence of disease was apparently not confirmed by biopsy, and follow-up was done only for patients attempting pregnancy.

Misinterpretation of published studies in favor of conventional dogma continues to be a problem. For example, a study published in 1977 recommended conservative surgery for endometriosis in younger patients, but oophorectomy in older patients if a hysterectomy was performed, since a high percentage of these patients required estrogen replacement therapy within 5 years postoperatively.[67] If the disease was resected and the ovaries were left in, only 6% of patients required reoperation for endometriosis. A recent study of GnRH agonist therapy[68] stated that: 'bilateral oophorectomy is the most effective treatment of endometriosis' and cited the 1977 study as the basis of this belief, although the earlier study said nothing of the kind. Nonetheless, it was proposed that GnRH agonists might therefore be effective treatment for endometriosis. Since the earlier study was cited out of context, and since there is no historical support for the concept of hypoestrogenic toxicity against endometriosis, it came as no surprise when the more recent study found that GnRH agonists do not eradicate endometriosis.[68] Other investigators have confirmed that GnRH agonists do not eradicate endometriosis.[69] Reversible reduction in trabecular bone accompanying the hypoestrogenic state has been reported,[70] and pain recurrence follows therapy by gonadotropin-releasing hormone.[71]

Current attempts at pseudomenopausal therapy share another feature which makes it impossible ever to mimic the menopausal state exactly. Menopause is characterized by low estrogen and high gonadotropin levels, whereas danazol and the GnRH agonists seek to lower the ovarian production of estrogen in part by reducing pituitary gonadotropin output. Thus, only a 'pseudo' pseudomenopause is achieved. The effect of high levels of gonadotropins on endometriosis is unknown.

It is becoming popular to subject women with pelvic pain to a three to six month trial of GnRH agonist therapy, the thinking being that if pain relief occurs, then endometriosis is likely to be present so medical therapy can be continued indefinitely. Actually, the evidence is clear that symptomatic response to such a trial of medical therapy will only narrow the field of possible diagnoses to at least six estrogen-mediated conditions that can cause pain: uterine fibroids, adenomyosis, primary dysmenorrhea, ovulation pain, endometriosis, and unknown. Trying to discriminate between these six conditions with diagnostic imaging tests such as ultrasound, computed tomography (CT) or magnetic resonance imaging (MRI) is difficult. Fibroids might be found if large enough, not all cases of adenomyosis or endometriosis would be evident, and none of the rest would be found. Thus, at the end of an expensive six months of treatment with its associated side-effects and after several types of scans, the clinician will still be unable to guarantee a diagnosis of endometriosis. Such a trial of therapy thus resolves down to whether or not to continue successful treatment of symptoms without a diagnosis.

Discussion

Berkson's fallacy seems to be affecting thought on endometriosis to this day. In the beginning, the weak pathoconsortive association between endometriosis and the symptom of infertility was observed in hospitalized patients, and it was inferred that endometriosis is causative of infertility, that it is promoted by voluntarily delayed childbearing, and that it can be cured or delayed by pregnancy. These unproven opinions are repeated to patients to the present time. Other authors, observing the rarity of symptomatic disease in hypoestrogenic women and perhaps not realizing the importance of estrogen to women, concluded that menopause, by its hypoestrogenic effect, cured or improved endometriosis and is good treatment, and this notion also persists to this day. These beliefs have indirect support from temporary symptom improvement, but for the most part are fueled by continuing errors in visual identification of disease as well as unreferenced hopes, beliefs, expectations and dogma all of which arise in part from the seductiveness of an unconfirmed belief.[72] Scientific studies based on these notions continue to be produced.

If either pregnancy or menopause resulted in the destruction of endometriosis, there should by now be abundant microscopic evidence of this effect in humans. Sadly, the simple studies which would have confirmed or denied the basis of all medical therapy have never been done. These studies would be simple to conduct: patients with surgically proven endometriosis would be surgically reinvestigated after pregnancy or menopause to see if their endometriosis was gone.

Since medical therapy cannot be used purposefully to eradicate endometriosis, there must be some other reason for its ethical use, such as relief of symptoms. However, hope of permanent relief of symptoms by medical therapy is misplaced because the cause of the symptoms is not eliminated, a permanent change in the disease is not induced, and it is unclear whether it can be suppressed forever. In the modern era of concern over medical costs and efficiency, consumer attention is toward a desire to get to the root cause of disease, not simply to mask symptoms. In this regard, current medical therapy is a cliché.

Emphasis on fertility as a cardinal symptom of the disease or endpoint of therapy has also contributed to continued disappointment and confusion, not only because infertility is a less common and less specific symptom than pain, but also because findings referable to patients with infertility may not be at all pertinent to the greater number with pain. It is poor medical practice to treat patients with one symptom based on study results of another symptom which may not be directly related to the disease. The presumed inherent 'goodness' of conservative medical management, the temporary improvement experienced by some patients during treatment, and the desire to avoid the morbidity of surgery with its ill-defined risk of postoperative adhesions are not necessarily convincing reasons to embrace current or future medical therapy of endometriosis.

References

1. Berkson J. Limitations of the application of fourfold table analysis to hospital data. Biometrics 1946;2:47–53.
2. Berkson J. The statistical study of association between smoking and lung cancer. Proc Mayo Clinic 1955;30:319–48.
3. Schenken RS. Pathogenesis. In: Schenken R (ed) Endometriosis: contemporary concepts in clinical management. Philadelphia: JB Lippincott, 1989:1–48.
4. Cullen TS. The distribution of adenomyomas containing uterine mucosa. Arch Surg 1920; 215–83.
5. Sampson JA. Perforating hemorrhagic (chocolate) cysts of the ovary. Arch Surg 1921;3: 245–323.
6. Meigs JV. Endometrial hematomas of the ovary. Bost Med Surg J 1922;187:1–13.
7. The American Fertility Society. Revised American Fertility classification system of endometriosis: 1985. Fertil Steril 1985;44:351–2.
8. Redwine DB. The visual appearance of endometriosis and its impact on our concepts of the disease. Prog Clin Biol Res 1990;323: 393–412.
9. Fallon J, Brosnan JT, Manning JJ, Moran WG, Meyers J, Fletcher EM. Endometriosis: a report of 400 cases. Rhode Island Med J 1950;33: 15–23.
10. Meigs JV. Etiologic role of marriage age and parity; conservative treatment. Obstet Gynecol 1953;2:46–53.
11. Meigs JV. An interest in endometriosis and its consequences. Am J Obstet Gynecol 1960;79: 625–35.
12. Haydon GB. A study of 569 cases of endometriosis. Am J Obstet Gynecol 1942;43:704–9.
13. Burns WN, Schenken RS. Pathophysiology. In: Schenken R (ed) Endometriosis: contemporary concepts in clinical management. Philadelphia: JB Lippincott, 1989:83–126.
14. Counsellor VS, Crenshaw JL. A clinical and surgical review of endometriosis. Am J Obstet Gynecol 1951; 62:930–42.
15. Beecham CT. Surgical treatment of endometriosis with special reference to conservative surgery in young women. JAMA 1949;139:971–2.
16. Hasson HM. Incidence of endometriosis in diagnostic laparoscopy. J Reprod Med 1976; 16:135–8.
17. Drake TS, Metz SA, Grunert GM, O'Brien WF. Peritoneal fluid volume in endometriosis. Fertil Steril 1980;34:280–1.
18. Strathy JH, Molgaard CA, Coulam CB, Melton LJ. Endometriosis and infertility: a laparoscopic study of endometriosis among fertile and infertile women. Fertil Steril 1982;38:667–72.
19. Counseller VS. Surgical procedures involved in the treatment of endometriosis. Surg Gynecol Obstet 1949;89:322–7.
20. Bennet ET. Endometriosis in the older age group. Am J Obstet Gynecol 1953;65:100–8.
21. Dougherty CM, Anderson MR. Endometriosis and adenomyosis. Am J Obstet Gynecol 1964;89:23–37.
22. Andrews WC, Larsen GD. Endometriosis: treatment with hormonal pseudopregnancy and/or operation. Am J Obstet Gynecol 1974;118:643–51.
23. Redwine DB. The distribution of endometriosis in the pelvis by age groups and fertility. Fertil Steril 1987;47:173–5.
24. McArthur JW, Ulfelder H. The effect of pregnancy upon endometriosis. Obstet Gynecol Surv 1965;20:709–33.
25. Hanton EM, Malkasian GD, Dockerty MB, Pratt JH. Endometriosis: symptomatic during pregnancy. Am J Obstet Gynecol 1966;95: 1165–6.
26. Norenberg DD, Gundersen JH, Janis JF, Gundersen AL. Early pregnancy on the diaphragm with endometriosis. Obstet Gynecol 1977;49:620–2.
27. Sampson JA. Heterotopic or misplaced endometrial tissue. Am J Obstet Gynecol 1925; 10:649–64.
28. Kistner RW. The use of newer progestins in the treatment of endometriosis. Am J Obstet Gynecol 1958;75:264–78.

29. Kistner RW. The treatment of endometriosis by inducing pseudopregnancy with ovarian hormones. A report of fifty-eight cases. Fertil Steril 1959;10:539–56.
30. Kistner RW. Infertility with endometriosis. A plan of therapy. Fertil Steril 1962;13:237–45.
31. Kistner RW. Current status of the hormonal treatment of endometriosis. Clin Obstet Gynecol 1966;9:271–92.
32. Kourides IA, Kistner RW. Three new synthetic progestins in the treatment of endometriosis. Obstet Gynecol 1968;31:821–8.
33. Bergqvist A, Rannevik G, Thorell J. Estrogen and progesterone cytosol receptor concentration in endometriotic tissue and intrauterine endometrium. Acta Obstet Gynecol Scand Suppl 1981;101:53–8.
34. Gould SF, Shannon JM, Cunha GR. Nuclear estrogen binding sites in human endometriosis. Fertil Steril 1983;39:520–4.
35. Janne O, Kauppila A, Kokko E, Lantto T, Ronnberg L, Vihko R. Estrogen and progestin receptors in endometriosis lesions: Comparison with endometrial tissue. Am J Obstet Gynecol 1981;141:562–6.
36. Andrews MC, Andrews WC, Strauss AF. Effects of progestin-induced pseudopregnancy on endometriosis: clinical and microscopic studies. Am J Obstet Gynecol 1959;78:776–83.
37. Goldstein DP, DeCholnoky C, Eman J. Adolescent endometriosis. J Adolesc Health Care 1980;1:37–41.
38. Sampson JA. Ovarian hematomas of endometrial type (perforating hemorrhagic cysts of the ovary) and implantation adenomas of the endometrial type. Bost Med Surg J 1922;186:445–56.
39. Cattell RB, Swinton NW. Endometriosis. With particular reference to conservative treatment. N Engl J Med 1936;214:341–6.
40. Cattell RB. Endometriosis of the colon and rectum with intestinal obstruction. N Engl J Med 1937;217:9–16.
41. Fallon J, Brosnan JT, Moran WG. Endometriosis. Two hundred cases considered from the viewpoint of the practitioner. N Engl J Med 1946:235:669–73.
42. Scott RB, TeLinde RW. External endometriosis – the scourge of the private patient. Ann Surg 1950;131:697–720.
43. Henriksen E. Endometriosis. Am J Surg 1955;90:331–7.
44. Kempers RD, Dockerty MB, Hunt AB, Symmonds RE. Significant postmenopausal endometriosis. Surg Gynecol Obstet 1960;3:348–56.
45. Montes M, Beautyman W, Haidak G. Cholesteatomatous endometriosis. Am J Obstet Gynecol 1961;82:119–23.
46. Reyniak JV, Lauersen NH. Danazol – a versatile pharmacologic agent. Fertil Steril 1982;37:475–7.
47. Dmowski WP, Cohen MR. Treatment of endometriosis with an antigonadotropin, danazol. A laparoscopic and histologic evaluation. Obstet Gynecol 1975;46:147–54.
48. Fraser IS, Markham R, McIlveen J, Robinson M. Dynamic test of hypothalamic and pituitary function in women treated with danazol. Fertil Steril 1982;37:484–8.
49. Schweppe K-W, Wynn RM, Beller FK. Ultrastructural comparison of endometriotic implants and eutopic endometrium. Am J Obstet Gynecol 1984;148:1024–37.
50. Evers JLH. The second-look laparoscopy for evaluation of the result of medical treatment of endometriosis should not be performed during ovarian suppression. Fertil Steril 1987;47:502–4.
51. Dmowski WP. Visual assessment of peritoneal implants for staging endometriosis: do number and cumulative size of lesions reflect the severity of a systemic disease? Fertil Steril 1987;47:382–4.
52. Fayez JA, Collazo LM, Vernon C. Comparison of different modalities of treatment for minimal and mild endometriosis. Am J Obstet Gynecol 1988;159:927–32.
53. Brosens IA, Verleyen A, Cornillie F. The morphologic effect of short-term medical therapy of endometriosis. Am J Obstet Gynecol 1987;157:1215–21.
54. Greenblatt RB, Borenstein R, Hernandez-Ayup S. Experiences with danazol (an antigonadotropin) in the treatment of infertility. Am J Obstet Gynecol 1974;118:783–7.
55. Seibel MM, Berger MJ, Weinstein FG, Taymor ML. The effectiveness of danazol on subsequent fertility in minimal endometriosis. Fertil Steril 1982;38:534–7.
56. Bayer SR, Seibel MM, Saffan DS, Berger MJ, Taymor ML. Efficacy of danazol treatment for minimal endometriosis in infertile women. J Rep Med 1988;33:179–83.

57. Telimaa S. Danazol and medroxyprogesterone acetate inefficacious in the treatment of infertility in endometriosis. Fertil Steril 1988;50:872–5.
58. Collins JA, Wrixon W, Janes LB, Wilson EH. Treatment-independent pregnancy among infertile couples. N Engl J Med 1983;309:1201–9.
59. Jepsen JM, Hansen KB. Danazol in the treatment of ureteral endometriosis. J Urol 1988;139:1045–6.
60. Fedele L, Arcaini L, Bianchi S, Baglioni A, Vercellini P. Comparison of cyproterone acetate and danazol in the treatment of pelvic pain associated with endometriosis. Obstet Gynecol 1989;73:1000–4.
61. Fedele L, Bianchi S, Viezzoli T, Arcaini L, Candiani GB. Gestrinone versus danazol in the treatment of endometriosis. Fertil Steril 1989;51:781–5.
62. Dmowski WP. Pseudomenopause: a new approach in treating endometriosis. Contrib Obstet Gynecol 1976;8:107–14.
63. Barbieri RL, Evans S, Kistner RW. Danazol in the treatment of endometriosis: analysis of 100 cases with a 4-year follow-up. Fertil Steril 1982;37:737–46.
64. Dmowski WP, Radwanska E, Binor Z, Tummon I, Pepping P. Ovarian suppression induced with Buserelin or danazol in the management of endometriosis: a randomized, comparative study. Fertil Steril 1989;51:395–400.
65. Lemay A, Maheux R, Faure N, Jean C, Fazekas ATA. Reversible hypogonadism induced by a luteinizing hormone-releasing hormone (LH-RH) agonist (Buserelin) as a new therapeutic approach for endometriosis. Fertil Steril 1984;41:863–71.
66. Henzl MR, Corson SL, Moghissi K, Buttram VC, Berqvist C, Jacobson J et al. Administration of nasal nafarelin as compared with oral danazol for endometriosis. A multicenter double-blind comparative clinical trial. N Engl J Med 1988;318:485–9.
67. Williams TJ, Pratt JH. Endometriosis in 1,000 consecutive celiotomies: incidence and management. Am J Obstet Gynecol 1977;129:245–50.
68. Steingold KA, Cedars M, Lu JKH, Randle D, Judd HL, Meldrum DR. Treatment of endometriosis with a long-acting gonadotropin-releasing hormone agonist. Obstet Gynecol 1987;69:403–11.
69. Nisolle-Pochet M, Casanas-Roux F, Donnez J. Histologic study of ovarian endometriosis after hormonal therapy. Fertil Steril 1988;49:423–6.
70. Dawood MY, Lewis V, Ramos J. Cortical and trabecular bone mineral content in women with endometriosis: effect of gonadotropin-releasing hormone agonist and danazol. Fertil Steril 1989;52:21–6.
71. Franssen AMHW, Kauer FM, Chada DR, Zijlstra JA, Rolland R. Endometriosis: treatment with gonadotropin-releasing hormone agonist Buserelin. Fertil Steril 1989;51:401–8.
72. Feinstein AR. Clinical epidemiology: the architecture of clinical research. Philadelphia: WB Saunders, 1985:408.

3

Modern medical therapy of endometriosis

David L Olive

The medical treatment of endometriosis has long played a major role in the therapeutic approach to this disorder. However, the approach to the design of medical therapeutics for endometriosis is evolving scientifically, as new strategies are aiding in the attack upon this disease. What once was an armamentarium of a handful of ovulation suppression agents is fast becoming a diverse array of finely directed treatment options.

The original development of medication to treat endometriosis was built upon several observations. First, endometriosis is infrequently encountered in the parous woman, but much more often in the nulliparous female, suggesting a protective effect of the hormonal milieu of pregnancy. Second, endometrium is known to be estrogen-dependent, with ectopic endometrium presumably behaving in much the same manner. Finally, endometriosis tends to occur nearly exclusively in menstruating, reproductive age women, again suggesting hormonal dependence. These findings suggested the potential benefits of hormonal therapy to alter the normal menstrual cyclicity of the reproductive years, the mainstay of medical treatment for endometriosis.

Recently, however, the approach has changed. We now have a much greater depth of understanding of the pathogenesis, growth, and maintenance of ectopic endometrium, particularly at the molecular level. This has provided drug developers with new, precise molecular targets for treatment of the disease. Currently under development, these newer agents hold the potential of greater efficacy and flexibility with fewer systemic effects.

This chapter will review those medications currently used as well as under development for the medical treatment of endometriosis. Results of treatment, when available, will be included and compared.

Established medical treatments of endometriosis

Danazol

The first drug to be approved for the treatment of endometriosis in the United States was danazol, an isoxazol derivative of 17-alpha-ethinyl testosterone. It was originally thought to produce a pseudomenopause, but subsequent studies have revealed the drug to act primarily by diminishing the midcycle luteinizing hormone (LH) surge,[1,2] creating a chronic anovulatory state. Additional actions include inhibitor of multiple enzymes in the steroidogenic pathology[3] and increase in free serum testosterone.[4] The recommended dosage of danazol for the treatment of endometriosis is 600–800 mg/day; however, these doses have substantial androgenic side-effects, such as increased hair growth, mood changes, adverse serum lipid profiles, deepening of the voice (possibly irreversible), and rarely, liver damage (possibly irreversible and life-threatening) and arterial thrombosis.[5,6] Studies of lower doses as primary treatment for endometriosis-associated pain have been uncontrolled or with small numbers and thus contain information of limited value.[7] However, due to the many side-effects of the drug, alternative routes of administration have been sought. Recently, the use of danazol vaginal suppositories[8] and danazol-impregnated vaginal rings[9] have been described in small, uncontrolled trials. Preliminary results suggest side-effects may be less severe with the transvaginal approach.

Progestogens

Progestogens are a class of compounds that produce progesterone-like effects upon endometrial tissue. A large number of progestogens exist, ranging from those chemically derived from progesterone (progestins), such as medroxyprogesterone acetate (MPA), to 19-nortestosterone derivatives, such as norethindrone and norgestrel. The proposed mechanism of action of these compounds is initial decidualization of endometrial tissue followed by eventual atrophy. This is believed due to a direct suppressive effect of progestogens upon the estrogen receptors of the endometrium. Recent evidence suggests that another mechanism of action at the molecular level is the suppression of matrix metalloproteinases, enzymes important in the implantation and growth of ectopic endometrium.[10]

The most extensively studied progestational agent for the treatment of endometriosis is medroxyprogesterone. The drug was originally used orally for the treatment of endometriosis, with doses ranging from 20 mg to 100 mg daily; published randomized studies are limited to 100 mg daily. However, the depot formulation has also been used, in a dose of 150 mg every three months. Side-effects of medroxyprogesterone are multiple and varied, yet even in high doses seems to be better tolerated metabolically than danazol. A common side-effect is transient breakthrough bleeding, which occurs in 38–47% of patients. This is generally well tolerated and, when necessary, can be adequately treated with supplemental estrogen or an increase in the progestogen dose. Other side-effects include nausea (0–80%), breast tenderness (5%), fluid retention (50%), and depression (6%).[11] In published trials, few patients have discontinued the medications secondary to side-effects. In contradistinction to danazol, all of the above-mentioned adverse effects resolve upon discontinuation of the drugs.

Norethindrone acetate has also been utilized as a treatment for endometriosis. This 19-nortestosterone derivative has only been analyzed in a retrospective, uncontrolled trial of 52 women.[12] Each was treated initially with 5 mg daily, with increases of 2.5 mg increments up to a maximum dose of 20 mg daily, until amenorrhea was achieved. Side-effects were similar to those seen with medroxyprogesterone.

Other progestational agents have also been used in the occasional study, including lynestrenol, a gestagen used primarily in Europe. Levonorgestrel, the active ingredient of Norplant, has also been utilized recently, via an intrauterine device delivery system.[13] The drug has been shown to effectively decrease vascular endothelial growth factor (VEGF) and blood vessel proliferation, providing a rationale for its use in endometriosis.[14] It has been touted recently as a desirable treatment for rectovaginal endometriosis, although evidence thus far is uncontrolled.[13]

Progestogens may adversely affect serum lipoprotein levels. The 19-nortestosterone derivatives significantly decrease high density lipoprotein (HDL), a change linked to an increased risk of coronary artery disease.[15] Data on medroxyprogesterone acetate are less clear, with studies demonstrating either no effect,[16] or a slight decrease.[17] It is likely that there is a decrement in HDL with all these agents, but the magnitude is related to the specific progestogen and the dose administered. Whether alterations in serum lipoprotein levels for 4–6 months have any clinical significance is unclear.

Oral contraceptives (combination estrogen-progestogen)

The combination of estrogen and progestogen for therapy of endometriosis, the so-called 'pseudopregnancy' regimen, has been utilized for 40 years. Like progestational therapy alone, pseudopregnancy is believed to produce initial decidualization and growth of endometrial tissue, followed in several months by atrophy. This has been observed in women,[18] but is in direct conflict with data from the rhesus monkey demonstrating larger implants with considerable local growth following such a therapeutic approach.[19]

Pseudopregnancy regimens have been administered both orally and parenterally. Combination oral contraceptive pills, such as norethynodrel and mestranol, norethindrone acetate and ethinyl estradiol, lynestrenol and mestranol, and norgestrel plus ethinyl estradiol have all been tried. Parenteral combinations have included 17-hydroxyprogesterone or depot medroxyprogesterone acetate paired with stilbestrol or conjugated estrogens.

Side-effects of pseudopregnancy are often quite impressive, and include those encountered with progestogens alone, as well as estrogenic- and androgenic-related effects. Estrogens may cause nausea, hypertension, thrombophlebitis, and uterine enlargement. The 19-nortestosterone-derived progestogens may cause androgenic effects, such as acne, alopecia, increased muscle mass, decreased breast size, and deepening of the voice. Noble and Letchworth, in a comparative trial of norethynodrel and mestranol versus danazol, found that 41% of the pseudopregnancy group failed to complete their course of therapy due to side-effects of the medication.[20] However, dosages generally involved more estrogen and progestogen than are found in modern contraceptive preparations. The oral contraceptives commonly prescribed today for combination therapy are most likely to produce a progestogen-dominant picture similar to that of progestogen alone.

Today, oral contraceptives are the most commonly prescribed treatment for endometriosis symptoms. Despite this, there are little data regarding mechanism of action. One recent investigation suggests that oral contraceptives suppress proliferation and enhance programmed cell death (apoptosis) in endometrial tissue, perhaps providing a mechanistic clue for the action of these drugs.[21]

GnRH agonists

Gonadotropin-releasing hormone agonists (GnRH agonists) are analogs of the hormone GnRH. This hypothalamic hormone is responsible for stimulating the pituitary gland to secrete follicle-stimulating hormone (FSH) and luteinizing hormone (LH), two hormones necessary for normal ovarian function. GnRH is secreted in a pulsatile manner; the correct pulse results in stimulation of FSH and LH release, while too high or too low a pulse rate results in a decrease in pituitary hormone secretion. GnRH agonists are modified forms of GnRH that bind to the pituitary receptors and remain for a lengthy period. Thus, they are identified by the pituitary as rapidly pulsatile GnRH and, after initial stimulation of FSH and LH secretion, result in a shutdown (down-regulation) of the pituitary, and no resulting stimulation of the ovary. The result is a hypoestrogenic state similar to that of menopause, producing endometrial atrophy and amenorrhea. It is also possible that the drug affects ectopic endometrium via additional mechanisms: animal studies have suggested alterations in plasminogen activators and matrix metalloproteinases, factors important in endometriosis development.[22]

The agonist can be given intranasally, subcutaneously, or intramuscularly depending upon the specific product, with frequency of administration ranging from twice daily to three-monthly. The side-effects are those of hypoestrogenism, such as transient vaginal bleeding, hot flashes, vaginal dryness, decreased libido, breast tenderness, insomnia, depression, irritability and fatigue, headache, osteoporosis and decreased skin elasticity; these are dose-dependent.[23]

A recent modification of GnRH agonist treatment is to 'add back' small amounts of steroid hormone in a manner similar to that used in the treatment of post-menopausal women. The theory is that the requirement for estrogen is greater for endometriosis than is needed by the brain (to prevent hot flashes), the bone (to prevent osteoporosis), and other tissues deprived of this hormone.[24] Interestingly, this 'threshold hypothesis' appears to be true, with estrogen-progestogen or progestogen only add back therapy resulting in an equivalent rate of pain relief with far fewer side-effects than GnRH agonist alone. Estrogen as a solitary add-back, however, is less effective and thus unindicated.[25] Currently, only levonorgestrel add-back therapy has been approved by the US Food and Drug Administration (FDA), although regimens of conjugated estrogens and medroxyprogesterone have also been demonstrated to be effective.

Gestrinone

Gestrinone (ethylnorgestrienone, R2323) is an antiprogestational steroid used extensively in Europe for the treatment of endometriosis, but not currently available in the United States. Its effects include androgenic, antiprogestogenic, and antiestrogenic actions, although the latter is not mediated by estrogen receptor-binding.

This steroid is believed to act by inducing a progesterone withdrawal effect at the endometrial cellular level, thus enhancing lysosomal degradation of the cellular structure. There is a rapid decrease in estrogen and progesterone receptors in normal endometrium following administration of gestrinone, as well as a sharp increase in 17-hydroxysteroid dehydrogenase. Interestingly, these cellular effects did not occur in samples of endometriotic tissue.[26]

Gestrinone may also inhibit ovarian steroidogenesis. A 50% decrease in serum estradiol level is noted after administration, perhaps related to the associated significant decline in sex hormone-binding globulin concentration (an androgenic or antiprogestogenic effect).[27] No effect on adrenal function or prolactin secretion has been noted.

Gestrinone is administered orally in doses of 2.5–10 mg weekly, on a daily, twice-weekly or thrice-weekly schedule. Side-effects include androgenic and antiestrogenic sequelae. Although most side-effects are mild and transient, several, such as voice changes, hirsutism, and clitoral hypertrophy, are potentially irreversible.

Experimental medical treatments of endometriosis

RU486 (mifepristone) and selective progesterone receptor modulators

Apart from its controversial role in pregnancy termination, mifepristone (RU486) may well prove to be of value in a wide variety of gynecologic disorders, including endometriosis. The drug is an antiprogesterone and antiglucocorticoid that can inhibit ovulation and disrupt endometrial integrity. Daily doses of the medication range from 50 mg to 100 mg, with side-effects ranging from hot flashes to fatigue, nausea, and transient liver transaminase changes. No effect upon lipid profiles or bone mineral density have been reported.

The ability of mifepristone to produce a regression of endometriotic lesions has been variable and apparently dependent upon duration of treatment. Trials of two months in the rodent model,[28] and three months in the human[29] failed to produce regression of disease. However, six months of therapy results in less visible disease in women.[30]

Uncontrolled trials suggest possible efficacy for endometriosis-associated pain, although numbers are small.[29] No data have yet been collected regarding fertility enhancement.

Selective progesterone receptor modulators (SPRMs) are partial antagonists of progesterone, but also behave like progesterone in some tissues. This mixed agonist – antagonist effect may prove valuable if a SPRM can inhibit endometrial growth while not producing other systemic effects of progesterone, such as breast tenderness, depression, and fluid retention. The mesoprogestin J867 is currently in phase III clinical trials; early studies have suggested efficacy in pain relief with minimal side-effects.

GnRH antagonists

Like GnRH agonists, the class of drugs called GnRH antagonists are analogs of GnRH that cause a down-regulation of the pituitary gland, a reduction of gonadotropin secretion, and suppression of ovarian steroid production. Thus, a hypoestrogenic state ensues, just as with GnRH agonists. Unlike GnRH agonists, however, these drugs do not cause an initial stimulation of gonadotropin and ovarian hormone release. Thus, they may have the advantage of working faster and more effectively, with better patient compliance due to earlier amelioration of symptoms. Studies in animal models of endometriosis have been quite promising,[31] and preliminary clinical trials suggest the drug to be safe and efficacious.[32] A recent investigation in women demonstrated a GnRH antagonist to improve the health-related quality of life in women with endometriosis.[33] Phase III clinical trials are currently ongoing to further validate the use of this medication for endometriosis, as questions regarding relative efficacy and rate of side-effects compared to GnRH agonists must be answered.

Aromatase inhibitors

Endometriosis appears to be dependent upon estrogen for growth and development. However, the estrogen does not have to come from elsewhere! Recent investigation has shown that endometriosis is capable of producing its own estrogen, due to the presence of an enzyme called aromatase.[34] This enzyme, not found in normal endometrium, is stimulated by prostaglandin E_2 (PGE_2); the resulting estrogen production then stimulates PGE_2, further enhancing estrogen. An obvious therapeutic target would thus be this aromatase enzyme. Aromatase inhibitors have now been tested in the rodent endometriosis model, with good success.[35] In addition, a case report of the use of anastrazole in a postmenopausal woman with severe endometriosis suggests the potential value of this treatment in women.[34] However, substantial bone loss in this woman emphasizes the need for caution with this class of medications, and reinforces the value of larger clinical trials to determine safety and efficacy.

TNFα inhibitors

Tumor necrosis factor-alpha (TNFα) is a cytokine that appears to be overproduced in endometriosis patients and may well be at least partially responsible for the influx of peritoneal macrophages known to occur in women with this disease. One therapeutic approach that has been considered is some type of blockade of this cytokine. This has been attempted in the baboon, where recombinant human TNF-binding protein-1 (TBP-1) was administered to menstrual endometrium prior to seeding the peritoneal cavity with the tissue.[36] In this scenario, endometriosis development was inhibited. Additionally, baboons with endometriosis were treated with TBP-1, GnRH antagonist, or placebo; significantly less endometriosis was noted with TBP-1 and GnRH antagonist treatment. These studies suggest TBP-1 is effective in treating the physical manifestations of endometriosis in the baboon, and may be of value in the human. Clinical trials, however, have not yet been conducted.

Angiogenesis inhibitors

According to the transplantation theory of endometriosis, when shed endometrium is placed in the peritoneal cavity, the establishment of a new blood supply is essential for the survival of the implant and development of endometriosis. Several angiogenic factors, that is, factors that aid in the development of new blood vessels, have been noted as present in endometrium and endometriosis. The most prominently studied of these factors is vascular endothelial growth factor (VEGF), which is responsible for inducing early vascular growth. This molecule has been noted in endometriosis lesions,[37] endometriomas,[38] and the peritoneal fluid[39,40] of endometriosis patients, although in the latter case it is unclear whether levels are the same as or increased over controls. In any event, one logical therapeutic step would be to attempt inhibition of these new vascular structures as a way of deterring the development of endometriosis. This has been attempted in the mouse model, where several angiogenic inhibitors (endostatin, TNP-470, celecoxib, and rosaglitazone) reduced the number and size of lesions.[41] No human trials have as yet been conducted with these or similar agents.

Matrix metalloproteinase inhibitors

Increased matrix metalloproteinase (MMP) activity has been described in endometriosis, and is believed to be integral in the ability of endometrium to invade tissue by breaking down extracellular matrix proteins. Inhibition of these enzymes might be effective in inhibiting the development of endometriosis. Only one study has been conducted to date: the MMP inhibitor ONO-4817 was used in the mouse model to deter the development of experimental adenomyosis.[42] The value and practicality of this approach in endometriosis remains to be tested.

Pentoxifylline

Pentoxifylline is a multisite immunomodulating drug. It inhibits phagocytosis and generation of toxic oxygen species and proteolytic enzymes by macrophages and granulocytes, stifles production of TNFα, and reduces the inflammatory action of TNFα and interleukin-1 (IL-1) on granulocytes.[43,44] Thus, this medication influences both the production of inflammatory mediators and the responsiveness of immunocompetent cells to inflammatory stimuli. Given the many immunologic abnormalities described in endometriosis, this medication has some rationale in an attempt to correct immune dysfunction. As it is not an inhibitor of ovulation, pentoxifylline has an advantage over ovulation suppressors when attempting to treat endometriosis-associated infertility: it can be administered throughout the time period of attempting conception. Doses have ranged from 400 mg to 1200 mg daily. The drug is extremely well tolerated, with the major adverse effects being gastric discomfort and dizziness; both are seen in few patients utilizing the recommended dose, and neither has been shown to occur more often in treated patients than placebo controls when giving commercial preparations of the drug.[45]

Results of medical treatment

Types of treatment trials

Although many studies have been published regarding the medical treatment of endometriosis, it is important to realize that not all are of equal importance. A hierarchy of clinical trial design exists that enables the discerning reader to determine which studies should be relied upon most heavily for validity and applicability.[46] These study designs, and their place in the hierarchy, are listed in Table 3.1.

Uncontrolled trials have limited value other than to suggest hypotheses to be tested by more rigorous designs. The same is true for historically controlled studies and concurrently controlled non-randomized trials, each of which introduces significant biases into the results. The gold standard today is the randomized clinical trial (RCT), where subjects are randomly allocated to one of several treatment groups, often in a blinded manner such that the assignment is unknown to the patient or physician until the conclusion of the trial. This design is the least biased of all approaches, and results in the most reliable conclusions.

Unfortunately, many RCTs are too small to reach a negative conclusion with any degree of confidence. The results of RCTs may also differ from one another, due to slight differences in study design, different patient populations, or even as a result of chance events. For these reasons, when multiple randomized trials exist they can often be combined into a single evaluation called a meta-analysis.[47] The meta-analysis allows us to gain a single, best answer to a question with a higher level of confidence than is usually possible with individual studies. However, it is important to keep in mind that a meta-analysis is only as good as the studies included in it; if poor quality trials are placed into a meta-analysis, the resulting conclusions are as tenuous as those of the component studies.

Assessing efficacy

The value of a particular medical treatment upon endometriosis will vary depending upon the therapeutic goal of the intervention. With regard to endometriosis, there are three outcomes that can be assessed to determine drug efficacy: (1) the anatomic manifestations of the disease; (2) pain symptomatology; and (3) infertility status.

The anatomic manifestations of endometriosis, implants and adhesions, can be assessed

Table 3.1 Hierarchy of evidence from clinical studies

  I. Meta-analysis or large randomized clinical trial
 II. Small randomized clinical trial
III. Non-randomized, concurrently controlled trial
 IV. Historically controlled trial
  V. Case-control study or cohort study
 VI. Time-series study or anecdotal case reports
VII. Expert opinion

before and after therapy to determine whether the intervention is of value. However, such a simple comparison makes two assumptions. First, it is assumed that endometriosis is an invariably progressive disease, never to regress on its own; this is unfortunately incorrect, as the disease has in fact been noted to regress in both baboons and humans.[48,49] Second, the above comparison presupposed that once regression has occurred via medical therapy, it is stable. This, too, is not the case, as implant and adhesion regrowth are both time-dependent phenomena. Thus, to adequately address the effect of a medical treatment upon endometriosis lesions, a proper control group for comparison is needed, with longitudinal follow-up.

A second outcome of interest is the effect upon pain. The first requirements of quality pain evaluation is the need for a valid method of assessing pain.[50] A second necessity in pain research is the need for longitudinal evaluation, as pain recurrence is a time-dependent phenomenon. Finally, to determine the efficacy of a drug in relieving pain, a large placebo effect must be accounted for. This phenomenon of relief by an inactive drug may occur in as many as 55% of women with endometriosis-associated pain.[51] Thus, placebo-controlled trials are needed to determine absolute efficacy; comparative studies between drugs will allow determination of relative efficacy.

The final outcome of interest is fertility enhancement. Unfortunately, it is rare that the woman with endometriosis-associated infertility has absolute infertility due to the disease, as is the case with bilateral tubal blockage or azoospermia. Instead, most women suffering from endometriosis-associated infertility have a relative reduction in fecundity.[49] Thus, they are able to conceive, albeit at a slower rate. To demonstrate improved fertility status after intervention, a comparison group of untreated women is clearly needed. Finally, as fertility is time-dependent, longitudinal assessment is again critical.

From the above discussion, it is clear that optimal trials are properly controlled and randomized. In addition, it is important to have studies that have lengthy follow-up so that we can determine the long-term course post-treatment. Studies such as these will be primarily relied upon in the subsequent discussion.

Medical treatment of endometriosis implants

The effect of medications on implant volume, number, and extensiveness has been examined for a number of drugs in a number of ways. Many are poorly controlled or uncontrolled investigations, and often the observation searching for effect is carried out while on the drug itself. Thus, what occurs after drug discontinuation is often a mystery.

An effect of danazol upon endometriotic implants has been consistently observed. Uncontrolled trials have demonstrated implant resolution in the vast majority of treated patients.[52,53] Questionable studies have shown a mean decrease of 61–89% of implant volume,[54,55] and a 43% decrease in classification score.[56] A single placebo-controlled RCT examined the effect upon implants six months following completion of drug therapy, with resolution of implants in 18% of the placebo group and 60% of the danazol treatment group.[57]

Although progestogens clearly affect ectopic endometrium, there is limited information on the histologic effect upon endometriosis. In the rhesus monkey, levonorgestrel has been shown to decrease lesion size. In the human, a single randomized prospective trial demonstrated that medroxyprogesterone acetate (MPA) 100 mg daily for six months produced complete resolution of implants in 50% of patients and a partial resolution in 13%, whereas corresponding figures for placebo were 12% and 6%, respectively.[57]

Several randomized trials have assessed the ability of gestrinone to decrease anatomic endometriosis. The drug has been shown to lower the amount of disease comparably to danazol,[58] and doses as low as 1.25 mg twice-weekly can accomplish this.[59,60]

GnRH agonists have been shown in numerous studies to decrease the classification score of endometriosis in patients on the drug; similar decreases were seen with the complete (rAFS) classification as well as a modified scoring system that excluded points for adhesions[61,62] (Fig. 3.1). Thus, the effect is limited to causing a lessening of implant volume. In comparative trials, the decreased AFS score is comparable to that seen with danazol treatment.[63] No study has evaluated the lingering effect of GnRH on implants after discontinuation of the drug, however. GnRH agonist plus add-back therapy has also been shown to decrease the AFS classification score, and to a degree similar to that seen with GnRH agonist alone.[64]

Currently, no published data exist for other forms of medical treatment.

Medical treatment of endometriosis-associated pain

Pain relief has also been well demonstrated with danazol, with 84–92% of women responding.[65] A placebo-controlled RCT proved danazol reduced pain significantly better than no treatment for up to six months following discontinuation of the drug.[57] No good data exists

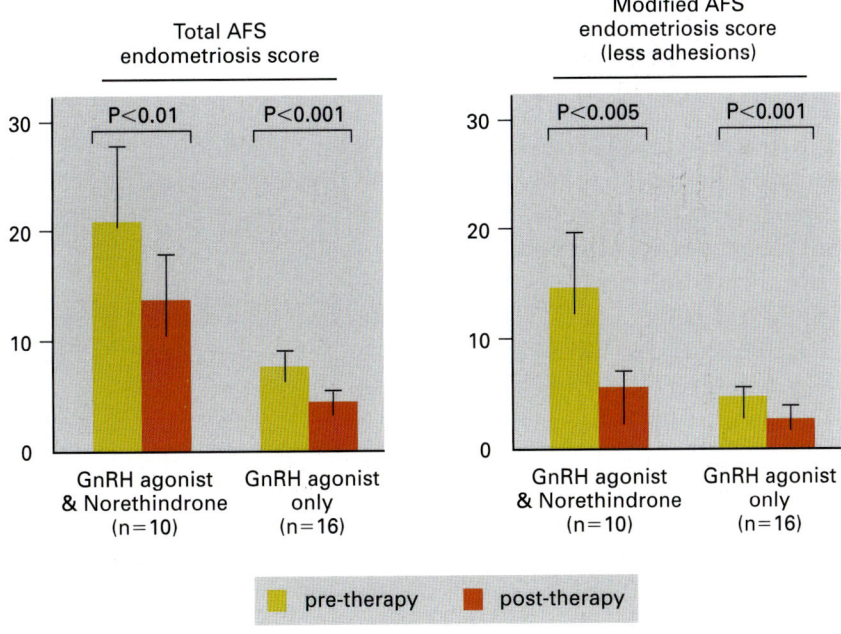

Figure 3.1
Decrease in point total from the AFS classification system with treatment of endometriosis by a GnRH agonist

for longer follow-up periods. Recent evidence suggests the median time to pain recurrence following discontinuation of the medication is 6.1 months.[66]

Few randomized trials exist to evaluate the effects of progestational agents on endometriosis-associated pain. Telimaa and colleagues evaluated the effect of medroxyprogesterone acetate, 100 mg/day for six months. The medication produced a significant and substantial improvement in pain scores while patients received the drug, as well as up to six months following discontinuation.[57] In fact, the relative attributable experimental effect (percentage decrease in pain severity attributable solely to treatment) was 50–74% at the conclusion of follow-up. Randomized comparative trials suggest medroxyprogesterone to be comparable in efficacy to danazol, although lynestrenol performed less well than a GnRH agonist for all aspects of endometriosis-associated pain.[67]

Numerous uncontrolled trials have evaluated pain relief with oral contraceptives, generally demonstrating improvement in 75–89%.[11] A recent randomized clinical trial compared cyclic low dose oral contraceptives to a GnRH agonist and found no substantial difference in the degree of relief afforded these women by the two drugs, except that the GnRH agonist provided greater relief of dysmenorrhea.[68] An uncontrolled trial of continuous oral contraceptive pills (OCPs) following failure of cyclic therapy suggested that this regimen may be superior, as 80% responded with pain relief.[69] However, no RCTs have as yet assessed continuous administration.

The effectiveness of GnRH agonists in the treatment of endometriosis-associated pain has been demonstrated in both placebo-controlled and comparative randomized trials. The one placebo-controlled study demonstrated greater effectiveness of the drug at three months, at which time those in the placebo group still suffering from pain were allowed to opt out of the study.[70] In comparative trials, GnRH agonists and danazol were equally effective in relieving pain.[63, 71–85] OCPs have also been compared with GnRH agonists: in a study of 57 women designed to have 80% power to detect a 35% difference in effect, cyclic oral contraceptive treatment was significantly less effective than GnRH agonist treatment for relief of dysmenorrhea, nearly as effective for relief of dyspareunia (statistically significantly different using one of two rating scales, but of questionable clinical importance), and equally efficacious in relieving non-specific pelvic pain.[68]

While the above studies randomize patients for initial therapy of endometriosis-associated pain, one study has examined the value of GnRH agonist in patients failing primary therapy. Ling and colleagues treated women having failed to obtain relief with OCPs with either GnRH agonist or placebo.[86] Those treated with active drug responded significantly better than those given placebo, with more than 80% experiencing pain relief in three months (Fig. 3.2).

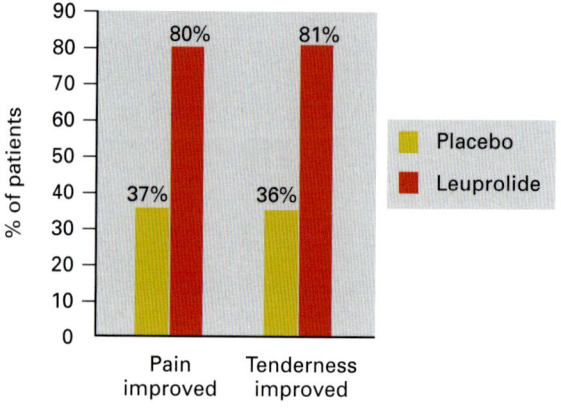

Figure 3.2
Subjective and objective pain relief with empiric treatment of GnRH agonist for presumed endometriosis following failure of other medical therapy

Of interest is the fact that the therapy seemed to be beneficial whether or not endometriosis was seen at laparoscopy.

Several trials have addressed the efficacy of combined add-back therapy and GnRH agonist treatment during six-month treatment periods.[87–92] In general, pain was relieved as effectively with the combination as with GnRH agonist alone, and it significantly reduced the side-effects of the GnRH agonist. The results were similar in three longer trials of approximately one year duration.[64,93,94] It seems clear that add-back therapy can be added to GnRH agonist treatment without loss of efficacy but with a substantial amelioration of hypoestrogenic symptoms (Fig. 3.3). This seems to be the case even when the add-back therapy is begun during the first month of treatment, suggesting that an 'add-back-free' interval at the beginning of a treatment cycle is unnecessary.[92]

Although not approved for use in the United States, gestrinone has been studied reasonably extensively. Comparative trials show gestrinone to be roughly equivalent in pain relief to danazol[58] and GnRH-agonists.[95] One study has even shown gestrinone to be slightly more efficacious than GnRH agonist for relief of dysmenorrhea six months after discontinuation of medication.[95]

Given the above data, a number of conclusions can be reached regarding treatment of endometriosis symptoms with medical therapy. It appears that most established medical treatments are effective for the primary treatment of endometriosis-associated pain, and all also seem to be roughly equivalent. Thus, for initial treatment the choice should probably be based on the cost and side-effect profile of the drug being considered. However, only GnRH agonists have been proven effective after the failure of a prior medical hormonal therapy. It remains to be seen what the value is for the newer, investigational therapies; the answers will await upcoming efficacy and comparative trials.

Medical treatment of endometriosis-associated infertility

Most of the established medical therapies used to treat endometriosis have been applied to the problem of subfertility in women with endometriosis. These medications inhibit ovulation, and thus are used to treat the disease for a period of time prior to allowing an attempt at conception. Five randomized trials with six treatment arms have compared one of these medical treatments directed at endometriosis to placebo or no treatment with fertility as the outcome measure[96–100] (Table 3.2). Another eight randomized clinical trials (RCTs) compared danazol to a second medication. These latter trials have been summarized recently by a meta-analysis by Hughes et al.[101] Clearly, no increase in fertility can be demonstrated with these medications when compared to expectant management; nor has any medication proven superior to danazol in this regard.

But wait! While some studies were placebo-controlled, others simply compared medication to no treatment. For this latter study design, follow-up of the patient was begun at the conclusion of therapy; thus those receiving no treatment began attempting to conceive immediately after the diagnostic laparoscopy, while those placed on drug therapy were not allowed attempted conception until after the medication course was completed (generally 6 months). These studies were analysed as if the time began at the conclusion of 'treatment', but for the patient, the clock begins ticking at the time of diagnostic laparoscopy. The real question is not who gets pregnant faster after therapy is completed, but rather who gets pregnant faster from the time of diagnosis?

If we reanalyse the above data, with follow-up proceeding from the time of diagnosis instead of

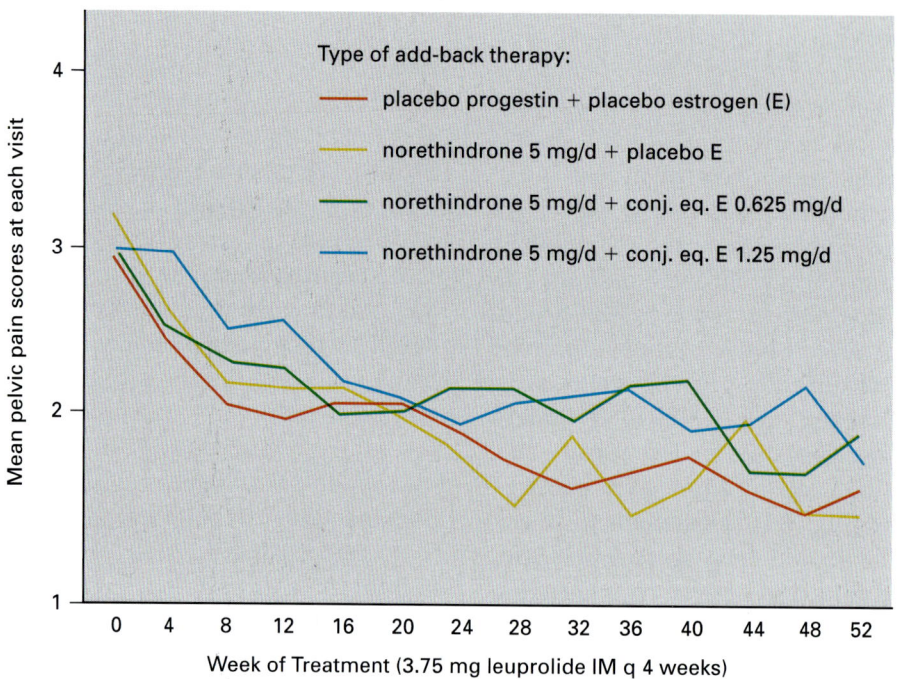

Figure 3.3
Pain relief with GnRH agonist with and without add-back therapy. Group 1, GnRH agonist alone; Group 2, GnRH agonist plus norethindrone; Group 3, GnRH agonist plus low dose conjugated estrogen/norethindrone; Group 4, GnRH agonist plus high dose conjugated estrogen/norethindrone

conclusion of treatment, a different image emerges (Table 3.3). Now, suppressive medical therapy proves significantly detrimental to fertility. In essence, the interval spent on medical therapy has been wasted time, merely serving to prolong the infertility in a number of couples. Thus, traditional medical therapy for endometriosis has not proven to be of value,

Table 3.2 Meta-analysis of medical therapy for endometriosis-associated infertility				
Study	Medical treatment	Placebo or no treatment	Relative risk	95% Confidence limits
Bayer[96]	11/37	17/36	0.63	0.32–1.22
Fedele[99]	17/35	17/36	1.03	0.60–1.76
Telimaa[97]	13/35	6/14	0.87	0.41–2.25
Thomas[100]	5/20	4/17	1.06	0.28–4.29
Harrison[98]	0/50	3/50	0.00	0.00–2.18
TOTAL	46/177	47/153	0.85	0.59–1.22

and in fact may be counterproductive, to the subfertile patient.

This is not to suggest that traditional medical therapy is incapable of playing a role in the treatment of the infertile couple with endometriosis. It is quite possible that a subgroup of infertile women exist who could be helped with drug therapy. However, this subgroup is thus far unidentified; advocates should focus future trials upon somehow stratifying endometriosis patients and then randomized to drug versus no treatment. Until that time, it is clear that these medications play no role in the treatment of endometriosis-associated infertility.

Of the experimental treatment for endometriosis, only pentoxifylline has been investigated as a treatment for endometriosis-associated infertility. This drug has the advantage of not inhibiting ovulation and thus can be utilized without delay of attempted conception. A single placebo-controlled RCT with 60 patients resulted in a 12 month pregnancy rate of 31% with pentoxifylline and 18.5% with placebo, a difference not statistically different but intriguing nonetheless.[102] It is hoped that additional, larger trials will further investigate this approach to help clarify the value of this and similar drugs.

Medical therapy following surgery

The use of medical therapy for endometriosis is not restricted to their use as stand-alone agents. Frequently, clinicians have used drugs in combination with surgical treatment of the disease. When this approach is utilized, the medical therapy may be administered either preoperatively or postoperatively.

Only one randomized trial has evaluated the value of preoperative hormonal therapy.[103] In this study, women with advanced endometriosis were either treated for three months with a GnRH agonist prior to surgery or with surgery alone. Surgery was noted to be easier (but not statistically significantly easier) by the surgeon, but surgical outcome was not assessed in terms of symptomatic relief.

Numerous RCTs have examined the issue of postoperative medical therapy as an effective adjunct for pain. Danazol was found not to enhance the results of surgery when administered for only three months,[104] but six months of postoperative administration reduced pain versus placebo for at least six months following discontinuation of the drug.[105] High dose medroxyprogesterone behaved similarly.[105] Three RCTs have examined the use of postoperative GnRH agonists: three months of treatment

Table 3.3 Meta-analysis of medical therapy for endometriosis-associated infertility: adjustment for follow-up from time of diagnosis

Study	Medical treatment	Placebo or no treatment	Relative risk	95% Confidence limits
Bayer[96]	11/37	17/36	0.63	0.32–1.22
Fedele[99]	10/35	13/36	0.79	0.36–1.68
Telimaa[97]	4/35	5/14	0.32	0.08–1.24
Thomas[100]	4/20	4/17	0.85	0.20–3.69
Harrison[98]	0/50	3/50	0.00	0.00–2.18
TOTAL	29/177	42/153	0.60	0.38–0.93

was ineffective at enhancing pain relief,[106] but six months of postoperative therapy significantly reduced pain scores and delayed recurrence of pain[107,108] (Fig. 3.4). The use of oral contraceptives for six months following surgery has been shown ineffective in improving the results of surgery.[109] Finally, an RCT compared postoperative use of a levonorgestrel-containing intrauterine device (IUD) versus surgery alone and found that all forms of pelvic pain were significantly reduced postoperatively by the addition of the IUD.[110]

One RCT has examined the use of a single postoperative medical therapy versus two sequential medical treatments following surgery. Morgante and colleagues compared the use of six months of postoperative GnRH agonist therapy to 6 months of GnRH agonist followed by six months of danazol, 100 mg/day.[111] Twelve months following surgery (at the conclusion of danazol for one group, and after six months of no treatment for the other) there was significantly less pain in those treated with the two sequential medical treatments.

Three studies have investigated the use of postoperative medical therapy for fertility enhancement, utilizing GnRH agonist[107,109] and raloxifene,[112] a selective estrogen receptor modulator. None has demonstrated any enhancement of fertility in women with endometriosis utilizing this approach.

While these studies suggest that postoperative medical therapy is of value when used for six months or more, a word of caution must be interjected. As is the case with all surgical trials, the degree of surgical skill and the technique used may be critical in determining the results. At least one retrospective trial has indicated that excision of endometriosis results in greater pain relief than ablation of lesions,[113] yet ablation is generally the treatment of choice with these studies (Fig. 3.5). Furthermore, we have no way of ascertaining the degree of surgical skill that was applied in the surgical treatment of these patients. Additional high quality studies are needed in a variety of settings by a larger number of surgeons to further examine this issue and confirm the above results.

Conclusions

The use of medical therapy in the treatment of endometriosis has a long and colorful history, with a wide variety of medications having been applied to the problems at hand. For decades we had little in the way of scientific information to guide us, but today the proliferation of randomized clinical trials in our literature provides the discerning clinician with excellent clues as to how best approach the treatment of symptomatic disease. One clear deficiency in the literature, however, is the lack of a direct comparison between medical and surgical therapy in the treatment of endometriosis-associated pain.

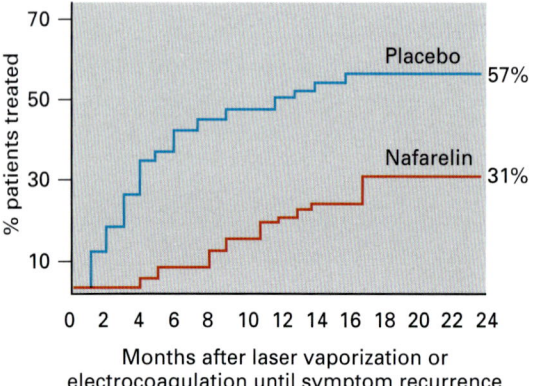

Figure 3.4
Rate of recurrence of pelvic pain following treatment with surgery alone versus surgery followed by GnRH agonist therapy

MODERN MEDICAL THERAPY OF ENDOMETRIOSIS

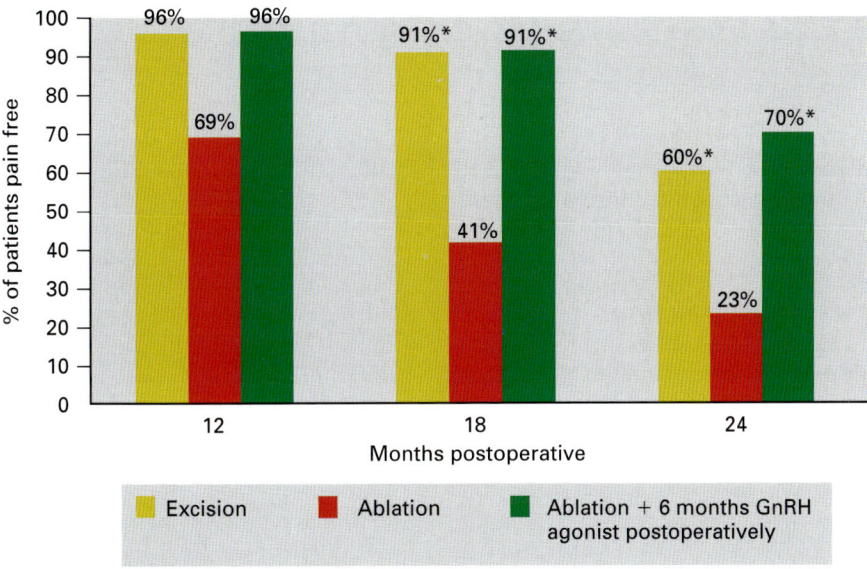

* P <0.05 compared to ablation

Figure 3.5
Pain relief with excision of endometriosis versus ablation of endometriosis versus ablation followed by medical therapy

Although several randomized trials have been attempted, none has ever been completed. Data from placebo and sham controlled studies suggest similar success rates, but these investigations have been carried out in different patient populations under differing conditions. Until a randomized clinical trial comparing medicine and surgery is carried out, the relative merits of each is purely speculative.

Nonetheless, what is clear from the above data is that medical therapy can be of value in the treatment of endometriosis, particularly with regard to pain symptomatology. Furthermore, with a wide variety of investigational medications being investigated, it is likely that the role of medication for this disease will expand in the future. As this occurs and our treatment options expand, we are likely to see an era of improved efficacy with fewer side-effects for more patients, a situation clearly advantageous to the many women suffering from the ravages of endometriosis.

References

1. Goebel R, Rjosk HK. Laboratory and clinical studies with the new antigonadotropin, danazol. Acta Endocrinol 1977;85(Suppl 212):134 (abstract).
2. Floyd WS. Danazol: endocrine and endometrial effects. Int J Fertil 1980;25:75–80.
3. Barbieri RL, Canick JA, Makris A, Todd RB, Davies IJ, Ryan KJ. Danazol inhibits steroidogenesis. Fertil Steril 1977;28:809–13.
4. McGinley R, Casey JH. Analysis of progesterone in unextracted serum: a method using danazol [17(-pregn-4-en 20 yno(2,3-d) osoxazol-17-ol] a blocker of steroid binding to proteins. Steroids 1979;33:127–38.
5. Buttram VC Jr, Belue JB, Reiter R. Interim report of a study of danazol for the treatment of endometriosis. Fertil Steril 1982;37:478–83.
6. Alvarado RG, Liu JY, Zwolak RM. Danazol and limb-threatening arterial thrombosis: two case reports. J Vasc Surg 2001;34:1123–6.
7. Vercellini P, Tresid L, Panazza S, Bramante T, Mauro F, Crosignani PG. Very low dose danazol for relief of endometriosis-associated pelvic pain: a pilot study. Fertil Steril 1994;62:1136–42.
8. Janicki TI. Treatment of the pelvic pain associated with endometriosis using danazol vaginal suppositories. Two year followup. Fertil Steril 2002;77:S52.
9. Igarashi M, Iizuka M, Abe Y, Ibuki Y. Novel vaginal danazol ring therapy for pelvic endometriosis, in particular deeply infiltrating endometriosis. Hum Reprod 1998;13:1952–6.
10. Bruner KL, Eisenberg E, Gorstein F, Osteen KG. Progesterone and transforming growth factor-beta coordinately regulate suppression of endometrial matrix metalloproteinases in a model of experimental endometriosis. Steroids 1999;64:648–53.
11. Olive DL. Medical treatment: alternatives to danazol. In: Schenken RS (ed). Endometriosis: contemporary concepts in clinical management. Philadelphia: JB Lippincott, 1989:189–211.
12. Muneyyirci-Delale O, Karacan M. Effect of norethindrone acetate in the treatment of symptomatic endometriosis. Int J Fertil Womens Med 1999;43:24–7.
13. Fedele L, Bianchi S, Zanconato G, Portuese A, Raffaelli R. Use of a levonorgestrel-releasing intrauterine device in the treatment of rectovaginal endometriosis. Fertil Steril 2001;75:485–8.
14. Lau TM, Affandi B, Rogers PAW. The effects of levonorgestrel implants on vascular endothelial growth factor expression in the endometrium. Mol Hum Reprod 1998;5:57–63.
15. Hamblen EC. Androgen treatment of women. South Med J 1957;50:743.
16. Hirvonen E, Malkonen M, Manninen V. Effects of different progestogens on lipoproteins during postmenopausal replacement therapy. N Engl J Med 1981;304:560.
17. Fahraeus L, Sydsjo A, Wallentin L. Lipoprotein changes during treatment of pelvic endometriosis with medroxyprogesterone acetate. Fertil Steril 1986;45:503.
18. Andrews MC, Andrews WC, Strauss AF. Effects of progestin-induced pseudopregnancy on endometriosis; clinical and microscopic studies. Am J Obstet Gynecol 1959;78:776.
19. Scott RB, Wharton LR Jr. The effect of estrone and progesterone on the growth of experimental endometriosis in rhesus monkeys. Am J Obstet Gynecol 1957;74:852.
20. Noble AD, Letchworth AT. Medical treatment of endometriosis: a comparative trial. Postgrad Med J 1979;55(Suppl 5):37.
21. Meresman GF, Auge L, Barano RI, Lombardi E, Tesone M, Sueldo C. Oral contraceptives treatment suppresses proliferation and enhances apoptosis of eutopic endometrial tissue from patients with endometriosis. Fertil Steril 2001;76:S47–48.
22. Sharpe-Timms KL, Zimmer RL, Jolliff WJ, Wright JA, Nothnick WB, Curry TE. Gonadotropin-releasing hormone agonist (GnRH-a) therapy alters activity of plasminogen activators, matrix metalloproteinases and their inhibitors in rat models for adhesion formation and endometriosis: potential GnRH-a-regulated

22. mechanisms reducing adhesion formation. Fertil Steril 1998;69:916–23.
23. Dmowski WP. The role of medical management in the treatment of endometriosis. In: Nezhat CR, Berger GS, Nezhat FR, Buttram VC Jr, Nezhat CH (eds) Endometriosis: Advanced management and surgical techniques. New York: Springer, 1995:229–40.
24. Barbieri RL. Endometriosis and the estrogen threshold theory. Relation to surgical and medical treatment. J Reprod Med 1998;43:287–92.
25. Hurst BS, Gardner SC, Tucker KE, Awoniyi CA, Schlaff WD. Delayed oral estradiol combined with leuprolide increases endometriosis-related pain. J Soc Laparoendosc Surgeons 2000;4:97–101.
26. Cornillie FJ, Brosens IA, Vasquez G, Riphogen I. Histologic and ultrastructural changes in human endometriotic implants treated with the antiprogesterone steroid ethylnorgestrenone (gestrinone) during 2 months. Int J Gynecol Pathol 1986;5:95.
27. Robyn C, Delogne-Desnoeck J, Bourdoux P, Copinschi G. Endocrine effects of gestrinone. In: Raynaud J-P, Ojasoot, Martini L (eds). Medical management of endometriosis. New York: Raven, 1984:207.
28. Tjaden B, Galetto D, Woodruff JD, Rock JA. Time-related effects of RU486 treatment in experimentally induced endometriosis in the rat. Fertil Steril 1993;59:437.
29. Kettel LM, Murphy AA, Mortola JF, Liu JH, Ulmann A, Yen SSC. Endocrine responses to long-term administration of the antiprogesterone RU486 in patients with pelvic endometriosis. Fertil Steril 1991;56:402.
30. Kettel LM, Murphy AA, Morales AJ, Ulmann A, Baulieu EE, Yen SSC. Treatment of endometriosis with the antiprogesterone mifepristone (RU486). Unpublished data.
31. Jones RC. The effect of a luteinizing hormone-releasing hormone antagonist on experimental endometriosis in the rat. Acta Endocrinol 1987;114:379–82.
32. Martha PM, Gray ME, Campion M, Kuca B, Garnick MB. Initial safety profile and hormonal dose response characteristics of the pure GnRH antagonist, Abarelix-depot, in women with endometriosis. Unpublished data.
33. Woolley JM, De Paoli AM, Gray ME, Martha PM. Reductions in health related quality of life in women with endometriosis. Abstract. Seventh Biennial World Congress of Endometriosis, London, 14–17 May 2000.
34. Bulun SE, Zeitoun KM, Takayama K, Sasano H. Molecular basis for treating endometriosis with aromatase inhibitors. Hum Reprod Update 2000;6:413–18.
35. Yano S, Ikegami Y, Nakao K. Studies on the effect of the new non-steroidal aromatase inhibitor fadrozole hydrochloride in an endometriosis model in rats. Arzneimittelforschung 1996;46:192–5.
36. D'Hooghe TM, Cuneo S, Nugent N, Chai D, Deer F, Mwenda J. Recombinant human TNF binding protein-1 (r-hTBP-1) inhibits the development of endometriosis in baboons; a prospective, randomized, placebo and drug controlled study. Fertil Steril 2001;76:S1.
37. Donnez J, Smoes P, Gillerot S, Casanas-Roux F, Nisolle M. Vascular endothelial growth factor (VEGF) in endometriosis. Hum Reprod 1998;13:1686–90.
38. Fasciani A, D'Ambrogio G, Bocci G, Monti M, Genazzani AR, Artini PG. High concentrations of the vascular endothelial growth factor and interleukin-8 in ovarian endometriomata. Mol Hum Reprod 2000;6:50–4.
39. Mahnke JL, Dawood MY, Huang JC. Vascular endothelial growth factor and interleukin-6 in peritoneal fluid of women with endometriosis. Fertil Steril 2000;73:166–70.
40. Barcz E, Kaminski P, Marianowski L. VEGF concentration in peritoneal fluid in patients with endometriosis. Gynekol Pol 2001;72:442–8.
41. Levine Z, Efstathiou JA, Sampson DA, Rohan RM, Folkman J, D'Amato RJ, Rupnick MA. Angiogenesis inhibitors suppress endometriosis in a murine model. J Soc Gynecol Investig 2002;9:264a.
42. Mori T, Yamasaki S, Masui F, Matsuda M, Sasabe H, Zhou YF. Suppression of the development of experimentally induced uterine adenomyosis by a novel matrix metalloproteinase inhibitor, ONO-4817, in mice. Exp Biol Med 2001;226:429–33.
43. Steinleitner A, Lambert H, Roy S. Immunomodulation with pentoxifylline abrogates macrophage-mediated infertility in an in vivo

model: a paradigm for a novel approach to the treatment of endometriosis-associated subfertility. Fertil Steril 1991;55:26–31.
44. Steinleitner A, Lambert H, Suarez M. Immunomodulation in the treatment of endometriosis-associated subfertility: use of pentoxifylline to reverse the inhibition of fertilization by surgically induced endometriosis in a rodent model. Fertil Steril 1991;56:975–9.
45. Physicians' Desk Reference. Medical Economics Company, Inc., Montvale, NJ, 2002:784.
46. Olive DL, Pritts EA, Morales AJ. Evidence-based medicine: study design for evaluation and treatment. J Am Assoc Gynecol Laparosc 1998;5: 75–82.
47. Hughes EG. Systematic literature review and meta-analysis. Sem Reprod Endocrinol 1996;14: 161–9.
48. Cooke ID, Thomas EJ. The medical treatment of mild endometriosis. Acta Obstet Gynecol Scand 1989;150(Suppl):27.
49. D'Hooghe TM, Bambra CS, Isahakia M, Koninckx PR. Evolution of spontaneous endometriosis in the baboon (Papio anubis, Papio cynocephalus) over a 12-month period. Fertil Steril 1992;58:409.
50. Jones G, Kennedy S, Barnard A, Wong J, Jenkinson C. Development of an endometriosis quality-of-life instrument: The Endometriosis Health Profile-30. Obstet Gynecol 2001;98: 258–264.
51. Kauppila A, Puolakka J, Ylikorkala O. Prostaglandin biosynthesis inhibitors and endometriosis. Prostaglandins 1979;18:655.
52. Dmowski WP, Cohen MR. Treatment of endometriosis with an antigonadotropin, danazol: A laparoscopic and histologic evaluation. Obstet Gynecol 1975;46:147.
53. Barbieri RL, Evans S, Kistner RW. Danazol in the treatment of endometriosis: Analysis of 100 cases with a 4-year follow-up. Fertil Steril 1982;37:737.
54. Doberl A, Jeppsson S, Rannevik G. Effect of danazol on serum concentrations of pituitary gonadotropins in post-menopausal women. Acta Obstet Gynecol Scand 1984;123(Suppl):95.
55. Buttram VC Jr, Reiter RC, Ward S. Treatment of endometriosis with danazol: Report of a six-year prospective study. Fertil Steril 1985;318: 485.
56. Henzl MR, Corson SL, Moghissi K et al. Administration of nasal nafarelin as compared with oral danazol for endometriosis. N Engl J Med 1988;318:485.
57. Telimaa S, Puolakka J, Ronnberg L, Kaupilla A. Placebo-controlled comparison of danazol and high-dose medroxyprogesterone acetate in the treatment of endometriosis. Gynecol Endocrinol 1987;1:13.
58. Fedele L, Bianchi S, Viezzoli T, Arcaini L, Cendiani GB. Gestrinone vs. danazol in the treatment of endometriosis. Fertil Steril 1989;51:781.
59. Worthington M, Irvine LM, Crook D, Lees B, Shaw RW, Stevenson JC. A randomized comparative study of the metabolic effects of two regimens of gestrinone in the treatment of endometriosis. Fertil Steril 1993;59:522.
60. Hornstein MD, Gleason RE, Barbieri RL. A randomized double-blind prospective trial of two doses of gestrinone in the treatment of endometriosis. Fertil Steril 1990;53:237.
61. Cedars MI, Lu JK, Meldrum DR, Judd HL. Obstet Gynecol 1990;75:641–5.
62. Surrey ES, Gambone JC, Lu JK, Judd HL. Fertil Steril 1990;53:620–6.
63. Henzl MR, Corson SL, Moghissi K, Buttram VC, Berqvist C, Jacobson J. Administration of nasal nafarelin as compared with oral danazol for endometriosis. A multicenter double-blind comparative clinical trial. New Eng J Med 1998; 318:485–9.
64. Surrey ES, Voigt B, Fournet N, Judd HL. Prolonged gonadotropin-releasing hormone agonist treatment of symptomatic endometriosis: the role of cyclic sodium etidronate and low dose norethindrone 'add-back' therapy. Fertil Steril 1995;63:747–55.
65. Bayer SR, Seibel MM. Medical treatment: Danazol. In: Schenkel RS (ed) Endometriosis: Contemporary concepts in clinical management. Philadelphia: JB Lippincott, 1989:169–87.
66. Miller JD, Shaw RW, Casper RF, Rock JA, Thomas EJ, Dmowski WP, Surrey E, Malinak LR, Moghissi K. Historical prospective cohort study of the recurrence of pain after discontinuation of treatment with danazol or a gonadotropin-releasing hormone agonist. Fertil Steril 1998;70:293–6.
67. Regidor PA, Regidor M, Schmidt M, Ruwe B, Lubben G, Fortig P, Kienle E, Schindler AE.

Prospective randomized study comparing the GnRH-agonist leuprorelin acetate and the gestagen lynestrenol in the treatment of severe endometriosis. Gynecol Endocrinol 2001;15: 202–9.

68. Vercellini P, Trespidi L, Colombo A, Vendola N, Marchini M, Crosignani PG. A gonadotropin-releasing hormone agonist versus a low-dose oral contraceptive for pelvic pain associated with endometriosis. Fertil Steril 1993;60:75.

69. Frontino G, Vercellini P, De Giorgi O, Zaina B, Pisacreta A, Crosignani PG. Continuous use of oral contraceptive (OC) for endometriosis-associated recurrent dysmenorrhea not responding to cyclic pill regimen. Fertil Steril 2002;77: S23–4.

70. Dlugi AM, Miller JD, Knittle J. Lupron depot (leuprolide acetate for depot suspension) in the treatment of endometriosis: a randomized, placebo-controlled, double-blind study. Fertil Steril 1990;419–27.

71. Anonymous. Goserelin depot versus danazol in the treatment of endometriosis. The Australian/New Zealand experience. Aus NZ J Obstet Gynaecol 1996;31:55–60.

72. Chang SP, Ng HT. A randomized comparative study of the effect of leuprorelin acetate depot and danazol in the treatment of endometriosis. Chin Med J (Taipei) 1996;57:431–7.

73. Cirkel U, Oochs H, Schneider HPG. A randomized, comparative trial of triptorelin depot (D-Trp6-LHRH) and danazol in the treatment of endometriosis. Eur J Obstet Gynecol Reprod Bio 1995;59:61–9.

74. Crosignani PG, Gastaldi A, Lombardi PL et al. Leuprorelin acetate depot versus danazol in the treatment of endometriosis: results of an open multicentre trial. Clin Ther 1992;14(Suppl A): 2936.

75. Dmowski WP, Radwanska E, Binor Z, Tummon I, Pepping P. Ovarian suppression induced with buserelin or danazol in the management of endometriosis: a randomized, comparative study. Fertil Steril 1989;51:395–400.

76. Fraser IS, Shearman RP, Jansen RP, Sutherland PD. A comparative treatment trial of endometriosis using the gonadotropin-releasing hormone agonist, nafarelin, and the synthetic steroid, danazol. Aus NZ J Obstet Gynaecol 1991;158–63.

77. Adamson GD, Kwei L, Edgren RA. Pain of endometriosis: effects of nafarelin and danazol therapy. Int J Fertil Med Stud 1994;39:215–17.

78. Wheeler JM, Knittle JD, Miller JD. Depot leuprolide versus danazol in treatment of women with symptomatic endometriosis: I. Efficacy results. Am J Obstet Gynecol 1992;167: 1367–71.

79. Dawood MY, Ramos J, Khan-Dawood FS. Depot leuprolide acetate versus danazol for treatment of pelvic endometriosis: changes in vertebral bone mass and serum estradiol and calcitonin. Fertil Steril 1995;63:1177–83.

80. The Nafarelin European Endometriosis Trial Group (NEET). Nafarelin for endometriosis: a large-scale, danazol-controlled trial of efficacy and safety, with 1-year follow-up. Fertil Steril 1992;57:514–22.

81. Rolland R, van der Heijden PF. Nafarelin versus danazol in the treatment of endometriosis. Am J Obstet Gynecol 1990;162:586–8.

82. Kennedy SH, Williams IA, Brodribb J, Barlow DH, Shaw RW. A comparison of nafarelin acetate and danazol in the treatment of endometriosis. Fertil Steril 1990;53:998–1003.

83. Rock JA. A multicenter comparison of GnRH agonist (Zoladex) and danazol in the treatment of endometriosis. Fertil Steril 1991;56:S49.

84. Shaw RW. An open randomized comparative study of the effect of goserelin depot and danazol in the treatment of endometriosis. Zoladex Endometriosis Study Team. Fertil Steril 1992;58:265–72.

85. Prentice A, Deery A, Goldbeck-Wood S, Farquhar C, Smith S. Gonadotropin-releasing hormone analogues for pain associated with endometriosis (Cochrane Review). In: The Cochrane Library, Issue 3, 1999. Oxford: Update Software.

86. Ling FW. Randomized controlled trial of depot leuprolide in patients with chronic pelvic pain and clinically suspected endometriosis. Obstet Gynecol 1999;93:51–8.

87. Surrey E, Judd H. Reduction of vasomotor symptoms and bone mineral density loss with combined norethindrone and long-acting gonadotropin-releasing hormone agonist therapy of symptomatic endometriosis: a prospective randomized trial. J Clin Endocrinol Metab 1992;75:558–63.

88. Makarainen L, Ronneberg L, Kauppila A. Medroxyprogesterone acetate supplementation diminishes the hypoestrogenic side-effects of gonadotropin-releasing hormone agonists without changing its efficacy in endometriosis. Fertil Steril 1996;65:29–34.

89. Tabkin O, Yakinoghe AH, Kucuk S, Uryan I, Buhur A, Burak R. Effectiveness of tibolone on hypoestrogenic symptoms induced by goserelin treatment in patients with endometriosis. Fertil Steril 1997;67:40–5.

90. Edmonds D, Howell R. Can hormone replacement therapy be used during medical therapy of endometriosis? Br J Obstet Gynecol 1994;101:24–6.

91. Kiiholma P, Korhonen M, Tuimala R, Korhonen M, Hagman E. Comparison of the gonadotropin-releasing hormone agonist goserelin acetate alone versus goserelin combined with estrogen-progestogens add-back therapy in the treatment of endometriosis. Fertil Steril 1995;64:903–8.

92. Moghissi KS, Schlaff WD, Olive DL, Skinner MA, Yin H. Goserelin acetate (Zoladex) with or without hormone replacement therapy for the treatment of endometriosis. Fertil Steril 1998;69:1056–62.

93. Hornstein MD, Surrey ES, Weisberg GW, Casino LA, Lupron Add-Back Study Group. Leuprolide acetate depot and hormonal add-back in endometriosis: a 12-month study. Obstet Gynecol 1998;91:16–24.

94. Lee PI, Yoon JB, Joo KY, Lee JK, Cho JY, Kim JS. Gonadotrophin releasing hormone agonist (GnRHa)-Zoladex (Goserelin) and hormonal add-back therapy in endometriosis: a 12 month study. Fertil Steril 2002;77:S23.

95. The Gestrinone Italian Study Group. Gestrinone versus a gonadotropin-releasing hormone agonist for the treatment of pelvic pain associated with endometriosis: a multicenter randomised, double-blind study. Fertil Steril 1996;66:911–19.

96. Bayer SR, Seibel MM, Saffan DS, Berger MJ, Taymor ML. Efficacy of danazol treatment for minimal endometriosis in infertile women: A prospective, randomized study. J Reprod Med 1988;33:179–183.

97. Telimaa S. Danazol and medroxyprogesterone acetate inefficacious in the treatment of infertility in endometriosis. Fertil Steril 1988;50:872–5.

98. Harrison RF, Barry-Kinsella C. Efficacy of medroxyprogesterone treatment in infertile women with endometriosis: a prospective, randomized, placebo-controlled study. Fertil Steril 2000;74:24–30

99. Fedele L, Parazzini F, Radici E, Bocciolone L, Bianchi S, Bianchi C, Candiani GB. Buserelin acetate versus expectant management in the treatment of infertility associated with minimal or mild endometriosis: A randomized clinical trial. Am J Obstet Gynecol 1992;166:1345–50.

100. Thomas E, Cooke I. Successful treatment of asymptomatic endometriosis: Does it benefit infertile women? Br Med J 1987;294:1117–19.

101. Hughes E, Ferorkow D, Collins J, Vandekerckhone P. Ovulation suppression for endometriosis (Cochrane Review). In: The Cochrane Library, Issue 1, 2000. Oxford, England: Update Software.

102. Balasch J, Creus M, Fabregues F, Carmona F, Martinez-Roman S, Manau D, Vanrell JA. Pentoxifylline versus placebo in the treatment of infertility associated with minimal or mild endometriosis: a pilot randomized clinical trial. Hum Reprod 1997;12: 2046–50.

103. Audebert A, Descampes P, Marret H. Pre or postoperative medical treatment with Nafarelin in stage III–IV endometriosis: a French multicentered study. Eur J Obstet Gynecol Reprod Biol 1998;79:145–8.

104. Bianchi S, Busacca M, Agnoli B. Effects of three month therapy with Danazol after laparoscopic surgery for stage III–IV endometriosis: a randomized study. Hum Reprod 1999;14:1335–7.

105. Telimaa S, Ronnberg L, Kauppila A. Placebo-controlled comparison of danazol and high dose medroxyprogesterone acetate in the treatment of endometriosis after conservative surgery. Gynaecol Endocrinol 1987;1:363–71.

106. Parazzini F, Fedele L, Busacca M et al. Post-surgical medical treatment of advanced endometriosis: results of a randomized clinical trial. Am J Obstet Gynecol 1994;171:1205–7.

107. Hornstein MD, Hemmings R, Yuzpe AA, Heinrichs WL. Use of nafarelin versus placebo after reductive laparoscopic surgery for endometriosis. Fertil Steril 1997;68:860–4.

108. Vercellini P, Crosignani PG, Fedini R. A gonadotropin-releasing hormone agonist compared with expectant management after conser-

vative surgery for symptomatic endometriosis. Br J Obstet Gynaecol 1999;106:672–7.
109. Muzii L, Marana R, Caruana P, Catalano GF, Margutti F, Panici PB. Postoperative administration of monophasic combined oral contraceptives after laparoscopic treatment of ovarian endometriomas: a prospective, randomized trial. Am J Obstet Gynecol 2000;183:588–92.
110. Frontino G, Vercellini P, De Giorgi O, Aimi G, Zaina B, Crosignani PG. Levonorgesterel-releasing intrauterine device (Lng-IUD) versus expectant management after conservative surgery for symptomatic endometriosis. A pilot study. Fertil Steril 2002;77:S25–6.
111. Morgante G, Ditto A, La Marca A, De Leo V. Low dose Danazol after combined surgical and medical therapy reduces the incidence of pelvic pain in women with moderate and severe endometriosis. Hum Reprod 1999;14:2371–4.
112. Alvarez-Gil L, Fuentes V. Raloxifene and endometriosis. Fertil Steril 2002;77:S37.
113. Winkel C. Unpublished data.

4

Patient preparation
David B Redwine

Successful treatment of endometriosis requires differentiating its symptoms from other sources of pain. Not all pelvic pain is due to endometriosis. If non-endometriotic sources of pain are ascribed to endometriosis, the results of treatment will seem confusing. While the interpretation of symptoms is part of the art of medicine, endometriosis is usually a disease that produces predictable symptoms.

Symptoms of endometriosis

A very common pattern of emergence of symptoms due to endometriosis is the occurrence of increasingly severe pain with menstruation beginning with menarche. Family and friends may offer the faint encouragement that such pain is 'normal' or 'part of being a woman'. However, it should be kept in mind that the youngest patient ever reported with endometriosis was 10.5 years of age and was diagnosed surgically five months after menarche.[1] Over-the-counter pain pills, heating pads and warm baths are commonly used in this age group. With the increase of symptoms comes absence from school and occasional trips to the emergency room where examination and tests are frequently non-conclusive, and the opinion is given to the patient that she may be overreacting. The young woman begins to doubt herself, thinking that perhaps it is 'all in her head' and tries to keep her pain to herself as best she can. The pain, however, may begin to occur earlier and earlier before the menstrual flow and become impossible to ignore. Many patients are bothered between ovulation and menses by increasingly severe pain which can be described with adjectives, such as 'sharp', 'shooting', 'burning' or 'knife-like'. With menses, severe uterine cramping may be superimposed on the endometriosis pain which has increased during the luteal phase of the ovarian hormonal cycle. Some patients will clench their fists as if holding a knife and make phantom thrusts of the weapon into their pelvis or display a twisting motion of their fists as they thrust toward the physician. Sports activities may be dropped because the pain can be aggravated by strenous, jarring activities. Sometimes, the pain may be aggravated by a bumpy automobile ride.[2] Invasive endometriosis with obliteration of the cul de sac may occasionally produce mild systemic flu-like symptoms and mild temperature elevation. Invasive disease of the uterosacral ligaments can sometimes radiate pain down the back of the leg into the thigh. If the doctor listens attentively to the patient, common patterns of descriptions will be heard which can frequently predict where endometriosis is located, or perhaps suggest that endometriosis is not a cause of pain.

Pelvic endometriosis

Endometriosis is a disease that occurs in recurring and predictable patterns, and specific symptoms can almost be predicted from the pattern of pelvic involvement. The cul de sac, uterosacral ligaments and medial broad ligaments are the sites most commonly involved by endometriosis. Disease in these areas can be affected by the function of adjacent structures including the rectum and the vaginal apex. Thus, with 'garden variety' peritoneal involvement of the cul de sac or uterosacral ligaments, bowel movements may be painful, especially during menses, as opposed to patients with obliteration of the cul de sac and rectal wall involvement who may complain of rectal pain with each bowel movement during the month, or rectal pain with flatus or sitting. Deep dyspareunia is extremely common in patients with superficial or deep disease of the cul de sac or uterosacral ligaments, and patients may complain that 'something is being hit' during intercourse. With obliteration of the cul de sac, deep penetration during intercourse may radiate pain into the rectum. Because of increasingly severe dyspareunia, intercourse is increasingly avoided, and the male partner becomes acutely aware that what should be an act of pleasure has become an act of pain and endurance for the woman.

Endometrioma cysts can cause pain in the area of the involved ovary especially if periovarian adhesions are put on stretch, although pain from adjacent pelvic areas may be present and confuse the issue. Occasionally, an ovarian cyst which is adherent to the pelvic sidewall may put pressure on an underlying ureter, which itself can further be entrapped in retroperitoneal fibrosis related to inflammation from the overlying cyst, or from invasive disease of a nearby uterosacral ligament which can send tendrils of fibrotic scarring around the ureter. Rarely, the ureter will be invaded by endometriosis spreading from invasive disease of the uterosacral ligament, with resultant hematuria or obstruction. Pressure on or invasion of the ureter by these processes may result in cyclic stricture of the ureter during menses with resultant hydroureteronephrosis that can cause renal flank pain. With slow stricture of the ureter, the kidney on the affected side may die a silent death.

Intestinal endometriosis

Isolated nodules of endometriosis of the sigmoid colon may be asymptomatic or cause vague left lower quadrant pain prior to a bowel movement. Endometriosis of the appendix and cecum is usually asymptomatic. Intestinal obstructive symptoms are rare when only the rectosigmoid colon or cecum is involved by endometriosis becaue of their relatively large diameters. When symptoms of bowel obstruction exist, they are almost always due to obstructive lesions of the distal ileum which obstructs more readily because of its smaller diameter.

Diaphragmatic endometriosis

Endometriosis of the diaphragm most commonly exists as a full-thickness lesion of the right hemidiaphragm.[3] Patients will complain of worsening right chest or shoulder pain with menses. Sometimes, the pain will radiate to the neck or upper arm and may be thought due to a muscular cause because it can possess an aching quality. Deep breathing may aggravate the pain and some patients must sleep upright during their episodes of diaphragmatic pain.

Umbilical endometriosis

This presents as a nodule in the inferior portion of the umbilicus which may grow slightly and become more painful with menses. Away from menses it can be smaller and less painful.

It is uncommon for a symptom of endometriosis to begin after the age of 30. In

PATIENT PREPARATION

such a patient, some other gynecological source of pain, such as adenomyosis uterii, should be remembered.

Endometriosis vs other causes of pain

It is important to try to distinguish endometriosis pain from other causes of pain, especially pain coming from the uterus. This can sometimes be difficult as endometriosis pain and uterine pain can coexist, especially during menses. Trying to discriminate the source of pain is important since uterine pain may not respond to endometriosis surgery, and pain due to endometriosis may not respond to uterine surgery. This is part of the art of medicine. In plying this art, it is important to remember that uterine pain occurs primarily with menses, although some cases of adenomyosis may cause pain throughout the month but with more extreme menstrual aggravation. Uterine pain is often described as a cramping that may resemble labor contractions and which seems to emanate from a central suprapubic location. The uterus is notorious for radiating pain to the low back (through the uterosacral ligaments), anterior thighs (through the round ligaments) and to the umbilicus (through the obliterated umbilical arteries or urachus).

Physical examination

Endometriosis of the umbilicus is rare and will be identified as a painful swelling less than 1.5 cm in diameter located within the umbilicus, usually in the inferior portion (Fig. 4.1). There may be a bluish/black discoloration due to the accumulation of surrounding bloody material. Occasionally, there may be frank bleeding seen.

Visualization of the vulva or cervix will rarely show endometriosis. The posteror fornix will

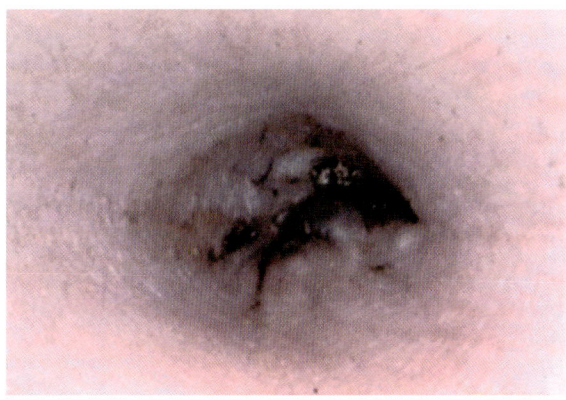

Figure 4.1
Endometriosis of the umbilicus. A small hemorrhagic nodule is present in the lower left quadrant of the umbilicus

occasionally show endometriosis which is invading from an underlying nodule of a uterosacral ligament or rectum (Fig. 4.2). Such a lesion may be missed unless the vaginal speculum is tilted posteriorly and opened so that the fornix can be displayed. Such vaginal endometriosis should

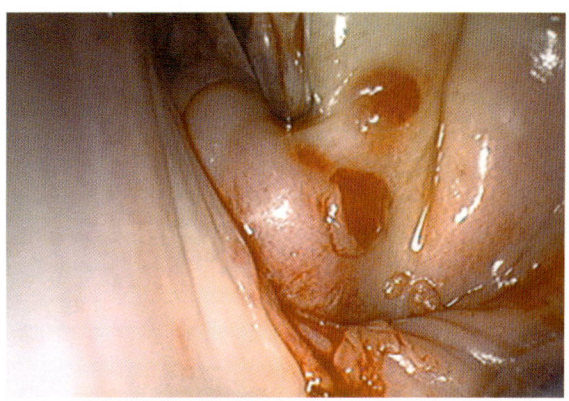

Figure 4.2
Endometriosis of the posterior vaginal fornix. A single-toothed tenaculum is holding the posterior lip of the cervix anteriorly. The vaginal mucosa immediately adjacent to the tenaculum shows epithelial piling and thickening with associated hemorrhagic changes. This presentation of endometriosis is commonly associated with obliteration of the cul de sac and invasive disease of the uterosacral ligaments

bring to mind the high likelihood of obliteration of the cul de sac and rectal involvement.

Bimanual examination is performed to determine if enlargement of the uterus or ovaries exists. If the uterus is anterior in the pelvis, it can be palpated between the fingers of the internal and external hands. It is very important to note whether the uterus is tender when compressed and whether this reproduces any component of the patient's pain. Pain of a uterine origin may not respond to treatment of endometriosis but may respond to presacral neurectomy if the patient refuses hysterectomy.

Digital examination of the posterior vaginal fornix is the most important part of the search for evidence of endometriosis and is best performed after bimanual examination of the uterus and ovaries is completed. This part of the examination is performed only with the internal fingers. The external hand is placed behind the examiner's back or on the patient's leg. The cul de sac is lightly palpated with the fingertips while the patient's face is observed, followed by light palpation of each uterosacral ligament, again observing the patient's reaction. Endometriosis in these areas typically will be very tender, causing the patient to wince or cry out and even move up and away on the examining table. The presence and size of nodularity is also noted in these regions. On rectal examination, an effort is made to see whether the mucosa will slide across any nodules, since this may predict the depth of rectal resection required. The patient is asked to estimate how much of her pain is reproduced by examination as this will predict the success of surgery in relieving pain.[4] In some cases of endometriosis involving the bladder, a nodule may be felt anterior to the uterus, or the anterior vaginal wall may display nodularity and tenderness if the trigone of the bladder is involved. Some authors have recommended pelvic examination during menses when tenderness and nodularity may be increased.[2,5]

Endometriosis of the higher intestinal tract or diaphragm exists without identifiable signs on physical examination.

Laboratory tests and imaging scans

There is no blood test that is specific for endometriosis. The CA125 level may be normal or elevated with ovarian or non-ovarian gynecologic cancer,[6] benign ovarian masses, infections, molar pregnancy or fibroids,[7] adhesions,[8] adenomyosis, endometriosis,[9] menstruation, or with a normal pelvis.[10]

Transrectal ultrasound for the diagnosis of rectal nodules[11] or magnetic resonance imaging (MRI) studies for bladder nodules[12,13] are used by some, but such scans appear to be unnecessary for the following reasons. Scans can frequently be negative. Scans do not treat the patient's pain. A negative scan in the presence of suggestive symptoms does not eliminate the need for surgical investigation with bowel preparation. The results of the scan do not alter how surgery is performed, since that is determined automatically by the surgical findings; if some type of bowel resection is seen to be necessary, it will be done regardless of the result of the scan. Scans add expense and no randomized controlled trial proves they are necessary or improve endometriosis surgical outcomes. Scans focus attention on themselves rather than on the patient. While scans may suggest involvement of an organ system which might alter the composition of the surgical team, endometriosis surgery by definition will require a multidisciplinary approach because of its ability to affect multiple organ systems. Thus, an endometriosis treatment program should be able to handle any surgical finding regardless of the presence or absence of preoperative scans.

Scans may be helpful in obese patients who are difficult to examine, or to determine if uterine fibroids or adenomyosis might be present, since the presence of a uterine abnormality may alter the surgical options presented to the patient. If the patient has uterine symptoms and an abnormal uterine scan, hysterectomy may be helpful.

Bowel preparation before surgery

Bowel preparation may be helpful for surgery on patients with known obliteration of the cul de sac since most of these patients will need some type of surgery on the rectum.[4] Patients with known intestinal involvement should receive a bowel prep. Patients with known or suspected presence of ovarian endometrioma cysts should have consideration of a bowel prep since the incidence of intestinal endometriosis is increased.[14] Bowel preparation should also be considered for patients with nodularity on examination which indicates more deeply invasive endometriosis possibly involving the rectum, as well as for patients with symptoms suggestive of intestinal involvement. Various osmotic or mechanical bowel prep regimens are available with or without the use of antibiotics and none is necessarily superior to others.

Bowel preparation is not without risks. At surgery, the colon will frequently be filled with fluid which may rush out and contaminate the pelvis and abdomen with a heavy bacterial innoculation (Fig. 4.3) resulting in the risk of postoperative abscess formation. The combination of prophylactic antibiotics and bowel preparation may result in postoperative overgrowth of *Clostridium difficile* which can cause low grade fever, intestinal cramping and watery diarrhea. This can be diagnosed with a *Clostridium difficile* toxin titer performed on a sample of the diarrhea, although false negatives are possible. Treatment is with oral metronidazole or vancomycin.

Surgical considerations

Uterine manipulation

It is virtually impossible to perform laparoscopic surgery for endometriosis without uterine manipulation. The patient's position is important for proper use of simple manipulators, such as a Hulka tenaculum. The patient's hips should be slightly off the end of the table so the handles of the manipulator can be pressed deeply into the crease of the buttocks, resulting in extreme anteversion of the uterus. The manipulator can then be pressed toward the ceiling, forcing the entire uterus anteriorly toward the abdominal wall and thus exposing the cul de sac for easy investigation and surgery. This is particularly vital during surgery for obliteration of the cul de sac, since such extreme uterine anteversion results in countertraction against

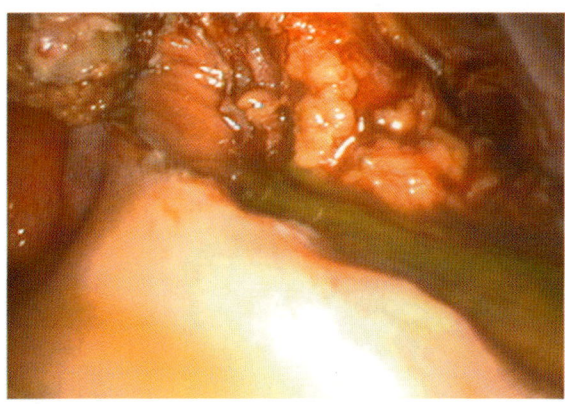

Figure 4.3
Greenish liquid bowel prep material pours out of a full thickness resection of the sigmoid colon, contaminating the pelvis

SURGICAL MANAGEMENT OF ENDOMETRIOSIS

the pull of the tissues posteriorly and will greatly help the dissection.

Patient positioning

The operating table should be able to tilt into extreme Trendelenburg position, which allows the bowel to fall superiorly out of the pelvis. Patients with endometriosis are typically young and healthy and can tolerate many hours in such a position without respiratory problems, although the anesthesiologist may notice a slight increase in required ventilatory pressures. Subcutaneous emphysema may occur and spread into the face (Figs 4.4, 4.5), particularly in thin patients, but other than a slight increase in end-expiratory carbon dioxide (CO_2) levels, this seems harmless.

The arms should be tucked to the sides and the elbows padded. Attention should be paid to maintaining patient temperature during surgery. The use of warm irrigation fluid during surgery, wrapping the legs and head in additional blankets and using warming devices for the upper torso and face or beneath the patient are all helpful. Leg stirrups should provide good padding for the popliteal and lower leg area,

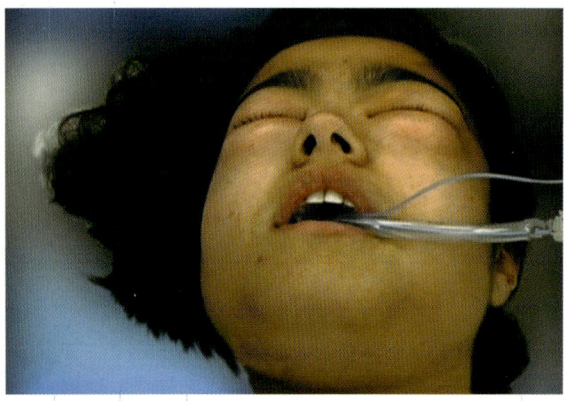

Figure 4.4
Massive subcutaneous emphysema extending to the face in a thin patient

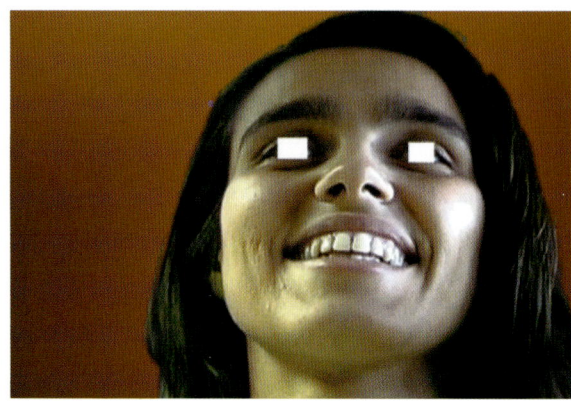

Figure 4.5
Complete resolution of subcutaneous emphysema several days after surgery

and the legs should be positioned so that the patient will not slide on the table toward the anesthesiologist since this will impair uterine manipulation.

Placement of trocars

Most surgeons use a laparoscope passed through a 10 mm sheath in the umbilicus. The umbilicus is the thinnest part of the abdominal wall, and a vertical incision within the inferior umbilicus or across its center will simultaneously allow the most efficient entry and the best cosmetic result following surgery. The trocar and sheath can be placed directly with or without initial insufflation of the abdomen with a Verres needle. Direct trocar insertion may be safer than the use of Verres needle insufflation followed by trocar insertion. Needle insufflation before insertion of the main trocar means that two blind trocar insertions are required instead of one if the umbilical trocar is placed directly, thus increasing, arithmetically, the possibility of damage to underlying structures. The tip of reusable trocars remain slightly dull, especially compared to disposable trocars, so their use is safer since there is less potential for a sharp surgical injury. Indeed, studies have found that the risk of unintentional injury with direct insertion is 1/1838 (0.05%),[15] as compared with a risk of 19/470 (4%),[16] associated with prior Veress needle insufflation before insertion of the main umbilical trocar.

For direct trocar insertion, the abdominal wall around the umbilicus should be elevated with hands or towel clips (Fig. 4.6). The tip of the trocar should be advanced toward the hollow of the pelvis. In obese patients, the bottom of the umbilicus may need to be grasped and everted with Allis clamps or hemostats since this area can be hidden beneath the enveloping fatty folds of the surrounding abdomen. An incision can be created across the center of the umbilicus and sometimes it is easiest to carry the incision into the peritoneal cavity for direct trocar placement. In obese patients, where the bottom of the umbilicus is visible, the trocar tip is advanced cautiously perpendicularly until it is felt biting into the fascia, then is directed toward the pelvis. Patients with endometriosis may have undergone many previous laparoscopies or laparotomies and alternate sites for insertion of an insufflating needle or initial trocar are sometimes recommended to avoid the theoretical complication of damage to bowel adherent around the umbilicus. However, the risk of damage to bowel with direct umbilical insertion has been found to be 1/2000 cases in the author's experience. It is more common to find light omental adhesions only around the umbilicus and these can be lysed either directly down the umbilical sheath or from an alternate direction through another port.

To perform laparoscopic surgery it is helpful to have other ports for graspers and suction-irrigators since this will decrease instrument changes and make surgery more efficient. A minimum of two additional ports is recommended. A triple-puncture technique consisting of insertion points at the umbilicus and a port

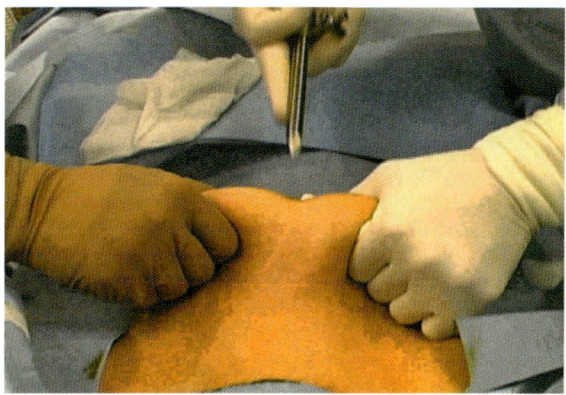

Figure 4.6
The abdominal wall is grasped and elevated before direct insertion of the 10 mm umbilical trocar

lateral to each inferior epigastric vessel bundle is adequate for all pelvic surgery and most intestinal surgery for endometriosis. Insertion of these accessory trocars can be done safely by using the laparoscope which has been inserted down the umbilical sheath to view through the parietal peritoneum the course of the inferior epigastric vessels (Figs 4.7–4.9). The tip of the laparoscope can be advanced lateral to these vessels and a skin incision can be placed across the end of the laparoscope. Transillumination of the abdominal wall (Fig. 4.10) will not reveal the

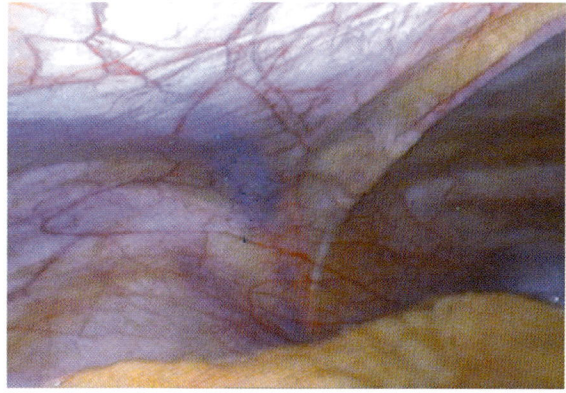

Figure 4.7
The left inferior epigastric vessels are visible as a bluish arc beneath the parietal peritoneum

SURGICAL MANAGEMENT OF ENDOMETRIOSIS

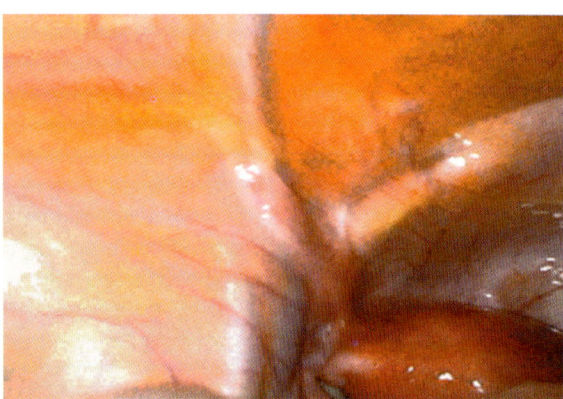

Figure 4.8
The left inferior epigastric vessels originate from the external iliac vessels near the internal inguinal ring

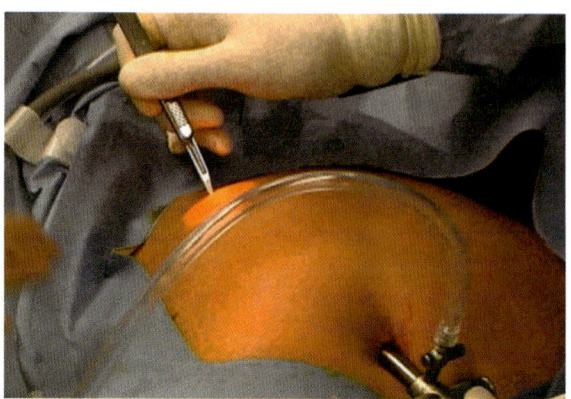

Figure 4.10
The tip of the laparoscope has been advanced under direct vision to a point lateral to the right inferior epigastric vessels. Now observing externally, the scalpel creates the left lower quadrant incision for insertion of an accessory trocar. Superficial epigastric vessels running in the subcutaneous fatty layer may be visible during transillumination of the abdominal wall, but not the deeper lying inferior epigastric vessels

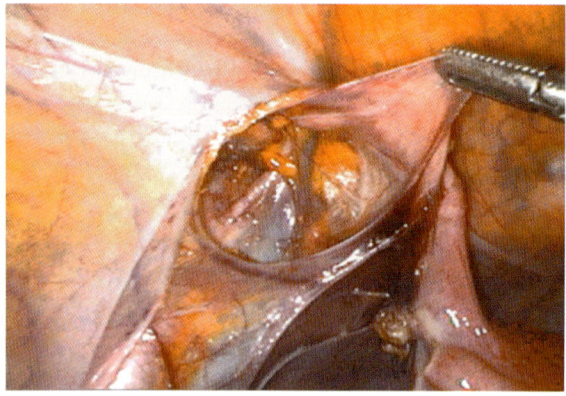

Figure 4.9
Retroperitoneal anatomy of the origin of the left inferior epigastric vessels

inferior epigastric vessels in most patients, but may instead reveal superficial epigastric vessels which are in the subcutaneous fat. It is important to try to avoid both sets of vessels.

After the skin incision has been made lateral to the inferior epigastric vessels in a transilluminated area without obvious vascular markings, the distal shaft of the laparoscope can be used to push anteriorly against the inferior epigastric vessels while the accessory trocar is inserted horizontally immediately beneath the laparoscope (Fig. 4.11). In this way, the trocar is never directed at the iliac vessels, but is instead directed into the middle of the pneumoperitoneum. The risk of bladder injury is decreased by such a port placement. Even if the accessory trocar does not injure the inferior epigastric vessels, vessels in the subcutaneous fat may be injured, particularly in obese patients where transillumination of the abdominal wall is useless. Blood dripping down the outside of the trocar (Fig. 4.12) should alert the surgeon to the possibility of injury to the inferior or superficial epigastric vessels.

Some surgeons may place only a single additional 5 mm port suprapubically in the midline. The bladder is the main organ at risk for such a port site. The placement of the skin incision for this port site is at the discretion of the surgeon based on training, experience, and the demands of the particular case. Depending on the direc-

PATIENT PREPARATION

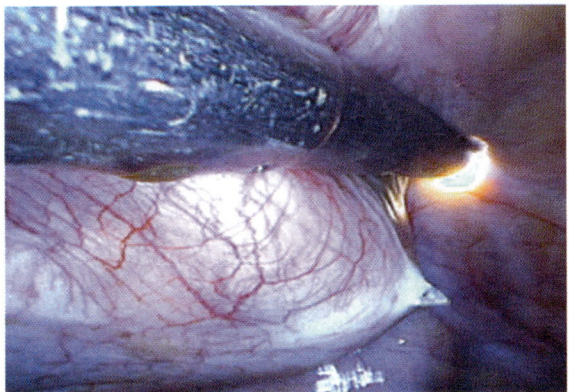

Figure 4.11
The abdominal wall is braced by the laparoscope while the trocar is advanced directly beneath the shaft of the laparoscope. The inferior epigastric vessels will lie immediately anterior or medial to the shaft of the laparoscope and thus are automatically protected from injury by the trocar. The accessory trocar is advanced in a horizontal direction parallel to the floor, entering the empty pocket of pneumoperitoneum beyond the laparoscope, thus avoiding risk of injury to the iliac vessels

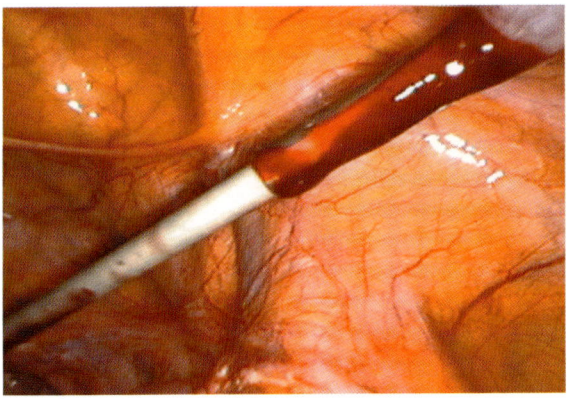

Figure 4.12
Blood dripping down the sheath of the accessory trocar is a sign of injury to a vessel of the abdominal wall

tion of insertion of the trocar, the bladder could be injured whether the skin incision is placed 1 cm or 10 cm above the pubic symphysis. The outline of the bladder cannot always be seen when the bladder is empty because of retroperitoneal fat and areolar tissue. While the balloon of a retention catheter may be visible as a round mass, this is usually positioned at the internal urethral meatus well away from the dome of the bladder. Because of this, insertion of the trocar under direct visualization will not guarantee that bladder injury will be avoided. If the bladder is injured by the suprapubic trocar, such injury may not be apparent during surgery. No bleeding may be seen laparoscopically or in the catheter bag, and any urine leaking down the trocar sheath will simply be lost in the irrigation fluid used during surgery. The catheter bag may not fill with CO_2 because the trocar sheath acts as a tamponade against CO_2 entering the bladder. Thus, it is entirely possible that a bladder perforation may go undetected during surgery.

Placement of incision for laparotomy

In patients with such overwhelming disease that requires laparotomy, a low transverse incision is adequate. Division of the rectus muscles is not necessary. This incision can be used to treat virtually any case of pelvic or intestinal endometriosis, and a vertical subumbilical incision is rarely called for. Endometriosis of the diaphragm requires upper abdominal laparotomy, either through a subcostal incision for unilateral disease, or a short vertical incision for bilateral disease.[3] If laparoscopy is abandoned for laparotomy, consideration should be given to taking the patient's legs out of the stirrups and placement in the supine position if a lengthy laparotomy is anticipated. Disease of the ileum is difficult to reach with typical laparoscopic port placements, and it is far easier to extend the right lateral port incision minimally and deliver the ileum onto the abdominal wall for surgery, or to extend the umbilical incision slightly if the sigmoid, ileum and cecum all require surgery (Fig. 4.13).

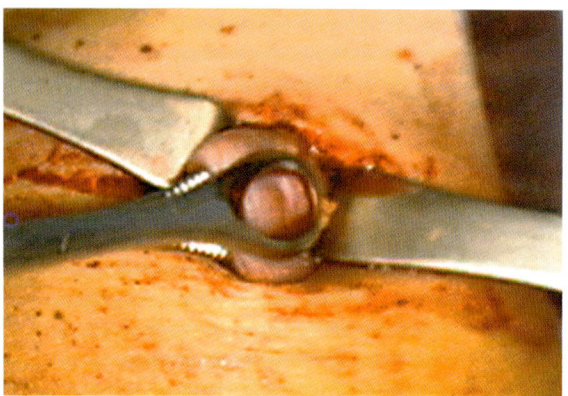

Figure 4.13
The right lower quadrant 5 mm trocar site has been enlarged slightly after all laparoscopic surgery has been completed so surgery on the ileum can be accomplished. The bowel can be grasped with atraumatic graspers and delivered onto the abdominal wall for easy surgery

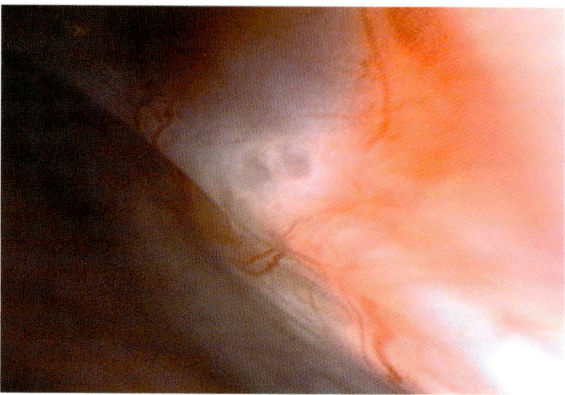

Figure 4.14
Subtle endometriosis can have the appearance of tapioca. Two individual glands of endometriosis surrounded by whitish stroma belie the concepts of invisible microscopic disease and hemorrhage as a constant companion of endometriosis

Visual identification of endometriosis

The visual appearance of endometriosis is important because every intellectual and therapeutic process concerning the disease starts with a surgeon identifying the disease in the pelvis. Protean visual appearances are possible with endometriosis. Young patients may have colorless lesions which can be identified as individual glands on close inspection (Fig. 4.14). With the passage of time, slight fibrosis may occur around these glands due to the irritating effect of their secretions (Fig. 4.15). Peritoneal blood painting[17] may be helpful in identifying subtle texture irregularities of the peritoneum which can be due to endometriosis (Fig. 4.16). Peritoneal pockets, sometimes with multiple underlying subpockets, may be present on either side of the rectum (Fig. 4.17) or occasionally on the pelvic sidewalls. These developmental peritoneal defects may contain endometriosis around their rims or in their depths.

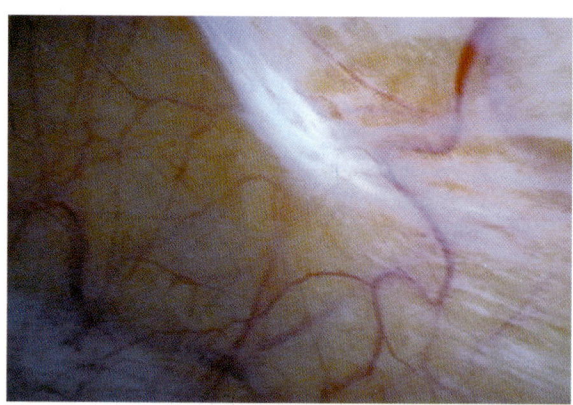

Figure 4.15
The glandular elements of endometriosis secrete an unidentified paracrine substance which can result in superficial fibrosis over and around subtle lesions. Note the complete lack of hemorrhage which is the hallmark of many endometriotic lesions

Carbon deposition from previous laser vaporization may masquerade as hemorrhagic endometriosis, although it should be remembered that most patients will have lesions that lack hemorrhagic coloration or neovascularity.[18] Laser vaporization may not burn deeply enough

PATIENT PREPARATION

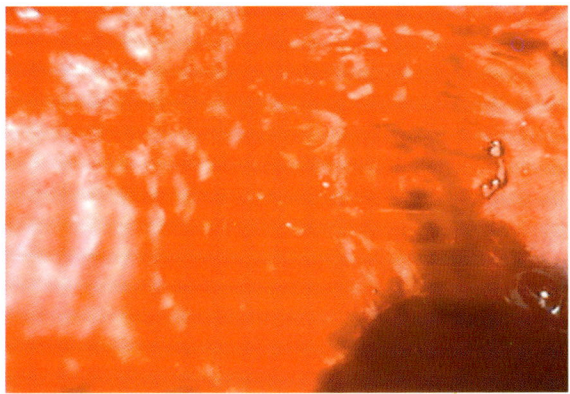

Figure 4.16
Peritoneal blood painting of the left broad ligament reveals innumerable peritoneal lesions of endometriosis which were not readily visible otherwise. The blood flows around the lesions, which are slightly elevated above the surrounding peritoneum, like water flowing around a rock in a stream

foreign body giant cell reaction which can be an iatrogenic cause of pain (Fig. 4.19).

Other forms of endometriosis can become increasingly obvious as the effects of the disease are manifest over time. These forms are amply illustrated in the chapters on surgical treatment. Dense yellowish or whitish fibrosis is a common finding that can hide underlying disease. While many surgeons may consider such an appearance to be 'burned out' disease, this morphology of endometriosis represents a biologically active form of the disease which is 'burned in'. The endometriosis surgeon's caveat must be: any peritoneal abnormality, no matter how subtle, must be considered possible endometriosis until proven otherwise by biopsy. Only after the disease has been completely identified can it be completely removed.

Once surgery has been completed, the umbilical incision should be closed with absorbable

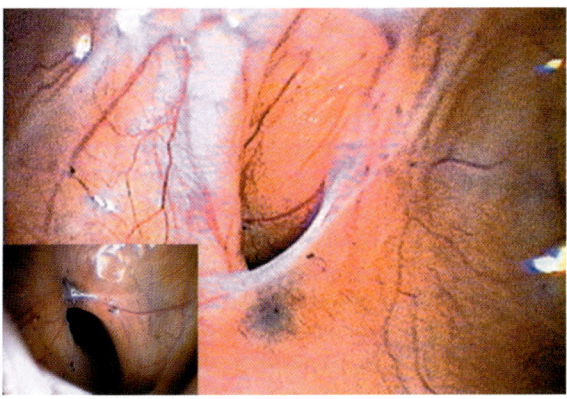

Figure 4.17
A peritoneal pocket of the left cul de sac medial to the left uterosacral ligament. (Inset) a subpocket hidden in the depths of the visible pocket with a lesion of endometriosis adjacent to its opening. The rectum is medial and immediately adjacent to such pockets and can be damaged during their removal

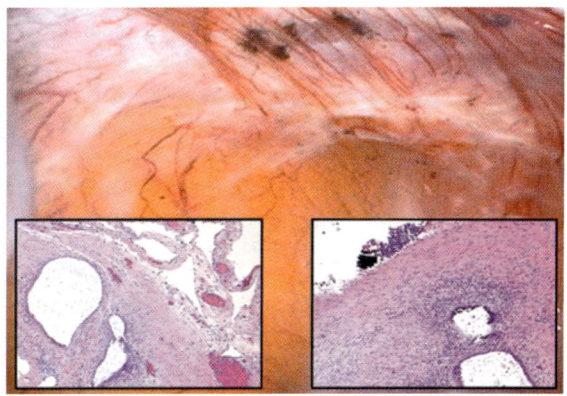

Figure 4.18
Superficial endometriosis which was not destroyed by laser vaporization performed too swiftly. Note the multiple sites of individual glands, some with fibrosis resulting from biologic activity of the disease. Superficial adhesions and carbon were left in the wake of treatment. (Left inset) endometriosis lies just beneath the peritoneal surface which has shaggy adhesions with congested vessels. (Right inset) Superficial endometriosis lies beneath carbon left on the peritoneal surface

to destroy even superficial endometriosis, and persistent disease can be present beneath the adhesions and carbon which laser leaves behind. (Fig. 4.18) Carbon within the tissue may incite a

57

SURGICAL MANAGEMENT OF ENDOMETRIOSIS

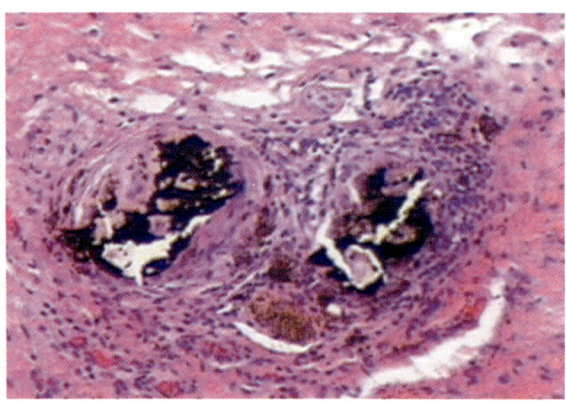

Figure 4.19
Carbon deposition within tissue following laser vaporization, with resulting foreign body giant cell reaction that can be a cause of pain in some women

suture placed in the umbilical fascia. Otherwise, omental prolapse may occur, especially in very thin patients. Smaller incisions can be closed with tape. Lengthy surgeries result in a larger volume of irrigation fluid left behind which will drain out of one or more of the laparoscopic puncture wounds. A drain left in the cul de sac will help keep bed-linen cleaner and also help detect postoperative bleeding.

Modern laparoscopic surgery can be very extensive and is not truly outpatient surgery. It is associated with a high incidence of postoperative nausea and vomiting. Most often, this is due to anesthesia, direct effects of surgery, or pain pills. Since postoperative vomiting can be a sign of a complication, it is unreasonable to send a patient home from the hospital while vomiting. Minimum criteria for discharge should include the ability to tolerate liquids and pain pills by mouth, ability to walk to the bathroom, and stable vital signs.

References

1. Goldstein DP, DeCholnoky C, Emans SJ. Adolescent endometriosis. J Adolesc Health Care 1980;1:37–41.
2. Counseller VS. Endometriosis: A clinical and surgical review. Am J Obstet Gynecol 1938;36:877–88.
3. Redwine DB. Diaphragmatic endometriosis: diagnosis, surgical management, and long-term results of treatment. Fertil Steril 2002;77:288–96.
4. Redwine DB, Wright J. Laparoscopic treatment of obliteration of the cul de sac in endometriosis: Long term followup. Fertil Steril 2001;76:358–65.
5. Fallon J. Endometriosis. Two hundred cases considered from the viewpoint of the practitioner. N Eng J Med 1946;235:669–73.
6. Niloff JM, Klug TL, Schaetzl E, Zurawski VR, Knapp RC, Bast RC. Elevation of serum CA125 in carcinomas of the fallopian tube, endometrium, and endocervix. Am J Obstet Gynecol 1984;148:1057–8.
7. Di-Xia C, Schwartz PE, Xinguo L, Zhan Y. Evaluation of CA 125 levels in differentiating malignant from benign tumors in patients with pelvic masses. Obstet Gynecol 1988;72:23–7.
8. Cheng Y-M, Wang S-T, Chou C-Y. Serum CA-125 in preoperative patients at high risk for endometriosis. Obstet Gynecol 2002;99:375–80.
9. Koninckx PR, Riitinen L, Seppala M, Cornillie FJ. CA-125 and placental protein 14 concentrations in plasma and peritoneal fluid of women with deeply infiltrating pelvic endometriosis. Fertil Steril 1992;57:523–30.
10. Molo MW, Kelly M, Radwanska E, Binor Z. Preoperative serum CA-125 and CA-72 in predicting endometriosis in infertility patients. J Reprod Med 1994;39:964–6.
11. Fedele L, Bianchi S, Zanconato G, Tozzi L, Raffaelli R. Gonadotropin-releasing hormone agonist treatment for endometriosis of the rectovaginal septum. Am J Obstet Gynecol 2000;183:1462–7.
12. Donnez J, Spada F, Squifflet J, Nisolle M. Bladder endometriosis must be considered as bladder adenomyosis. Fertil Steril 2000, 74:1175–81.
13. Vercellini P, Frontino G, Pisacreta A, De Giorgi O, Cattaneo M, Crosignani PG. The pathogenesis of bladder detrusor endometriosis. Am J Obstet Gynecol 2002; 187:538–42.
14. Redwine DB. Ovarian endometriosis: A marker for more severe pelvic and intestinal disease. Fertil Steril 1999;73:310–15.
15. Kaloo P, Cooper M, Reid G. A prospective multicentre study of laparoscopic complications related to the direct-entry technique. Gynaecol Endosc 2002;11:67–70.
16. Jones KD, Fan A, Sutton C. Safe entry during laparoscopy: a prospective audit in a district general hospital. Gynaecol Endosc 2002;11:85–9.
17. Redwine DB. Peritoneal blood painting: an aid in the diagnosis of endometriosis. Am J Obstet Gynecol 1989; 161:865–6.
18. Redwine DB. Age related evolution in color appearance of endometriosis. Fertil Steril 1987;48:1062–3.

5

Principles of monopolar electrosurgery
David B Redwine

Electrosurgery is a useful, inexpensive, and a sometimes misunderstood form of surgical energy. A better understanding of the principles of electrosurgery can lead to more widespread use with greater safety. This chapter discusses monopolar electrosurgery as used by the author. Other forms of monopolar electrosurgery, such as argon beam coagulation and fulguration, will not be discussed.

Background

Any form of surgery imparts energy to living tissue, which reacts in some way. All forms of surgery can impart varying levels of energy to a tissue. Because of this, all forms of surgery have the potential of producing equivalent surgical endpoints, depending on the equivalence of the concentration of energy applied. A scalpel concentrates cutting power on a very narrow cutting surface, resulting in clean separation of tissue on each side of the blade. Firmer pressure on the scalpel results in an increase of cutting power, producing a cut which is deeper than if lighter pressure is used. A quick motion applied lightly produces a shallow cut, while a sustained pressure produces a deeper cut. The effect of the scalpel can be further modified by scraping or shaving tissue with a blade held at an oblique angle, so that relatively more metal is in contact with the tissue, thus blunting the effects of a sharp blade by reducing the cutting power. Thus, any surgeon using a scalpel is intuitively aware of the concept of surgical power density because it is felt directly through the fingers and hand. All forms of surgery have their effects as a result of power density delivered to tissue and all forms of surgical energy depend on the same basic features of power application:

1. *Power*. This is the force behind the surgical energy. With a scalpel, it is the pressure applied with the hand to the cutting edge. With electrosurgery, it is a number that can be set on a dial in watts but which is actually measured in volts. With lasers, it is also a wattage set on a dial.
2. *Effective surface area*. This is the area of the energy source which affects the tissue, or its 'footprint'. With a scalpel or electrosurgery, it is the area of metal in touch with the tissue. With lasers, it is the diameter of the spot of laser light.
3. *Power density*. This is the energy which is delivered to the tissue and is the result of the effects of (1) and (2) above. The formula for calculating electrosurgical power density is straightforward: power (in watts) divided by effective surface area, or $PD = W/A$. A higher power density will produce a more concentrated effect than a lower power density, resulting in a 'sharper knife'. In electrosurgery, power density is sometimes referred to as current density.

Electrosurgery is the performance of surgery using electricity, which is the flow of electrons. Many surgeons use electrosurgery exclusively, while some surgeons use photons, very commonly delivered by carbon dioxide (CO_2) lasers. Electrons and photons share several common characteristics that are important in surgery. Both travel at the speed of light. Both have a tiny mass. Both carry energy that can be modulated by substances in their paths. Both can impart their energy to a receiving surface. Both can cut or coagulate tissue. There are important differences. Electrons are channeled within a simple electrical conductor, while photons can be carried in air or in a vacuum, or modulated by reflecting or refracting surfaces. Machines to generate electrons are relatively inexpensive while machines to generate useful photons are not. Photons cannot be used to palpate, retract, grasp, or rearrange tissue, unlike the electrical conductors which carry electrons. Because of these facts, in a world that places a premium on multipurpose, inexpensive technologies, electrosurgery has an advantage.

The monopolar circuit

Monopolar electrosurgery begins with an electrosurgical generator. Electricity (in the form of traveling electrons) flows out through a wire which is connected to some type of metal-tipped surgical tool (which is called the 'active electrode'). Since the metal in the wire and in the active electrode are good conductors of electricity, no heat is generated in the metal by the flow of electrons. Living tissue is not a particularly good conductor of electricity, so when the active electrode is touched to tissue and the electrons enter that tissue from the electrode, tissue resistance to electron flow produces heat. It is important to realize that the tip of the active electrode is not what gets hot (that would be 'endocoagulation'), it is the tissue beneath that gets hot, although heat in the tissue can eventually warm the active electrode tip. Heat in the tissue is what produces the various effects possible with electrosurgery. On this point, the tissue effects of electrosurgery are very similar to the tissue effects seen with the CO_2 laser, since the collimated beam of photons produced by the laser also heats tissue. Once the electrons enter the tissue, they disperse rapidly away in all directions from the tip of the active electrode and find their way to the grounding pad (properly termed the 'return electrode') attached to the patient's skin. The circuit is completed as the electrons find their way back to the electrosurgical generator. Electrosurgical generators produce alternating voltage, so as soon as the circuit is completed, it begins flowing in the opposite direction, although for practical purposes the concept of electrons flowing out of the tip of the active electrode is accurate.

Instrumentation for electrosurgery

There are too many instruments for any one surgeon to master them all. In fact, using too many instruments during surgery will slow its pace because of all the instrument changes that are required. A surgeon would do better to use one, two or at most three separate instruments exclusively and adapt their use as required to solve the surgical problem at hand. Another advantage comes if a single instrument can perform more than one function. For example, a 3 mm hook scissors (Fig. 5.1) allow the surgeon to palpate tissue, retract, grasp or rearrange tissue, cut sharply, cut with electrosurgery, coagulate bleeders and retrieve pathology specimens. If one of these functions was served by a separate instru-

PRINCIPLES OF MONOPOLAR ELECTROSURGERY

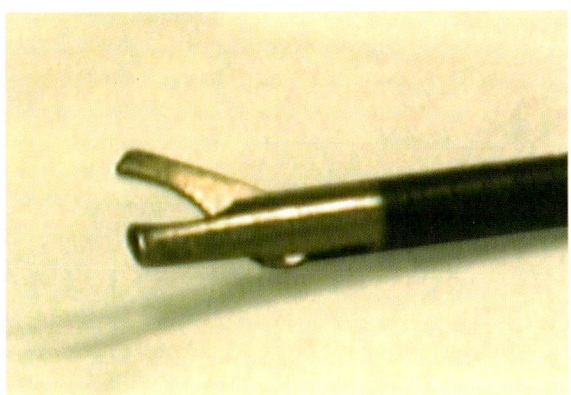

Figure 5.1
Laparoscopic 3 mm hook scissors allow fine, meticulous dissection

ment (such as a bipolar coagulator to control bleeders), the pace of surgery would slow down.

Size matters. The larger the instrument, the less precise surgery becomes. Small instruments bring the possibility of greater precision because of the ability to bring mechanical or electrosurgical energy to almost a pinpoint focus. The focus of equipment manufacturers on 5 mm shafted instruments is unfortunate because surgery for endometriosis is extremely exacting when operating around all the various vital structures that can be affected by the disease. It would be very difficult to do precise electrosurgery with a relatively huge 5 mm instrument with its much larger area of exposed metal. This focus on 5 mm instrumentation is one of the reasons most gynecologists will not be great laparoscopic surgeons.

Power density in electrosurgery

Power density determines the tissue effect seen with electrosurgery. From the power density formula PD = W/A, we see that power density varies inversely with footprint of the electrode which is in touch with the tissue and varies directly with the wattage set on the electrosurgical generator. It should also be apparent that the same power density can be achieved with almost any combination of any watt setting and any electrode footprint, although most electrosurgeons use a specific range of watt settings that works for their style of surgery and the size of the footprints of the active electrodes they are using.

The size and shape of the active electrode is very important in electrosurgery. For a given watt setting on the electrosurgical generator, the power density will be lower with a larger active electrode footprint. Examples of tools having a large footprint would be ball electrodes or almost any instrument with a 5 mm shaft. At very low power densities, intracellular water and cells themselves will be slowly cooked, and the visual effect will be one of slow coagulation with sometimes significant lateral thermal spread indicated by white desiccated tissue. Examples of the use of lower power densities include tubal coagulation for permanent sterilization in females and hemostasis. If a surgical instrument with a smaller footprint is used, the power density will be higher. Examples of instruments with small footprints would be needle electrodes and 3 mm scissors. Higher power density results in the instant boiling of intracellular water which causes the cell to explode. This results in a clean cut with little or no lateral thermal spread. Examples of the use of high power density would be making precise cuts into bowel, bladder or ureter.

Power density can be varied by varying the footprint in touch with the tissue. For example, at a watt setting of 90, the power density delivered through the same 3 mm scissors might vary from about 10 000 W/cm^2 if just the point of a scissors tip is used, to about 139 W/cm^2 if the broad side of the metal tip is buried into the tissue (Fig. 5.2). Thus, cutting and coagulation

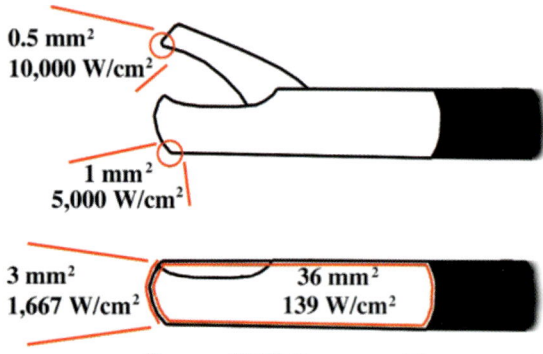

Figure 5.2
Schematic diagram showing approximate surface areas in square millimeters (top number of each number pair) and resultant current densities in watts per square centimeter (bottom number of each number pair) possible at a constant wattage using various presentations of the scissors to the tissue. The tissue effects will be different with different current densities

can occur at the same watt setting by varying how the electrode is presented to the tissue.

Electrosurgical waveforms

There are two main types of current used in electrosurgery. These are popularly called 'cutting current' and 'coagulating current', although these names do not restrict their use. Cutting current can be used to coagulate (by burying the metal electrode into or against tissue) and coagulation current can be used to cut (by using only a very small footprint).

Cutting current is always 'on' and has a never-varying sawtooth type of pattern alternating continuously between the maximum positive voltage of about +500 V and the minimum negative voltage of about −500 V (Fig. 5.3). This results in a peak-to-peak voltage of about 1000 V. Since the waveform of the current as seen on an oscilloscope does not vary, the current is 'unmodulated' or 'undamped'.

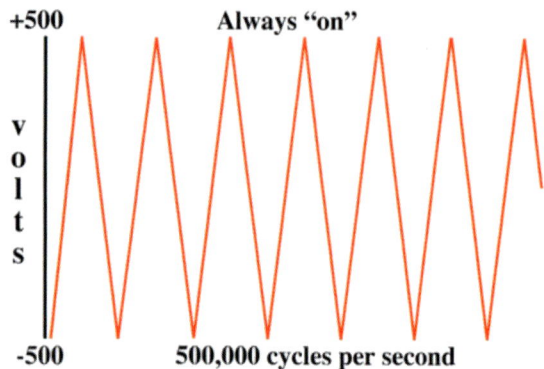

Figure 5.3
Waveform of pure cutting current, also known as unmodulated current

Coagulation current is 'on' only about 6% of the time and has a peak-to-peak voltage of about 5000 V (Fig. 5.4). The higher voltage results in a greater generation of tissue heat which is clinically useful for coagulation of bleeders during surgery. Since the waveform of the current varies from usually 'off' to occasionally 'on', synonyms for coagulation current are 'modulated' or 'damped'.

Blended waveforms are combinations of these two main waveforms. Just as there are too many

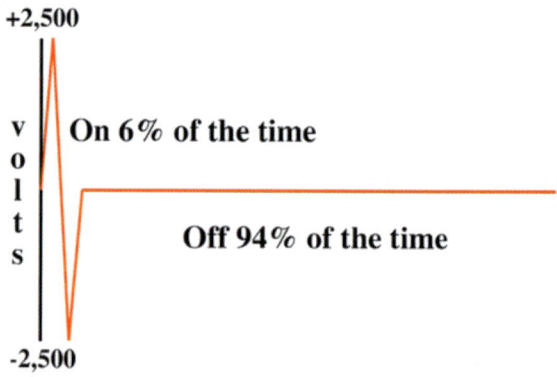

Figure 5.4
Waveform of coagulation current, also known as modulated current

instruments to become familiar with all, a surgeon who tries to use all waveforms will never master them all. It would be better to become familiar with the two main waveforms and adapt them to the surgeon's style and requirements.

Monopolar electrosurgical safety

Power settings

Sufficient power should be used to have the desired tissue effect as quickly as possible, just as a surgeon would favor a sharp scalpel over a dull one. Since low wattage settings result in low power density, electrosurgery will more closely resemble surgery with scalpel and scissors if it is used with higher power settings. Lower wattage settings can be associated with a greater degree of lateral thermal spread that not only can damage adjacent vital structures, but which can also distort local anatomy because of coagulation. Higher power settings will produce quick clean cuts when delivered through instruments with small tips. It is easier to repair a small clean hole than a large coagulated area.

With 3 mm hook scissors, 90 W of pure cutting current and 50 W of coagulation current are power settings that will accomplish almost all electrosurgical tasks.

Dwell time

The length of time an activated electrode is presented to tissue is the dwell time. Monopolar electrosurgery can be made safer by using short bursts of energy delivered with superficial grazing strokes, almost as if the tissue is being sanded away. This is particularly true when the higher voltage coagulation current is being used.

Safety can be increased even further if irrigation fluid is used to bathe tissue intermittently while it is being treated. Bathing the tissue is most commonly done during coagulation of bleeders, when the dwell time is intentionally longer. Monopolar scissors rarely would be used to gnaw through tissue mechanically while activated since this would present a greater footprint with a reduction of power density and degradation of the desired surgical effect. The 3 mm scissors can be used most usefully as a point electrode (Fig. 5.5), resulting in an increased power density and quick, certain tissue effects.

Capacitive coupling

Just as a radio transmitting tower emits electromagnetic radiation which induces electrical energy in the receiving antenna of an automobile, so does the active electrode and its wiring emit unseen electromagnetic radiation that may be picked up by surrogate metal 'antennae' inside or around the patient. Fortunately, such energization of nearby metal objects occurs to a fraction of the level that is generated within the

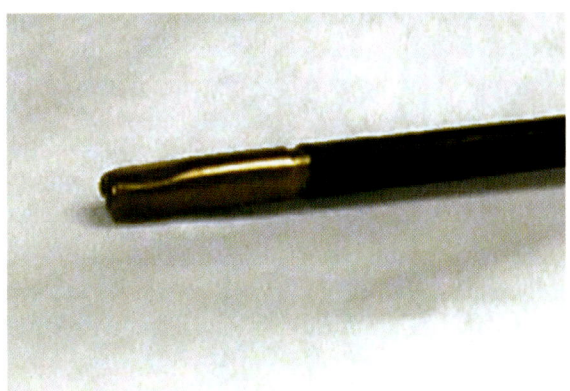

Figure 5.5

Laparoscopic 3 mm scissors in the closed position for use as a point electrode

active electrode itself, and the level of energization falls as the distance increases between the active electrode transmitter and the passive antenna receiver. Since a capacitor is represented by two conductors separated by an insulator, secondary energization of an accessory metal instrument is called capacitive coupling. In laparoscopic surgery, the conductors consist of the active electrode and the wire supplying it and any other nearby metal. Capacitive coupling seems to occur primarily when the active electrode is energized, and the capacitor system does not seem to store up a dangerous charge which can then be discharged even when the active electrode is not energized. Capacitive coupling poses a risk that is almost exclusive to bowel, particularly small bowel because it is so thin-walled.

In the case of laparoscopic surgery, there are several possible forms capacitive coupling can take. The most obvious case is when the conductors are the active electrode and its supplying wire and an accessory metal instrument, while the insulator is whatever insulation is around the conductors as well as the gas distending the abdomen. In this case, the metal tip of the accessory instrument could theoretically become energized and transmit electrical energy into tissue which is being held or retracted. Since the footprint of the accessory instrument on the tissue may be rather large, and since it would be energized only to a fraction of the active electrode, unintended injury would be uncommon because the power density delivered to the tissue would be low. Occasionally, if the accessory instrument is inserted lateral to the inferior epigastric vessels, secondary energization of the instrument will stimulate a nerve which results in a spasm of muscular activity causing jerking of a leg. While this does not appear to injure a nerve, muscle sprain could occur with repeated episodes, so electrosurgery should be cautiously used if this happens.

Another form of capacitive coupling occurs if trocar sheaths contain metal. Even if there is no active electrosurgical instrument within such a sheath, the metal in the sheath can become energized by a nearby transmitter. Since capacitatively stored energy is inversely proportional to the distance from the transmitter, this would rarely be a problem. If the sheath is entirely metal, then there will be a relatively large footprint of the sheath as it passes within the abdominal wall. This large metal footprint will cause dispersion of capacitatively stored electrical energy into the abdominal wall at a low power density, so unintended injury is unlikely to occur. If the sheath has a plastic component (which may be threaded) that passes through the abdominal wall and a metal component which extends beyond the plastic portion within the abdomen, the metal part of the sheath will have no way to discharge its energy back into the abdominal wall because the plastic component is not a conductor. If such an isolated metal sheath comes into contact with bowel during use of the active electrode, it could become energized and represent a potential risk to the bowel.

A special form of capacitive coupling exists when an active electrode is inserted down the operating channel of an operating laparoscope since the metal of the laparoscope itself can become energized. If the laparoscope is passed through a metal umbilical sheath, any charge within the laparoscope will be dispersed through the metal sheath's large footprint into the abdominal wall. If a plastic sheath were to be used, then the laparoscope could theoretically become energized, in which case, if small bowel were to touch a portion of the tip of the laparoscope out of sight of the surgeon, it could be burned if the power density were sufficient.

Insulation breaks represent a potential for unsafe laparoscopy. Even if the insulation on an instrument is inspected before surgery begins, an insulation break can occur during surgery while the shaft of the instrument is out of view within a laparoscope or secondary sheath. While active electrode monitoring devices exist which can detect insulation breaks and automatically shut off the electrosurgical generator, not all hospitals have such equipment and it is not available for instruments with 3 mm shafts. Nonetheless, there are three signs that appear during use of the active electrode that can alert the surgeon to the possibility of an insulation break: (1) Static on a TV monitor. (2) Twitching of abdominal wall muscles. (3) Declining efficiency of electrosurgery at a particular power setting. If any of these occur, the insulation of the active electrode should be checked.

Monopolar vs bipolar electrosurgery

Any form of surgery has rules for safe use which the surgeon must understand. If a surgeon were to make an unintended cut with a sharp scalpel, a dull blade would not be substituted as a superior alternative simply because it would not make an unintended cut. He would understand that the problem was not the sharpness of the blade, but the way it was used. He would continue to use the sharp scalpel because it is more useful than the dull one. He would simply use it in the proper way.

While it is claimed that bipolar electrosurgery is safer than monopolar, this is not necessarily true. Bipolar instruments require larger heads than monopolar devices, so mechanical or electrosurgery using bipolar devices will rarely be as precise as is surgery with smaller monopolar devices, such as 3 mm scissors. Bipolar electrocoagulation can continue to drive electrons across the adjacent paddles in some circumstances even when the tissue is coagulated and completely desiccated, resulting in continued heat production. Many bipolar instruments are designed primarily to coagulate tissue by constant use over several seconds, which increases the duration of time required for their use and which can result in relatively wide thermal spread.

One of the relatively unknown intrinsic safety features of monopolar electrosurgery is the increasing insulating effect of tissue during desiccation. Electron flow diminishes, then effectively ceases when complete tissue desiccation has occurred. Thus, there is an ultimate limit to damage that can occur from monopolar electrosurgery, even if an electrode were activated in a single location for a long period of time. In surgical practice, monopolar electrosurgery is used in short bursts, which increases its safety because the dwell time in any specific location is kept to an absolute minimum. Accordingly, monopolar electrosurgery can be used safely on or around the ureter, bowel, bladder, or vascular structures. Just as a hand can pass quickly through the intense flame of a blowtorch, so can virtually any vital structure withstand a short burst of electrosurgery.

One of the myths of electrosurgery is that electrons will pass through the body in unintended and unpredictable ways, possibly following paths of least resistance which can cause unanticipated injury. This notion has no basis in reality. With electrosurgery, 'what you see is what you get'. If there is no visual sign of damage or thermal spread, then none has occurred. It must be remembered that although the current density or power density immediately beneath the tip of the active electrode may be quite high, the effect will be propagated in a hemispheric pattern in all directions away from the tip. This means that away from the tip the power density will drop off rapidly, as will the chance for any electrosurgical effect. The surface area (A) of a hemisphere is given by the formula $A = 2\pi r^2$. The formula for the power density (PD) at a radius, r, from the tip of the electrode becomes $PD = W/(2\pi r^2)$. So for a power setting of 50 W of pure cutting current, the power density at the very tip of a 3 mm scissors may be 5000 W/cm^2 (Fig. 5.2), but 1 cm away in any direction the power density would be less than 8 W/cm^2 (Fig. 5.6). This is too low a power density to cause harm, especially if electrosurgery is used in short bursts.

Monopolar electrosurgery in endometriosis

While many surgeons treat endometriosis by monopolar or bipolar electrocoagulation, this represents a crude and imprecise form of electrosurgery. The footprint of the active electrode is intentionally large. The dwell time is necessarily increased. The visual endpoint of surgery is uncertain since the depth of destruction is uncertain. Electrocoagulation of endometriosis suffers a much more serious problem, however, since it has never been described in the literature! For a surgeon to be able to effectively duplicate electrocoagulation of endometriosis, several pieces of information are necessary: (1) the type of electrosurgical generator used; (2) the power settings; (3) the type of active electrode used; (4) how that electrode is used; (5) visual endpoints of complete surgery. Since none of the influential papers on electrocoagulation of endometriosis provides these details, it seems impossible for any surgeon to use this modality consistently effectively. Most surgeons using it are probably simply using a technique handed down to them in training, or which they have seen in passing. Furthermore, there is insufficient evidence from systematically studied reoperated patients to gauge the efficacy of electrocoagulation of endometriosis. Given that endometriosis can invade several centimeters beneath the visible surface, the use of electrocoagulation violates common sense, since it would truly be a fantasy to imagine that electrocoagulation could treat all endometriosis effectively. In this sense, electrocoagulation of endometriosis converts all disease into superficial disease in the surgeon's mind, since the application of electrocoagulation to endometriosis must be accompanied by some hope that it is completely eradicating all disease. It is unlikely that surgeons are obtaining complete informed consent from their patients before using electrocoagulation of endometriosis, since it is highly unlikely that any woman would agree to a treatment which has never been fully described in the literature, whose efficacy is unknown and which violates common sense.

Monopolar electroexcision of endometriosis suffers none of the problems associated with electrocoagulation. The technique has been described in detail in the literature.[1–9] It is intuitively obvious that excision can treat any manifestation of endometriosis, of any depth of invasion, in any area of the body. Its efficacy has been published.[10] The technique of

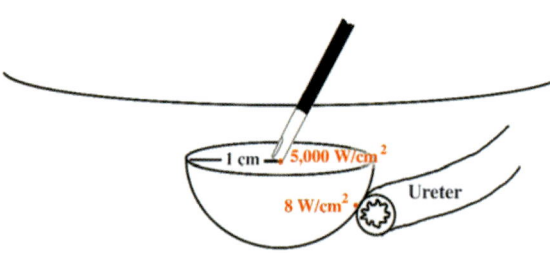

Power: 50 Watts pure cutting current

Figure 5.6

As electrons enter the tissue from the tip of the active electrode, the current density is very high immediately beneath the electrode tip. As the electrons spread throughout the tissue in a hemispherical pattern away from the active electrode, the current density becomes much lower. This, along with the use of monopolar electrosurgery in brief bursts, makes this surgical energy form very safe in the hands of those who understand its use

monopolar electroexcision of endometriosis is based largely simply on blunt dissection with the inactive electrode, separating healthy tissue from diseased tissue. Perhaps 75% of the surgery is performed by blunt or sharp dissection, with electrosurgery used for peritoneal incisions, bleeders, or for severing the remaining tendrils of tissue between endometriosis and healthy tissue. Using electrosurgery in short bursts is another key to its safe use. The higher voltage of coagulation current can cut through almost any tissue with good hemostasis and little lateral thermal spread *if* the active electrode is moved rapidly. The lower voltage of pure cutting current can cut through vital structures, such as the bowel, bladder or ureter with very little lateral thermal spread (Fig. 5.7). Again, the active electrode must be kept in constant motion. If a 5 mm instrument is used the 'footprint' will be larger and the power settings may need to be increased slightly to obtain tissue effects similar to those achieved with 3 mm instruments. An additional consideration when using 5 mm shafted instruments is that the larger size of the instrument can hide the surgical field from view, leading to imprecise and possibly dangerous surgery.

While monopolar electroexcision offers many advantages, chief of which is complete removal of endometriosis anywhere in the body, laser excision of endometriosis, by carbon dioxide (CO_2), yttrium-aluminum garnet (NdYAG), potassium titanyl phosphate (KTP) laser, or harmonic scalpel, offer the possibility of the same complete removal of the disease. Excision of endometriosis is the only treatment that can eradicate superficial as well as invasive disease. Laser vaporization or electrocoagulation cannot be considered equivalent to excision for this reason.

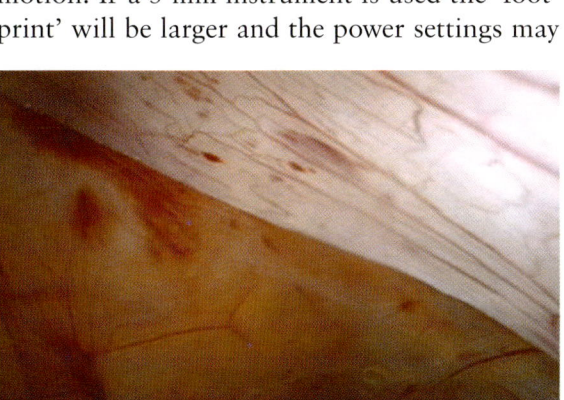

Figure 5.7
An area of peritoneum involved by endometriosis in the bottom half of the frame has been excised using 90 W of pure cutting current. Residual shiny normal peritoneum remains in the top half of the frame. Notice the cut edge which has no sign of lateral thermal spread

References

1. Redwine DB. Laparoscopic excision of endometriosis with 3 mm scissors: Comparison of operating times between sharp excision and electro-excision. J Am Assoc Gynecol Laparosc 1993;1:24–30.
2. Redwine DB. Excising endometriosis. OBG Management. Dec 1998;10:24–40.
3. Redwine DB. Laparoscopic diagnosis of endometriosis. Surgery for endometriosis. Operative techniques in gynecologic surgery. Philadelphia: WB Saunders, 1997, Ch 2:58–66.
4. Redwine DB. Non-laser resection of endometriosis. In: Sutton CA, Diamond MP (eds) Endoscopic surgery for gynaecologists. London: WB Saunders, 1993:220–8.
5. Redwine DB. Treatment of endometriosis of the cul-de-sac. In: Nezhat CR, Berger GS, Nezhat FR, Buttram VC Jr, Nezhat CH (eds) Modern surgical management of endometriosis. New York: Springer, 1995:105–115.
6. Redwine DB. Surgical treatment of endometriosis by electroexcision. In: Motoshaw ND, Dave S (eds) Endometriosis. Hyderabad, India: Orient Longman, 1997:24–44.
7. Redwine DB. Laparoscopic electroexcision of endometriosis, 2nd edn. In: Soderstrom RA (ed) Operative laparoscopy, the masters' techniques. New York: JB Lippincott-Raven, 1997:105–10.
8. Redwine DB. Monopolar electroexcision of endometriosis. In: Sutton CA, Diamond MP (eds) Endoscopic surgery for gynaecologists, 2nd edn. London: WB Saunders, 1998:369–79.
9. Redwine DB. Laparoscopic treatment of endometriosis. In: Tulandi T (ed) Atlas of laparoscopic technique for gynecologists, 2nd edn. London: WB Saunders, 1998:77–84.
10. Redwine DB. Conservative laparoscopic excision of endometriosis by sharp dissection: life table analysis of reoperation and persistent or recurrent disease. Fertil Steril 1991;56:628–34.

6

Electrosurgical resection of endometriosis
Ray Garry

No single therapeutic strategy has been shown to be completely effective in the management of the symptoms of endometriosis. Therapeutic options range from observation alone through a host of medical therapies to surgical ablation or excision to performing hysterectomy with or without bilateral oophorectomy. After carefully reviewing the literature we decided that we would adopt complete surgical excision of all extrauterine disease as the therapeutic approach most likely to benefit patients suffering from this most challenging disease.

Selection of excisional modality

There are a number of excisional modalities available and each has proponents and each has a spectrum of advantages and disadvantages. We have selected electrosurgical scissors as our primary excisional tool for a combination of practical and theoretical reasons. From a conceptual point of view, we instinctively favor the simplest and least complex tool that will effectively complete the task. As surgical operations mature and develop, it is the aim of most surgeons to gradually simplify their techniques. It is axiomatic that the fewer tools that are required to effectively complete an operation, the better. In laparoscopic procedures this will not only significantly reduce the cost of the procedure but also the complexity and time required by reducing the number of instrument changes.

A laparoscopic instrument table loaded with multiple complex sources of energy, each designed to facilitate minor variations of the essential surgical processes of tissue division and haemostasis, often betokens a lack of skill with a single source rather than indicating the immense complexity of the task to be performed. We have observed that the most experienced laparoscopic surgeons tend to use the least number and simplest instrumentation. The use of multiple tools will not mask surgical ineptitude.

I began this type of work using a carbon dioxide (CO_2) laser but was never convinced that in my hands the increased complexity (and cost) of the equipment was reflected in a superior outcome. Certainly, electrosurgical scissors are the most generally available devices and are most suitable for surgeons like myself who are called on to operate in many different locations. Electrosurgical scissors allow tissues to be divided with either scissor blades or electrosurgery and also allows an element of haemostasis to be achieved with a single instrument. Although we would prefer the use of reusable scissors the practical reality is that the repeated use of electrosurgery rapidly blunts these instruments destroying the cold cutting capability. Thus, for routine work we either use the completely disposable scissors manufactured by Ethicon and AutoSuture or semi-disposable models, such as those produced by Microline. We only use cutting current and no coagulation current with our scissors at settings as low as possible and usually between 30 and 60 watts.

The extent of endometriosis and the morphology likely to be found at surgery can frequently be deduced simply from an appropriate history combined with a careful vaginal and combined rectovaginal examination. During physical examination, each uterosacral ligament should be carefully palpated throughout its length and the presence of nodules and/or tenderness noted. This can be facilitated on a rectovaginal examination by placing the index finger in the vagina behind the cervix and pushing it forwards. This will place the uterosacral ligaments on stretch and any induration or nodules can then be detected by the middle finger placed simultaneously in the rectum. The thickness and feel of the posterior vaginal vault should also be defined and the presence of irregularities, increased thickness or nodules carefully noted. Watching the patient's face during examination can be helpful in detecting tender areas, even in stoical patients.

With more advanced endometriosis there is considerable evidence to support the concept that local tenderness on examination is positively associated with deposits of endometriosis that can be found at surgery.[1,2]

Complementary investigations include transvaginal and transabdominal ultrasound to help detect endometriomata and adenomyosis. Rectal ultrasound is being investigated as a means of determining the degree of rectal muscularis involvement preoperatively. Computed axial tomography (CAT) scans are of little benefit but magnetic resonance imaging (MRI) scans may help in localizing extrauterine nodules of the diseases or in detecting adenomyosis of the uterus. Intravenous pyelogram (IVP) will determine if there is ureteric stricture and may be of medicolegal value. Barium enemas may reveal a lower bowel stricture (Fig. 6.1) but are frequently negative even in the presence of significant bowel disease, as are preoperative sigmoidoscopies. At the end of the day, however, the results of any test are not always helpful. Tests surely do not treat the disease, and tests may be negative even in the face of severe and symptomatic endometriosis or uterine adenomyosis. The surgeon will be forced to handle disease as it is found at surgery regardless of the results of scans. The depth of excision required during surgery will be determined by the degree of invasion of organs, not the results of preoperative tests. The history, physical examination, and the patient's desire for pregnancy remain the most important determinants of where the disease might be and what type of surgery might be required. The need for general surgical or urological assistance during surgery will usually be apparent beforehand.

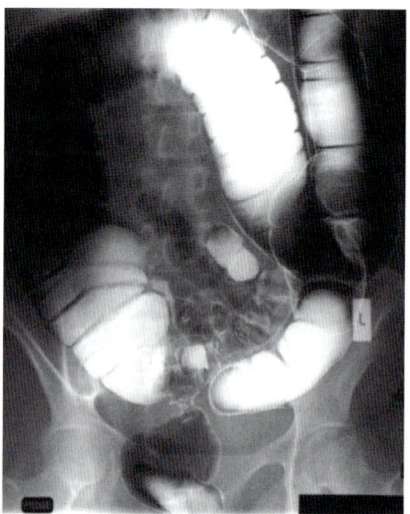

Figure 6.1

Barium enema demonstrating an 'apple core' stricture due to endometriosis. Symptoms of subacute large bowel obstruction were present. By courtesy of Ray Garry

Preoperative preparation

When preparing a patient for extensive laparoscopic excision of endometriosis it is essential that the surgeon and the patient share the same goals and that she be fully aware of the implications of these goals. The patient must be fully appraised of the risks and consequences of excising bowel, ureteric and bladder endometriosis. They must have a formal bowel preparation of the surgeon's choice, such as a low residue diet three days before surgery and cleaning enemas the evening before surgery. The patient must be made aware that sometimes it will be necessary to convert from the laparoscopic to the laparotomy mode of access during the case. This is particularly likely in the rare instances that formal excision of segments of colon or ureter is required.

A realistic amount of time should be made available for the surgery. Attempting to squeeze a case that may take several hours to complete into a surgical slot appropriate to a more minor procedure produces tension amongst all members of the operative team. Realistic timing can only come with experience. The author would recommend pessimism as the guiding attitude when arranging the timing of an extensive laparoscopic case.

Laparoscopic excision of endometriosis involves working in all areas of the pelvis. Some of these areas are vascular but relatively far from vital structures. In such places the liberal use of electrosurgery with cutting current delivered by the tips or the edges of the scissor blades can produce a relatively bloodless dissection. Other areas are very close to structures, such as the bowel and ureter, where lateral spread of thermal energy may provoke severe complications. In these areas, cold cutting with the scissors will minimize the risk of such collateral tissue damage. When bleeding occurs from smaller vessels, haemostasis can often be achieved using the scissors by slightly opening their blades and placing then firmly in contact with the tissues before discharging cutting current. This set-up will produce a superficial, effective coagulation effect. Large vessel bleeding cannot be controlled in this manner and an effective pair of bipolar forceps or suturing is required for such circumstances.

Laparoscopic entry technique

Although there are many techniques for safely entering the abdomen I prefer a high pressure Veress needle technique. The umbilicus is grasped, elevated and slightly rotated with the left hand. The primary 10 mm incision is made along the base of the umbilicus. The Veress needle is held like a dart someway down its shaft and is carefully inserted through the layers of the abdominal wall. Two distinct 'pops' are felt, first, when the needle passes through the sheath, and second, when it pierces the peritoneum and enters the abdominal cavity. The needle is not inserted further and is not rotated or rocked. Correct positioning is checked with Palmer's saline test and then by observing a good flow/low pressure reading when the gas insufflator is connected. The gas is insufflated until a pressure of 25 mmHg is established. A short barrel-length trocar is then palmed in the right hand with the index finger extended down the shaft of the cannula to within 1 cm of the tip. With a large air bubble under high pressure it is then safe to insert the trocar vertically down through the layers of the abdominal wall until it just enters the abdominal cavity. The direction of thrust is then changed towards the bowl of the pelvis while the trocar is secured. Three secondary ports are inserted with combined transillumination and laparoscopic direct visualization. The two lateral trocars are placed outside the line of the inferior epigastric vessels and the

SURGICAL MANAGEMENT OF ENDOMETRIOSIS

midline trocar is placed in suprapubically 2 cm above the hairline. The intraabdominal pressure is reduced to 15 mmHg after the trocars have been safely inserted.

Anatomic distribution of severe disease

A prerequisite for complete surgical excision is precise definition of the extent and distribution of the endometriotic lesions. I believe that failure to do this accurately is one of the most common reasons for the subsequent failure of surgical approaches. My increasing experience with surgical excision of endometriosis has led me to revise my opinions about the distribution and nature of the disease. Despite pelvic chaos, with the disease apparently distributed at random throughout the pelvis, I have found that most endometriotic lesions (particularly in patients who have not had previous pelvic surgery) demonstrate a remarkably consistent distribution. My change of perception has been facilitated by the routine use of vaginal and rectal probes in addition to the invariable use of a Valchev uterine manipulator during my operative assessment (Fig. 6.2).

Pushing the uterus firmly cephalad with the Valchev puts the uterosacral ligaments on stretch and makes the appreciation of the extent of their involvement with endometriosis more obvious (Fig. 6.3). Similarly, pushing and opening a pair of sponge-holding forceps placed in the posterior fornix of the vagina clearly demonstrates the occurrence of nodular endometriosis in the tissues in the region of the posterior vaginal vault.

Endometriosis of the peritoneum overlying the cervix and posterior vaginal fornix (Fig. 6.4) frequently coexists with extensive involvement of one or both uterosacral ligaments and can

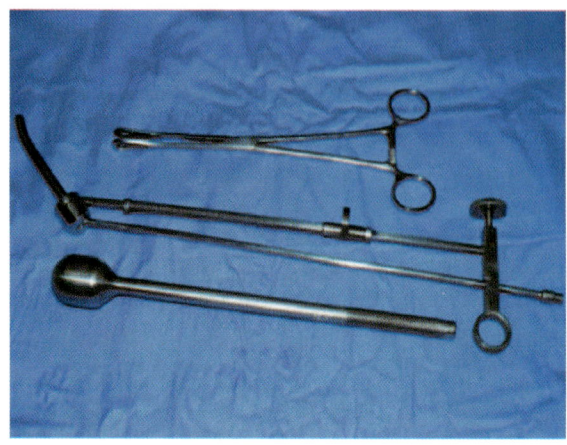

Figure 6.2
Essential equipment for radical excision of endometriosis. (Top) a sponge-holding forceps to define the posterior vaginal fornix. (Middle) a Valchev uterine mobilizer to manipulate the uterus and ensure sharp anteversion and good vision of the pouch of Douglas. (Bottom) a rectal probe to demark boundaries of the rectum and exclude major stricture. By courtesy of Ray Garry

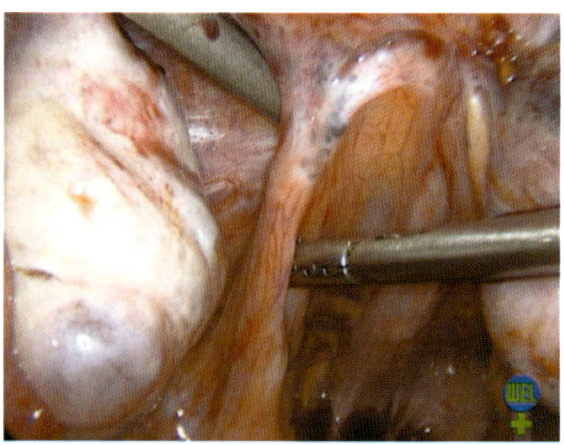

Figure 6.3
The uterosacral ligaments are being stretched by extreme uterine elevation anteriorly to demonstrate the extent of their involvement with endometriosis. The instruments are displaying the left uterosacral ligament. By courtesy of Ray Garry

appear as a sheet of abnormal tissue that spreads from one lateral pelvic sidewall and its uterosacral ligament across the posterior vaginal

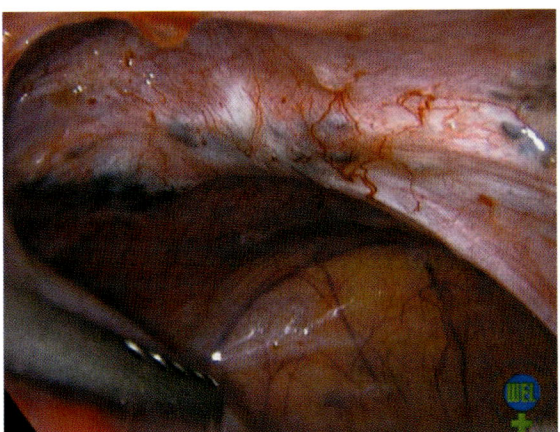

Figure 6.4
Endometriosis spread across the posterior vaginal fornix. By courtesy of Ray Garry

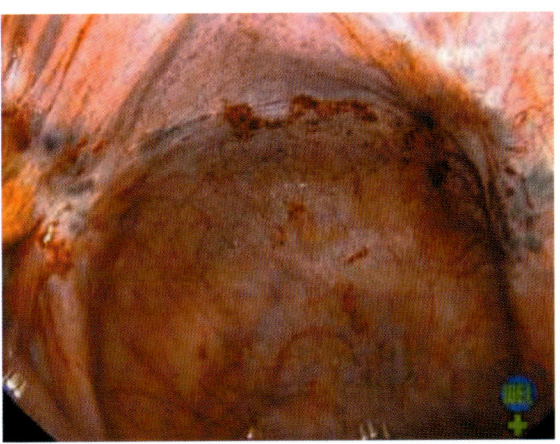

Figure 6.5
Endometriosis involving both uterosacral ligaments and the area above the posterior vaginal fornix between. By courtesy of Ray Garry

fornix to the other uterosacral ligament (Fig. 6.5). Such disease can be associated with severe vaginal and rectal symptoms. Endometriosis in this area is frequently incorrectly described as being endometriosis of the rectovaginal septum[3] because the septum itself is infrequently involved. These lesions are frequently associated with exquisitely tender nodules palpable on vaginal examination of the posterior fornix. Pressure on these lesions may reproduce much of the patient's symptoms, particularly dyspareunia. Reproduction of symptoms during examination increases the chance for pain relief following surgery.[4] Such lesions may also fix the uterus, reducing its normal mobility. While uterine retroversion may be present, it is not always because the uterus is being pulled to the rear by fibrosis due to endometriosis. The uterus may be in a normal anterior position in many patients.

Endometriosis and its associated peritoneal fibrosis may also extend upwards to involve the peritoneum of the ovarian fossa, often in conjunction with an ovarian endometrioma. The lesion above the posterior vaginal vault may also frequently extend posteriorly and attach to the anterior surface of the rectum. This then pulls the rectum forward and fixes it to the back uterus. In doing so, the cul de sac is obliterated and the rectum distorted and kinked (Fig. 6.6). Such anatomical kinking of the lower bowel

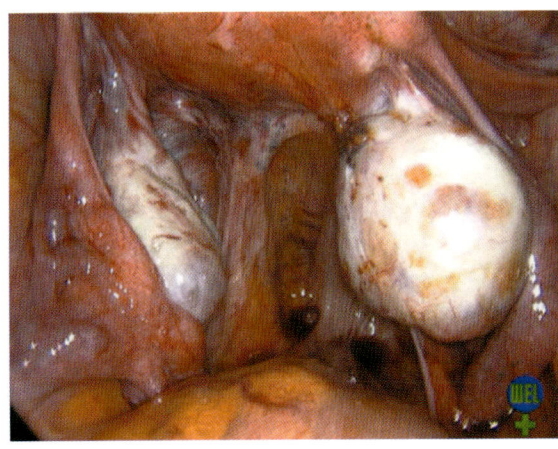

Figure 6.6
A typical, moderately severe case, of deep endometriosis with involvement of both uterosacral ligaments and the tissue between them over the posterior vaginal fornix. The rectum is also drawn up and fixed to the back of the cervix and there is a right-sided endometrioma in continuity with the right uterosacral lesion. By courtesy of Ray Garry

contributes to the dyschezia that is such a frequent component of the endometriosis symptom complex.

Cul de sac obliteration almost invariably occurs at the level of the posterior vaginal vault and occasionally is not readily obvious to the naked eye. Observation of the blades of the sponge forceps in the vaginal vault will help identification in some cases. In a normal situation, the vaginal tissues are remarkably thin and the outline of the ring of the forceps can easily be appreciated beneath the tented vaginal tube. When a sheet of endometriotic tissue is present the crisp outline of the forceps is lost. The thickness of this rectovaginal deposit may vary from a few millimetres to several centimetres. Failure to identify and remove this common and extensive area of endometriosis is a frequent cause of failure of surgical excision.

From this 'standard' distribution, endometriosis can be observed to invade surrounding structures in all directions. Most problematically, lesions that cause obliteration of the cul de sac may spread posteriorly and invade the rectum and/or sigmoid colon musculature. Such colonic invasion may produce cyclical rectal bleeding, dyschezia, rectal stenosis and rarely large bowel obstruction. It may also spread caudally and invade through the whole thickness of the vaginal epithelium. This will produce lesions that often have blue-colored areas (Fig. 6.7) and that may be a source of vaginal bleeding with or without the presence of a uterus.

Endometriosis may also spread laterally to involve the structures of the pelvic sidewall including the ureter (Figs 6.8, 6.9). The symptoms and signs of hydronephrosis may develop and one or both kidneys may be destroyed if the lesions are not effectively managed.

More recently, we have also come to appreciate that these extrauterine lesions might invade the outer surface of the uterus. In this situation, the lesions are by definition adenomyosis but

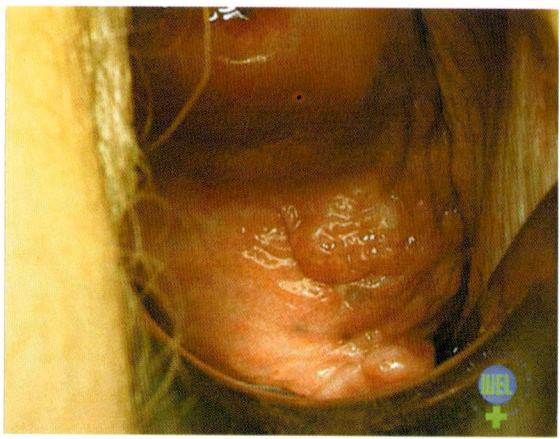

Figure 6.7
A view of the posterior vaginal mucosal epithelium showing the features of a full-thickness vaginal endometriotic lesion with characteristic blue-domed lesions, scarring and induration. By courtesy of Ray Garry

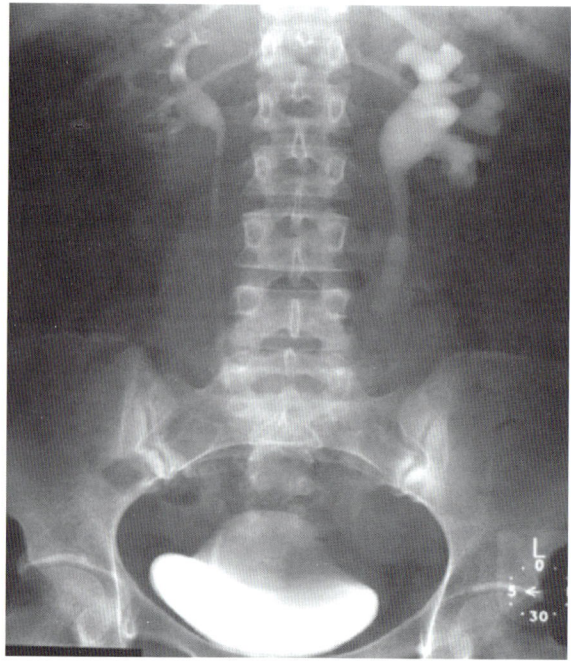

Figure 6.8
Intravenous pyelogram (IVP) showing hydronephrosis due to endometriosis obstructing the left ureter. By courtesy of Ray Garry

ELECTROSURGICAL RESECTION OF ENDOMETRIOSIS

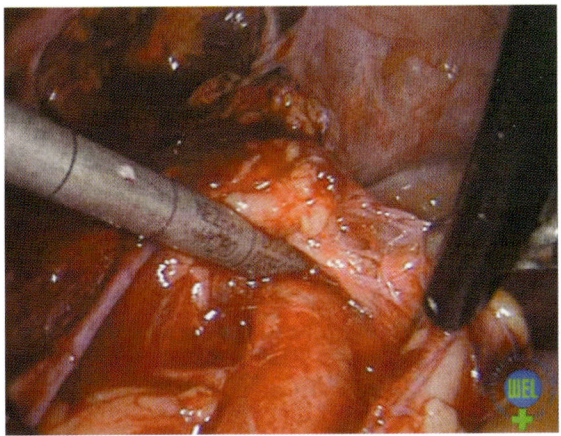

Figure 6.9
The same hydroureter being dissected to reveal the band of endometriotic tissue surrounding the ureter. By courtesy of Ray Garry

appear to be associated with lesions outside the uterus spreading in rather than intrauterine pathology spreading out.

Radical laparoscopic excision of endometriosis (RLEE)

Our principle for the management of endometriosis is excision with disease-free margins around the excised specimens in the manner pioneered by oncological surgeons. Due to the 'invasive' nature of the disease we do not always succeed in these aims despite aggressive attempts. Excision can frequently be best achieved by undertaking an 'en bloc' excision, whereby all the abnormal material is removed in one single piece, similar to reports almost a century old.[5] Such an en bloc excision need not include the uterus if conservative surgery is undertaken but will usually contain the proximal portions of both uterosacral ligaments as well as the tissues over the vaginal vault and from the front of the rectum. We regard such an en bloc resection as the standard surgical treatment for cases of severe, invasive endometriosis.[6]

When the endometriosis is confined to the bottom of the pelvis, the en bloc excision (Fig. 6.10) begins in the uninvolved peritoneum lateral to and above the most posterior lesion on the left pelvic sidewall (Fig. 6.11). The peritoneum is elevated and incised. The cut edge is grasped by the assistant with forceps and pulled medially. The retroperitoneal space is developed by blunt dissection aided by insufflation gas entering the space. The course of the ureter is identified, and the surgeon, using a suction-irrigator or grasping forceps, displaces the ureter laterally while the peritoneum and endometriosis is teased away medially (Fig. 6.12). All of the involved uterosacral ligaments on the left is excised starting posteriorly and progressively mobilizing it towards its insertion into the back of the cervix. The uterosacral ligament is transected at its origin, taking care to avoid the adjacent uterine vessels. After this, the incision is extended medially across the uterus above the lesions (Fig. 6.13).

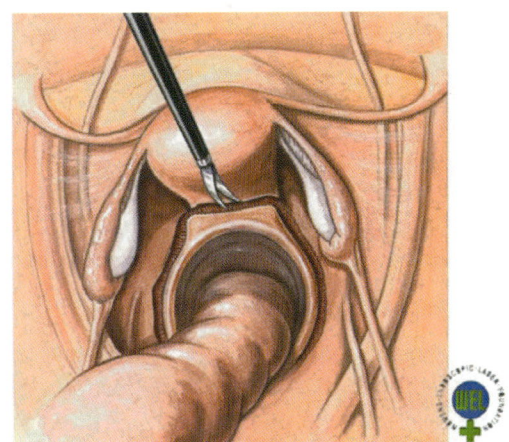

Figure 6.10
Diagrammatic representation of the field to be removed with an en bloc excision. By courtesy of Ray Garry

SURGICAL MANAGEMENT OF ENDOMETRIOSIS

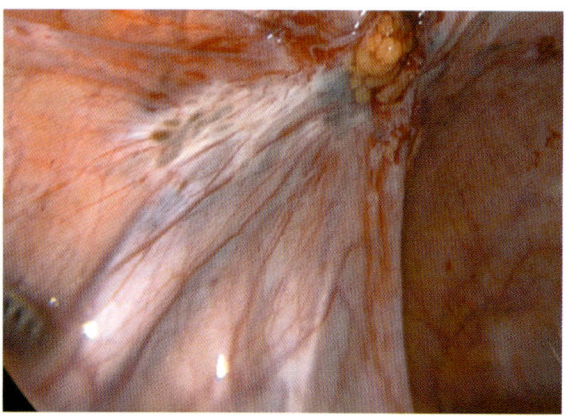

Figure 6.11
Lesion on the left pelvic sidewall overlying the ureter before dissection begins. By courtesy of Ray Garry

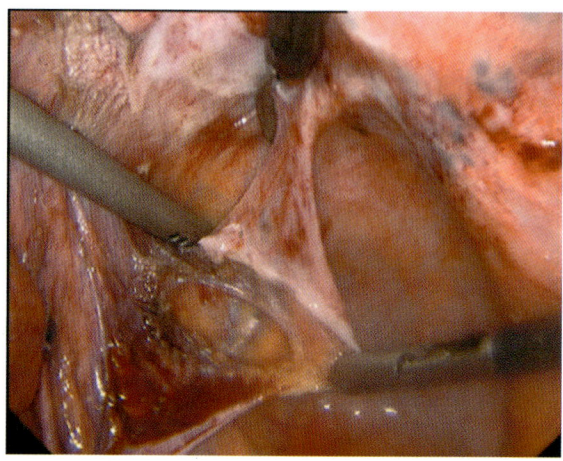

Figure 6.13
The next stage of the en bloc excision with the incision being extended across the back of the uterus above the lesion. By courtesy of Ray Garry

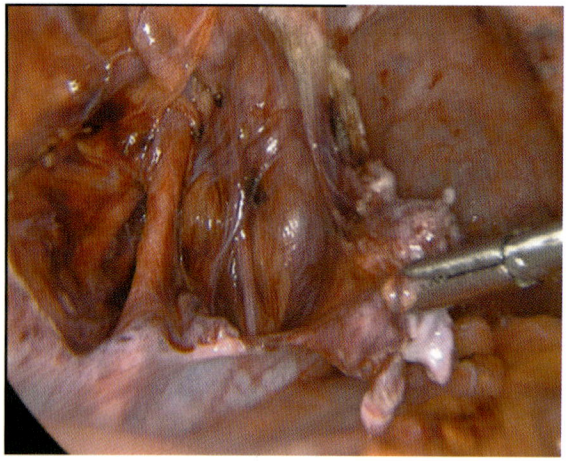

Figure 6.12
View of the same case after mobilizing the left pelvic sidewall peritoneum and demonstrating the course of the left ureter. By courtesy of Ray Garry

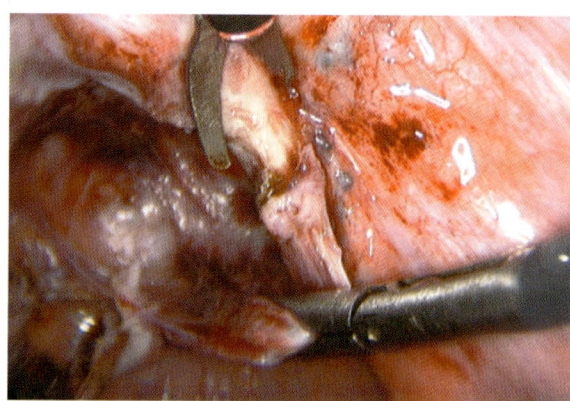

Figure 6.14
The right uterosacral ligament is now divided from its origin in the back of the uterus. Note the chocolate-colored material escaping from glands located deep in the structure of the ligament. By courtesy of Ray Garry

The right uterosacral ligament is next excised in the reverse manner, that is, starting from its insertion into the uterus (Fig. 6.14) and removing it until all involved material is freed from the pelvic sidewall. On this side, the right-handed surgeon is pulling the disease attached to the pelvic sidewall peritoneum medially with a grasper in his left hand while the assistant guards and displaces the ureter laterally (Fig. 6.15). The incision now resembles an inverted U.

Often, endometriosis extends from the pelvic sidewalls onto one or both lateral borders of the rectum. The disease must be freed from its lateral attachments so that the prerectal spaces can be defined. Placing the ring forceps in the

ELECTROSURGICAL RESECTION OF ENDOMETRIOSIS

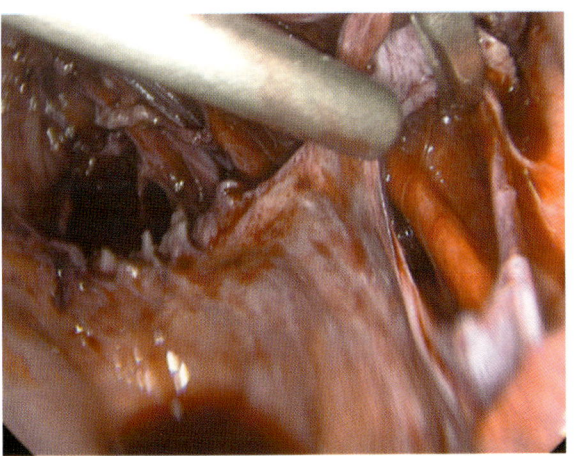

Figure 6.15

The incision is now extended down the right pelvic sidewall above and lateral to the uterosacral ligament and medial to the ureter. By courtesy of Ray Garry

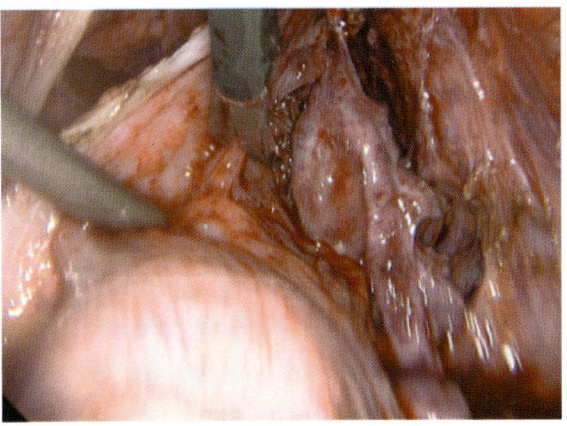

Figure 6.16

The incision is now extended across the front of the rectum to free the lesion. By courtesy of Ray Garry

posterior vaginal fornix and opening and pushing them firmly towards the patient's head will define the outline of the posterior vaginal vault. If the rings of the forceps are easily seen, the posterior vaginal wall is not involved, but in most cases a sheet of tissue of varying thickness will be seen between the forceps and the peritoneum. The left lateral edge of this is identified and progressively excised from the normal vaginal structures. The dissection is continued down towards the vagina until the shiny white appearance of the vaginal fascia is seen. The dissection continues down the back of the vagina until the entire firm abnormal block of tissue has been mobilized. When this occurs we will have usually entered the prerectal space lateral to rectovaginal septum, and normal tissue planes will again be encountered below the lesion but above the pelvic floor.

The right posterior margin of the incision is once again grasped by the assistant and pulled medially. The surgeon then extends the incision carefully over the anterior surface of the rectum (Fig. 6.16). Sometimes, a plane of cleavage between the disease and the rectum will be identified and when this is present the whole lesion can be fairly simply removed. In a substantial percentage of cases, however, there is no plane since the endometriosis is invading through the serosa and into the muscularis layers of the rectum or sigmoid colon. When no plane is identified the surgeon must elect either to cut through the lesion and knowingly leave endometriosis behind in the rectal wall or follow the disease through part or the whole thickness of the rectal wall. The latter course should only be contemplated in patients who had preoperatively been consented and prepared for such an eventuality. When the incision reaches the left pelvic sidewall the remainder of the specimen is undercut until it can be removed in an en bloc manner in its entirety (Fig. 6.17). After removal of the fibrotic disease, the jaws of a ring forceps spreading the posterior vaginal fornix will be clearly seen laparoscopically (Fig. 6.18).

Variations to the standard 'en bloc excision'

In addition to our standard procedure for the removal of deep endometriosis it is often

SURGICAL MANAGEMENT OF ENDOMETRIOSIS

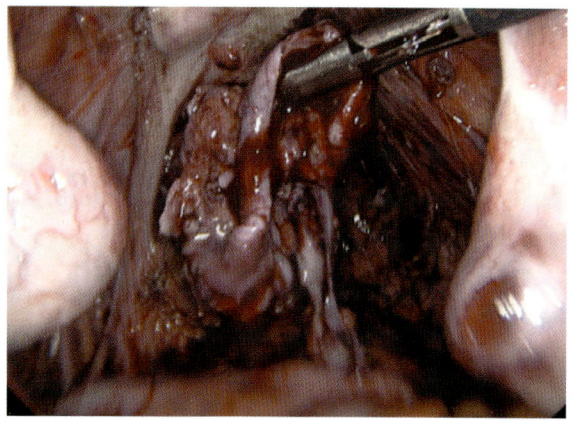

Figure 6.17
The whole lesion is now freed and then removed through a port to be analysed histologically. By courtesy of Ray Garry

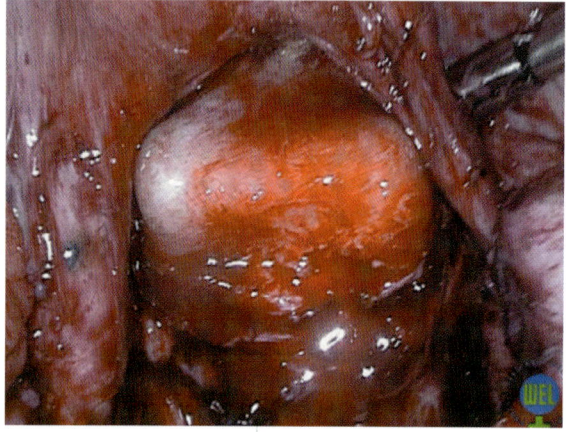

Figure 6.18
The blades of a ring forceps are being spread in the posterior vaginal fornix. After removal of the fibrotic lesion in this area, the outline of the blades is clear. By courtesy of Ray Garry

Usually, these adhesions are of a different nature to the hard retroperitoneal lesions characteristic of deep pelvic endometriosis. These are often filmy in nature and divide easily. Great care must be taken to avoid bowel that is frequently surrounded by this type of adhesion (Fig. 6.19).

Ovarian endometriomata

The optimal treatment of endometriomata remains controversial. The preliminary step is invariably mobilizing the enlarged ovary from the adhesions that hold it to the pelvic sidewalls. This inevitably releases the viscid chocolate-coloured material that must be carefully aspirated. I then favor widely opening the endometrioma and washing the cavity. The ovary is then biopsied and the capsule treated with argon beam coagulation, laser or electrosurgical energy, depending on availability. It is important to remember that ovarian endometriosis is a necessary to modify the technique to manage variations in the presentation of this enigmatic disease. Frequently patients have had previous surgery or may have tubo-ovarian endometriosis that fills the upper pelvis with adnexal adhesions and adherent bowel. These adhesions must of course be taken down before the pouch can be defined and the lesions deep in the pelvis treated.

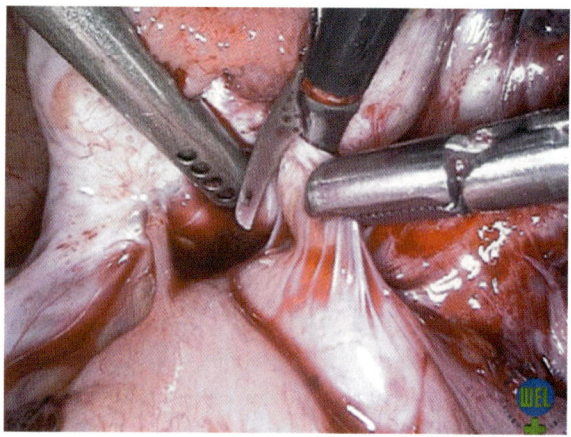

Figure 6.19
Some adhesions of the posterior pelvis are relatively filmy and of a different character to the firm and hard endometriotic adhesions. These probably represent adhesions forming as a consequence of previous surgery. By courtesy of Ray Garry

ELECTROSURGICAL RESECTION OF ENDOMETRIOSIS

marker for more severe pelvic and intestinal disease.[7]

Isolated nodules

Occasionally, the endometriotic lesion in the pelvis is not buried within a sheet of abnormal tissue but is present as an isolated nodule. Such nodules can invariably be defined with careful vaginal palpation but can be missed on laparoscopic inspection because they are not associated with the peritoneum stigmata of classic endometriosis. Such nodules should be defined, dissected and removed in a standard manner which will often require opening the vagina, as such lesions are often full thickness (Figs 6.20–6.23).

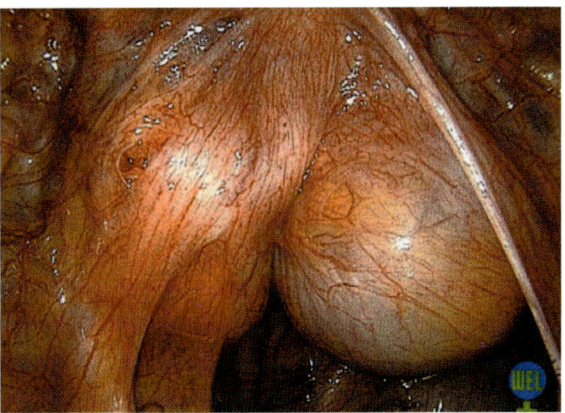

Figure 6.21
The same lesion with a probe in the rectum (the bulge to the right) that also clearly demonstrates a large retroperitoneal lesion on the left side of the vaginal apex. By courtesy of Ray Garry

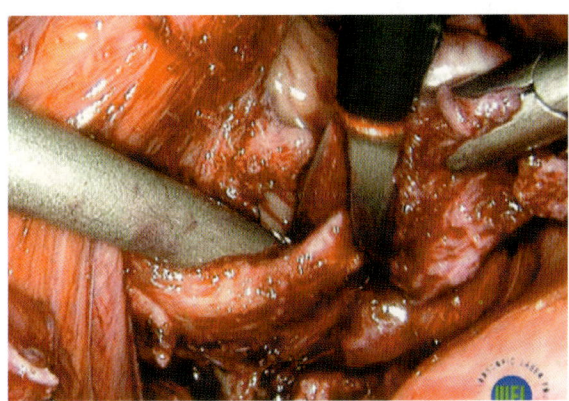

Figure 6.22
Excising the lesion that requires entering the vagina. By courtesy of Ray Garry

Colorectal endometriosis

More technical difficulties occur when the rectum or sigmoid colon is involved with endometriosis. These lesions should be excised, but this often requires the cooperation of an informed colorectal surgeon and may require the intraoperative conversion to laparotomy. All levels of colorectal involvement may occur.

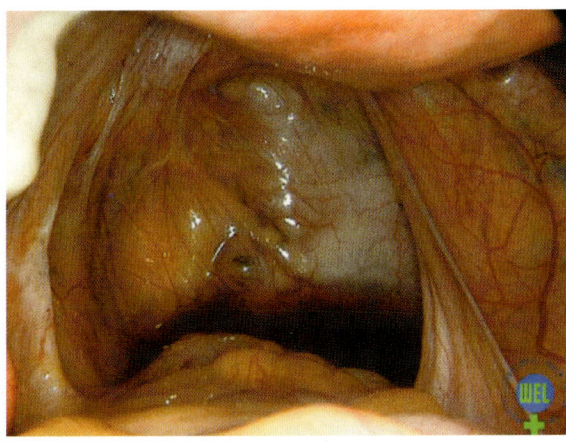

Figure 6.20
Many major lesions are missed on laparoscopic inspection because they are not associated with classic powder-burn lesions. Here, a patient with a superficially normal pelvis has, in fact, a golf ball size lesion that was readily palpable on vaginal examination. By courtesy of Ray Garry

SURGICAL MANAGEMENT OF ENDOMETRIOSIS

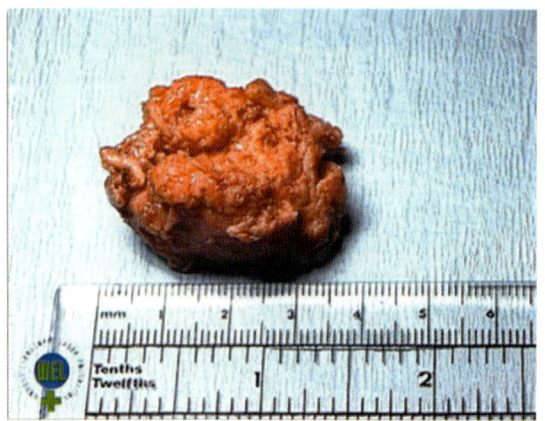

Figure 6.23
The excised nodule. By courtesy of Ray Garry

Many lesions can be shaved off the serosal surface of the colon. On occasion, such as illustrated, the lesion extends some distance into the muscularis layer and it may be possible to shell out the endometriosis without penetrating the mucosa. In these circumstances, the muscularis can be reinforced with laparoscopic sutures (Fig. 6.24). More often, however, the bowel lumen

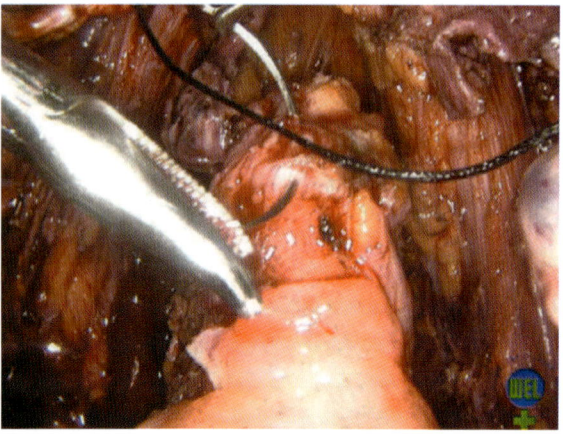

Figure 6.24
Repairing laparoscopically a partial-thickness rectal lesion caused by the shelling out of a nodule that had invaded the rectal muscularis layer. By courtesy of Ray Garry

must be entered to ensure complete excision. Subsequent management depends on the size of the lesions. Very small 'holes' may be repaired with laparoscopic sutures. Somewhat larger lesions may be removed with the help of intrarectal circular staplers as described by Harry Reich. Not infrequently, however, large lesions are encountered that require a formal anterior resection. This is particularly indicated when there is a frank stricture of the lower bowel. Some laparoscopic surgeons are able to complete even this type of surgery laparoscopically but I prefer to convert to laparotomy and use the skills of my colorectal surgeon to complete this procedure.

Results

Previous reports on aggressive laparoscopic excision of endometriosis have detailed the favourable response of disease extent[8] and symptoms.[9–13]

My unit has recently completed two studies to demonstrate the effectiveness of this type of approach in managing this condition.[14]

We followed 135 patients for up to 5 years after treatment: 19 of these patients had Stage I disease, 39 had Stage II, 23 Stage III and 54 had Stage IV disease. Each parameter of pain was highly significantly improved by the surgery and this improvement was maintained for a mean of 3.2 years (Table 6.1). There were significant improvements in European Quality of Life (EuroQoL) and the Sexual Activity Questionnaire (SAQ) instruments along with a non-significant trend to improvement in the SF12 scores (Tables 6.2, 6.3).

Despite these encouraging results one third of the patients required further surgery within 5 years (Fig. 6.25) and perhaps not surprisingly the risk of reoperation was greater in those with severe (rAFS>70) endometriosis (Fig. 6.26).

Table 6.1 The changes in various visual analogue pain scores following RLEE (maximum possible pain = 10)

	Baseline median pain score (SD)	2–5 yrs postop median pain score (SD)	Z-score	P-value
Dysmenorrhoea	9 (7–9)	3.3 (2–7)	7.9	<0.0001
Non-menstrual	8 (6–9)	3.0 (0–5)	7.6	<0.0001
Dyspareunia	7 (5.5–9)	0 (0–4)	6.8	<0.0001
Dyschezia	7 (4–8)	2 (0–2)	7.1	<0.0001

RLEE, Radical laparoscopic excision of endometriosis.

Table 6.2 Changes in EuroQoL instruments following RLEE

	Baseline mean score (SD)	2–5 yrs mean score (SD)	t-test	P-value
EQ-5Dvas	68.8 (19)	74.9 (14.8)	2.1	0.03
EQ-5Dindex	0.6 (0.31)	0.7 (0.29)	2.7	0.008

EuroQol, European Quality of Life.

Table 6.3 Changes in sexual activity questionnaire following RLEE

	Baseline median score (IQR)	2–5 yrs median score (IQR)	Baseline vs 2–5 yrs Z-score	P-value
Pleasure (max 18)	10 (5–12)	12 (9–16)	3.1	0.001
Habit (max 3)	1 (0–1)	1 (1–1)	2.5	0.012
Discomfort (max 6)	3 (1.5–5)	2 (1.5–3)	3.2	0.001

IQR,

As part of a placebo-controlled randomized clinical trial (RCT) we were able to observe the progress of the disease both after and without radical laparoscopic excision of endometriosis (RLEE). In nine of 16 (56%) women who had a second look operation 6 months after definitive surgery there was no evidence of residual endometriosis. Of the remainder, four had decreased their rAFS score and stage, two had remained at Stage IV and one had progressed from Stage II to Stage IV, despite our best efforts at complete surgical excision. In contrast, eight of 18 women (45%) who had a second-look operation 6 months after a purely diagnostic laparoscopy had disease that had got worse, of whom three had increased a stage and two had gone from Stage II to Stage IV. In six (33%) others the disease remained the same and in four (22%) the disease had improved. This study again demonstrated that RLEE improved all aspects of pain and quality of life 6 months after definitive surgery. It also demonstrated that

SURGICAL MANAGEMENT OF ENDOMETRIOSIS

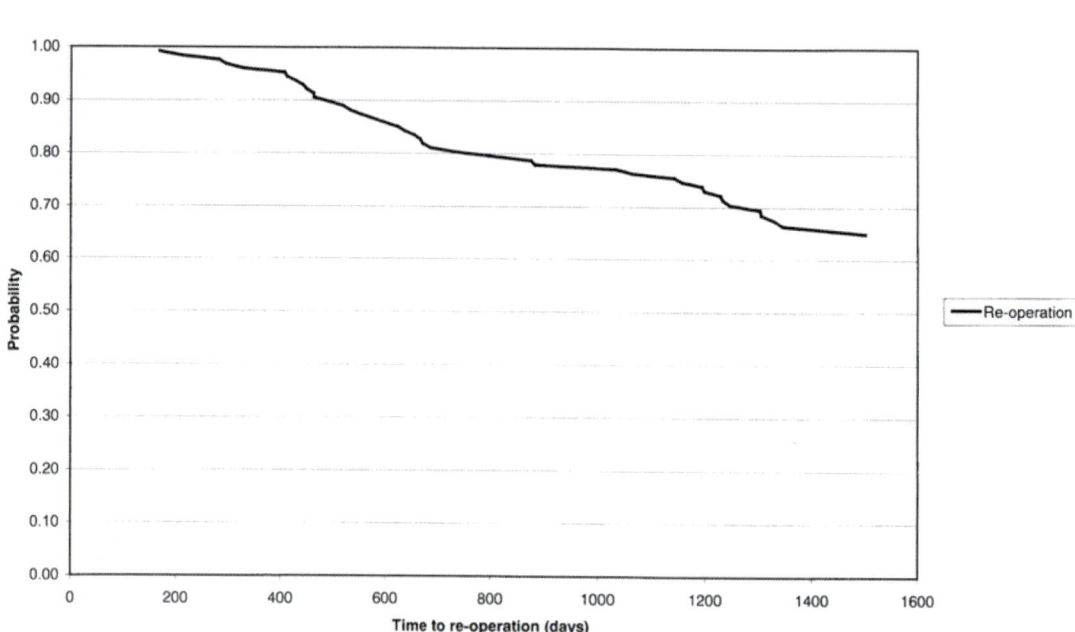

Figure 6.25
Survival curve estimating the probability of reoperation (–) at 5 years after initial surgery. By courtesy of Jason Abbot and Ray Garry

there was also a very significant placebo effect that persisted for 6 months. However, no pregnancy occurred in the placebo group but 50% of those actively trying, conceived within 6 months of primary surgery.

Conclusions

We can conclude from these two studies that RLEE is effective in relieving pain and infertility and improving aspects of the quality of life of many patients with severe endometriosis. This effect is in addition to the powerful placebo effect that this treatment for this intractable condition also provides. These welcome results are sustained for 5 years in two thirds of the patients. We have also documented that, at least in our hands, there is persistence and even progression of the disease despite surgery within 6 months in a small proportion of cases. One third of our patients will require further surgery within 5 years of our initial treatment and this risk is higher in those with severe initial disease. We are certainly reviewing the role of the uterus and hysterectomy as part of the management plan in some cases. We may also be undertreating those with bowel lesions. Not all patients with persistent symptoms have evidence of persistent endometriosis and in at least some

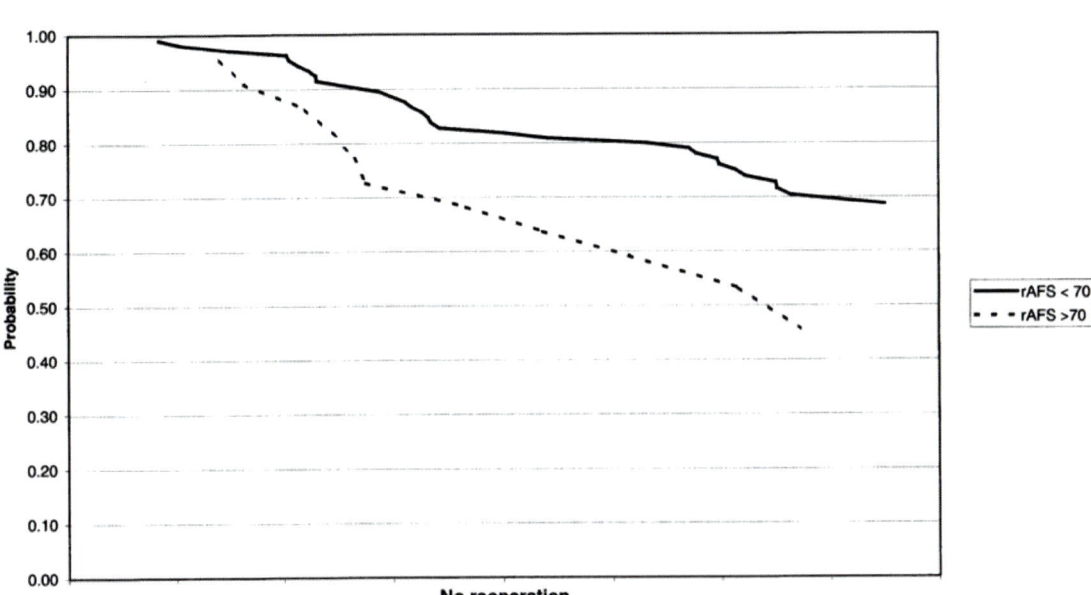

Figure 6.26
Survival curves estimating the probability of no reoperation. By courtesy of Jason Abbott and Ray Garry

of these women the cause of persistent pain must be other than endometriosis. In general, however, we believe that at this time extensive laparoscopic excision is the best treatment for endometriosis, although this will not relieve non-endometriotic symptoms. The role of effective adjuvant therapies against other causes of pain associated with endometriosis remains to be explored.

Acknowledgements

I would like to express my appreciation to David Redwine and Harry Reich for 'pointing me in the right direction'. Thanks are also due to my research fellows and to Jason Abbott, in particular, who collected and collated much of the data in this chapter.

References

1. Fallon J. Endometriosis. Two hundred cases considered from the viewpoint of the practitioner. N Engl J Med 1946;235:669–73.
2. Ripps BA, Martin DC. Focal pelvic tenderness, pelvic pain and dysmenorrhea in endometriosis. J Reprod Med 1991;36:470–2.
3. Martin DC, Batt RE. Retrocervical, rectovaginal pouch, and rectovaginal septum endometriosis. J Am Assoc Gynecol Laparosc 2001;8:12–7.
4. Redwine DB, Wright J. Laparoscopic treatment of obliteration of the cul de sac in endometriosis: Long term followup. Fertil Steril 2001;76:358–65.
5. Lockyer C. Adenomyoma in the recto-uterine and recto-vaginal septa. Proc Roy Soc Med 1913; 4:112–6 (plus Discussion).
6. Redwine DB. Laparoscopic en bloc resection for treatment of the obliterated cul de sac in endometriosis. J Reprod Med 1992;37:695–8.
7. Redwine DB. Ovarian endometriosis: A marker for more severe pelvic and intestinal disease. Fertil Steril 1999;73:310–5.
8. Redwine DB. Conservative laparoscopic excision of endometriosis by sharp dissection: life table analysis of reoperation and persistent or recurrent disease. Fertil Steril 1991;56:628–34.
9. Wood C, Maher P, Hill D. Laparoscopic removal of endometriosis in the pouch of Douglas. Aust NZ J Obstet Gynecol 1993;33:295–9.
10. Wood C, Maher P. Peritoneal surgery in the treatment of endometriosis – Excision or thermal ablation? Aust NZ J Obstet Gynecol 1996; 36:190–7.
11. Garry R, Clayton R, Hawe J. The effect of endometriosis and its radical laparoscopic excision on quality of life indicators. Br J Obstet Gynaecol 2000; 107:44–54.
12. Chapron C, Dubisson J-B, Fritel X, Fernandez B, Poncelet C, Beguin S, Pinelli L. Operative management of deep endometriosis infiltrating the uterosacral ligaments. J Am Assoc Gynecol Laparosc 1999;6:31–7.
13. Busacca M, Bianchi S, Agnoli B, Candiani M, Calia C, De Marinis S, Vignali M. Follow-up of laparoscopic treatment of stage III–IV endometriosis. J Am Assoc Gynecol Laparosc 1999; 6:55–8.
14. Abbot J, Hawe J, Clayton RD, Garry R. The effects and effectiveness of Laparoscopic excision of endometriosis: a prospective study with 2–5 year follow up. Human Reproduction 2003; 18:1922–1927.

7

Laser vaporization and electrocoagulation of endometriosis

Christopher Sutton

History of lasers in surgery

The basis for laser physics can be traced back to Albert Einstein when he published his treatise on the quantum theory of radiation in 1917.[1] In this paper, he theorized the existence of a phenomenon by which a photon can stimulate an atom or molecule and produce multiple identical photons. The process by which electricity is converted into light is called 'stimulated emission' and microwaves were the first portion of the energy spectrum used to demonstrate this effect. It was not until the mid 1950s that Gordon and colleagues[2] developed the laser based on Einstein's principles, and three years later Schawlow and Townes[3] developed the theory of light amplification by the stimulated emission of radiation, which is more simply referred to by the acronym 'laser'. In this context, radiation merely refers to light, not the ionizing radiation associated with x-rays. Lasers are essentially devices that produce intense beams of light energy which have three physical characteristics that differentiate them from normal light: (1) monochromaticity; (2) collimation; and (3) coherence. In other words, the light of any particular laser is of the same wavelength and the waves are in phase both temporally and spatially.

The first laser beam was produced by Maiman in 1960 by using a high voltage current to stimulate a synthetic ruby rod.[4] He used strobe light energy producing a red laser beam with a wavelength of 0.69, and this beam was then used experimentally before eventually becoming the first surgical laser. This was used to precisely photocoagulate lesions at the back of the retina without the need for an external incision. This laser was later replaced by an argon laser, which was developed in the mid 1960s and had more useful absorption properties.

The helium-neon laser (he-ne) was introduced in 1961 and is mainly used as an aiming beam for invisible light lasers, such as the carbon dioxide (CO_2) and neodymium-yttrium-aluminium garnet (Nd:YAG) lasers.

The CO_2 laser, which is probably the most commonly used laser in gynaecology was developed at Bell Laboratories by Patel and colleagues in 1964 for use in the communications industry.[5]

Lasers used in endoscopic surgery

Carbon dioxide laser

The carbon dioxide (CO_2) laser provides energy at a wavelength of 10 600 nm, which is within the infrared area of the spectrum, and was first used laparoscopically in 1979 by Bruhat and his team at the University of Clermont-Ferrand in France.[6] The safety and precision of this laser relies on the fact that the energy is maximally absorbed by water, and as the majority of biological tissue volume is water, the penetration of the CO_2 laser is very superficial: 99.9% of the incident power is absorbed in the first 0.1 mm of soft tissue. The superficial cells are vaporized by energy which is converted to heat. Carbonization then occurs as a result of ignition of the debris coming out of the laser crater, causing a plume of smoke which has to be evacuated. Because of this laser–tissue interaction the CO_2 laser is a tool of considerable cutting and vaporizing precision. Average power densities can be varied from 10 W/cm² to 150 000 W/cm² but greater power density results in improved surgical precision and speed, at the expense of reduced haemostasis.

The other variable that influences tissue penetration and destruction is fluence: the speed of transit of the beam over the target tissue. The Swiftlase™ (Sharplan Laser Industries, Tel Aviv, Israel) employs two mirrors rotating at speed, which allows a greater rate of fluence than would be possible with the human hand and allows a technique of using high power densities to ablate large areas of tissue accurately, virtually layer by layer, with great precision and very little charring.

Super-pulse and ultra-pulse systems

The CO_2 laser is usually operated in continuous mode to ablate tissue and coagulate small vessels. In order to ablate tissue more precisely, super-pulse systems were introduced in the late 1980s, with the advantage of high peak powers providing the laser surgeon with a greater degree of precision. Pulse energy is an important measure of pulse laser performance. When the length of the pulse is short, pulse energy determines the amount of tissue removed by the laser and the amount of heat energy left in the tissue.

A more recent development in CO_2 laser technology is the ultra-pulse mode whereby the laser beam is delivered as very high pulse energy bursts of up to 250 MJ and average powers of 950 MW. Again, this is a method of producing char-free, extremely precise cutting with minimal damage to surrounding tissue. Unfortunately, ultra-pulse lasers are extremely expensive and a similar tissue effect can be achieved much more cheaply with the rotating mirror delivery system described above.

Beam distortion

Apart from misalignment of the mirrors in the articulated arm as a cause for beam distortion, the CO_2 laser beam can also be distorted as a result of condensation on the lens, and it is important to avoid large temperature gradients between the lens and room air. Additionally, the laser plume itself may absorb or defocus the beam and it is important to insufflate gas through the operating channel of the laparoscope to minimize the smoke and debris, but this gas can itself cause the blooming effect that defocuses the beam.[7] This is because the CO_2 in the centre of the laparoscope channel is heated up more than the dense gas at the edges, creating a divergent gas lens which effectively defocuses the beam. A cunning way to get round this problem is to use an isotope of CO_2 – the CO_2-13-C laser – which circumvents this problem.[8] In practice, the blooming effect almost disappears at a gas flow of 8 L/min, which can be achieved by modern high flow insufflators.[9]

Neodymium-yttrium-aluminium garnet (Nd:YAG) laser

The Nd:YAG laser penetrates tissue much more deeply than the CO_2 laser, and also generates significant back scatter from the tissue impact. As a result of its greater depth of tissue penetration, it can seal blood vessels of up to 5 mm in diameter. Because it penetrates water, the Nd:YAG laser should not be chosen for vaporization or cutting, and it is generally accepted that the standard bare fibre is unsafe for use in the abdominal cavity for laparoscopic gynaecological surgery,[10] although it is excellent for hysteroscopic surgery. This deficiency has led the laser manufacturers to introduce sculpted quartz fibres (Sharplan Laser Industries, Tel Aviv, Israel) or artificial sapphire tips (Surgical Laser Technologies, Pennsylvania, USA) which effectively concentrate the beam as it leaves the fibre. The advent of these probes has resulted in the production of a laparoscopic 'laser scalpel', restoring a tactile sense to what was previously 'no touch' surgery. Unfortunately, these devices have a limited life, or are disposable, and add considerably to the cost of laser surgery. This is no longer 'laser surgery' because the cutting is similar to that achieved by a hot wire. Experiments have shown that these devices do not work until they are contaminated with tissue debris which ignites, causing the temperature of the tip to rise to as much as 600°C, and cutting is achieved by a purely thermal effect.[11] A similar effect may be achieved by an electrodiathermy needle at a fraction of the cost, as both the laser and the artificial sapphire tips and sculpted quartz fibres are expensive and need to be replaced frequently.

A further refinement was the introduction of the 'fibretom' (Medilas MBB, Munich, Germany). Laser manufacturers have completed the circle by realizing that they have produced a sophisticated 'hot needle' and have introduced an optoelectronic control system to regulate the heating mechanism. A sensor in the laser measures the temperature of the fibre tip during cutting, and the laser power is automatically controlled by a servomechanism to keep the temperature at the tip at an effective safe level below the meltdown threshold.

Potassium titanyl phosphate (KTP) and argon lasers

The potassium titanyl phosphate (KTP) laser (Laserscope, Cwmbran, UK) is probably the most advanced of the visible light lasers, and represents the state of the art in flexible fibre laser technology. The energy is generated from an Nd:YAG laser and the beam is then passed through a crystal of KTP, which results in a halving of the wavelength from 1064 nm to 532 nm, which is in the visible part of the spectrum and produces an emerald green light. This avoids the need for an aiming beam and, although it does require a safety filter to be incorporated into the eyepiece of the endoscope, it nevertheless avoids the need for all operating room personnel to have to wear safety goggles, which is the case with the invisible beam of the Nd:YAG laser.

The KTP laser penetrates soft tissue to a depth between that of the CO_2 and the Nd:YAG lasers, and because lateral scatter occurs to only a small degree it is much safer to use the bare fibre within the abdominal cavity. As there is no need for sapphire tips or sculpted fibres, one can use a single fibre many times, making it a much more economical laser to use.

As with all fibre lasers, the tissue cuts much more effectively when stretched by grasping forceps, and the small 300 μm fibre is the most effective for cutting. This is, however, a thermal effect, and care must be taken with any fibre lasers if used close to the bowel. This laser does cut more effectively than the argon laser, which is a mixture of wavelengths between 488 nm and 515 nm, which produces a blue light and is ideal for coagulation. The KTP laser will photovaporize tissue, if it is held in contact with the tissue, and photocoagulate tissue if it is pulled slightly away from the tissue. Both KTP and argon lasers have the advantage that the wavelength at which they operate is close to the absorption peak for haemosiderin and haemoglobin, and their energies are selectively absorbed by tissue of this colour – which is particularly useful when using the KTP or argon laser for diffuse endometriosis. As it works in the presence of fluid and blood, it is particularly effective in the treatment of ovarian endometriomas and for the drilling of polycystic ovaries without causing troublesome bleeding, although this is achieved much more simply and cheaply using an electrosurgical needle.

Tissue effects of the carbon dioxide laser

Tubal microsurgery and the treatment of endometriosis appeared to be excellent applications for the introduction of the carbon dioxide (CO_2) laser into gynaecology. Initial studies of wound healing on the peritoneal surface of New Zealand white rabbits showed that laser wounds healed more satisfactorily than those inflicted by electrocautery.[12] All tissue debris is evacuated as smoke in the laser plume, so that healing occurs with very little tissue oedema, and therefore less pain, with minimal scarring, wound contracture and anatomical distortion.[13]

The strong absorption of CO_2 laser energy by the water molecule limits the zone of irreversible tissue damage to 70 µm,[14] although there is some cellular damage 200 µm beyond that.[15] Thus, using a CO_2 laser beam with a TEM ∞ mode and a spot size of 200 µm, it is possible, given a rapid speed of beam transit and high power density, for the surgeon to make a 350 µm incision.[16]

The advantage of the ultra-pulse mode is char-free, extremely precise cutting with irreversible adjacent tissue damage of only 50 µm.[17] This is not possible with other techniques currently available. Microelectrocautery will make an incision of less than 1 mm lateral on either side resulting in an incision that is 2–3 mm in width.[16] For these reasons, together with the attraction of a destructive force that utilized a 'no touch' surgical technique, the CO_2 laser appeared to be the ideal physical energy mode available to create precise incisions that would heal easily; nowhere were these properties sought more desperately than in the field of fertility surgery and endometriosis.

The CO_2 laser is the laser of choice for the treatment of peritoneal endometriosis. We use it via a second portal cannula in the right or left iliac fossa to try to get the beam at right angles to the area to be vaporized.

Initial experience with the carbon dioxide laser

We started using the CO_2 laser down the laparoscope in Guildford in October 1982, and this was the first gynaecology centre to use it in the UK. The idea of trying to vaporize the endometriosis implants endoscopically was based on the premise that, since the woman required a laparoscopy to establish the diagnosis, it would be preferable to perform ablative surgery at the same time, rather than put her through the inconvenience and discomfort of a second laparoscopic procedure.

Initially, we used the prototype instrumentation designed by Yoni Tadir in Israel for Sharplan Laser Industries (Tel Aviv, Israel) and used a specially designed operating laparoscope with a sidearm for viewing. This allowed the laser energy to pass from the laser generator down the central channel of the laparoscope (Fig. 7.1). Unfortunately, this meant that most of the diameter of the laparoscope was taken up by the laser channel resulting, in those days, in inferior optics. Also the long focal length meant that it was necessary to continually adjust and

LASER VAPORIZATION AND ELECTROCOAGULATION OF ENDOMETRIOSIS

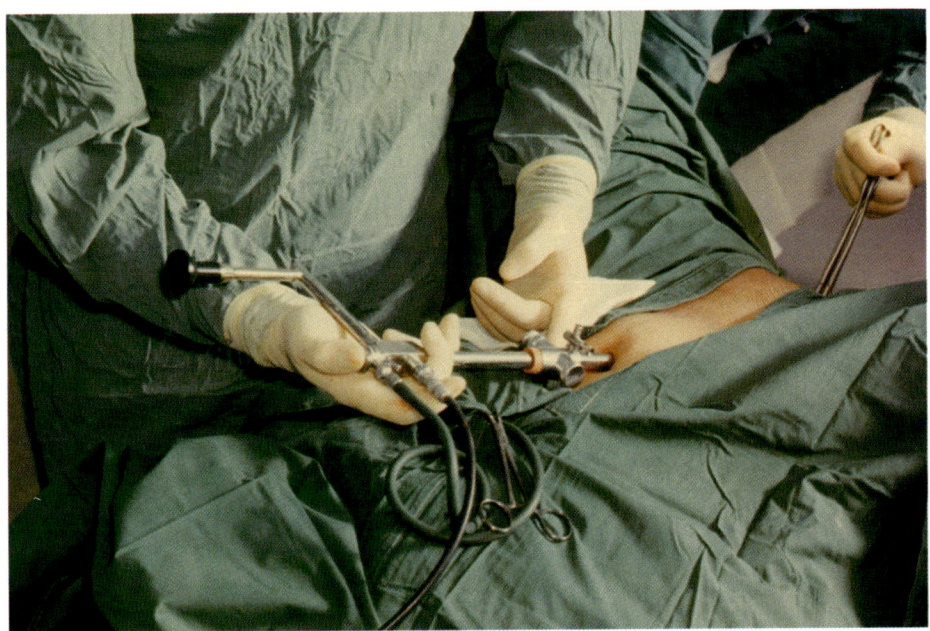

Figure 7.1
Operating laparoscope with sidearm for viewing. The operator's right thumb is over the laser channel to prevent leakage of carbon dioxide prior to attachment of laser mirrors

centralize the aiming beam to stop it reflecting off the sidewalls of the operating channel of the laparoscope. However, an advantage of this single puncture approach was that the camera could be held by the operating surgeon. However, at that time, the original cameras for endoscopic surgery were extremely heavy, making the equipment cumbersome and difficult to use.

We preferred the second puncture cannulae but those that were commercially available were much too long and also had a micromanipulator which had to be constantly adjusted to centralize the aiming beam. We therefore designed our own laser cannulae (Rocket, London, UK). These were much shorter and were attached to a fixed-focus lens, so that the laser beam was sharply focused about 10 mm to 20 mm beyond the end of the probe. The cannulae were short and easy to use and allowed the surgical procedure to be visualized with a standard diagnostic laparoscope with a camera attached to a television monitor. These second puncture cannulae are now available from several laser manufacturers and, in practice, any laser that was originally purchased for colposcopy but has been replaced by simpler and cheaper electrosurgical devices, can be easily modified for laparoscopic use. The cannulae come in three designs: (1) open-ended for vaporization of peritoneal endometriosis; (2) constructed with a back-stop for safe division of adhesions; and (3) has a 45 degree mirror to direct the beam at a right-angle for deposits in difficult to reach areas.

Our major concern when we began this procedure was the possible adverse effects of accidentally perforating the large bowel. We conducted a series of experiments using freshly obtained colonic specimens provided by general surgeons and bathed them in an atmosphere of carbon dioxide. We were relieved to find that deliberate puncture with the laser beam did not result in an explosion caused by the ignition of methane. It soon became apparent that, provided that one adhered to rigid safety rules, laser energy was not dangerous and the simpler optical physics avoided the hazards of 'stray energy', always inherent in the early devices used in electrosurgery. We ensure that the laser is never activated unless the aiming beam is clearly seen and targeted on a safe area in the pelvis. When it is not being used, the laser technician always ensures that it is placed on 'standby' to avoid an accident occurring if the surgeon inadvertently depressed the laser pedal when he was intending to use electrosurgery to achieve haemostasis.

It later became apparent that the CO_2 laser, which is strongly absorbed by the water molecule limiting the zone of irreversible tissue damage to about 50 μm, is an extremely safe surgical tool. During the past 20 years we have used it on well over 12 000 patients without a single adverse event attributable to the use of the CO_2 laser during laparoscopy. Clearly, with this number of patients we have had the occasional accident during the introduction of trocars.

Early clinical results of the carbon dioxide laser

By the summer of 1984 we had accumulated sufficient cases to publish our initial results and we were certain that Guildford was the only centre using laparoscopic laser surgery on a routine basis. We were therefore disappointed to discover a publication from James Daniell of Tennessee,[18] which indicated that he had used this procedure slightly earlier. In addition, it was also clear from one of his references that the French team from Clermont-Ferrand, under the leadership of Professor Maurice Bruhat had already been performing this procedure on women as long ago as 1978.[6] However, our initial results were published in *Lasers in Medical Science* in 1986.[19] (Our paper had been rejected by the Editor of the *British Journal of Obstetrics and Gynaecology* who, not unreasonably, said that he would not consider publication of a new technique unless it had at least five years follow-up.) We therefore conducted a longitudinal follow-up of the first 228 patients over five years.[20] Relatively few of the patients were lost to follow-up, since at that time most of them came from our local Health District in South West Surrey. Only 12 were lost to follow-up, 6 from the pain group and 6 from the infertility group. Although the results reflected the success of the procedure, it clearly did not work in all cases, since 38 out of the 187 complaining of pelvic pain were no better and also during that five year period, 17 patients relapsed due to recurrent endometriosis. The vast majority of patients in these two latter groups, who had second look laparoscopy, were found either to have no endometriosis at all, or it was found in different places. The original site of the laser surgery could be identified by some carbon granules beneath the surface, but usually there was no recurrent disease in these sites, except in three patients, where clearly we had not vaporized deeply enough. In these two groups it was clear that there were two obvious problems: first, endometriosis was not necessarily the correct diagnosis for pelvic pain; second, it was evident that we were dealing with a recurrent disease and although we could remove all the deposits of endometriosis seen at the time of initial ablative surgery, there was no guarantee that implants would not reappear in the future. Nevertheless, we were encouraged by the fact that 70% of the patients were pain-free. Also, if there were no other infertility factors, 80% of the patients who were infertile became pregnant.

Early retrospective results of laser laparoscopic surgery

During the 1980s there were many published studies on the use of laser laparoscopy for the treatment of endometriosis, which claimed a success rate in relieving pain in 60–70% of patients with a pregnancy rate of 55–80%.[18,20–25]

Although these studies demonstrated very low morbidity, they were either retrospective or not controlled and were therefore of no true scientific value, in particular, because the alleviation of pain in endometriosis is highly subjective and symptoms are difficult to evaluate. In such a retrospective study, it is all too easy for the surgeon to influence the patient to provide an answer that she has benefited from his surgery. Such a doctor–patient dialogue could severely alter the interpretation of the results.

We therefore realized that it was necessary to prove that laparoscopic laser surgery was effective. This can be done in much the same way as medical treatments are evaluated, and that is, by a prospective, randomized, double-blind controlled trial (RCT). This would compare laser laparoscopy with diagnostic laparoscopy alone, to see whether removal of these implants did, in fact, result in statistically significant improvements or resolution of pain and also determine whether there was an increased pregnancy rate.

The allure to patients of a high-tech treatment such as laser made it difficult to recruit subjects for this study, since patients believed that laser surgery would help them. We had to explain that we did not know ourselves what contribution the vaporization of endometriosis played in the alleviation of pelvic pain and infertility. However, the study was approved by the Hospital Ethics Committee, but it was felt that it was unethical to withhold treatment from patients with Stage IV disease, particularly since our previous experience had shown 80% pain relief in this group and a 57% pregnancy rate, most of whom had failed to respond to medical therapy.[26]

The Guildford double-blind, prospective, RCT of laser laparoscopy[27]

The study population was recruited from women seen in the gynaecological outpatient clinic with pain suggestive of endometriosis, who had been advised to undergo a diagnostic laparoscopy. To be included in the study, the women were required to be neither pregnant nor lactating, between 18 and 45 years of age, and had not received any medical or surgical treatment for endometriosis in the previous 6 months. Patients were asked to record the intensity of their pain on a linear analogue scale and also to give a subjective score to their pain symptoms. Although 74 women entered the study, only 63 completed the trial to the 6 month follow-up visit, since two became pregnant, five, against our advice, began hormonal contraception, and three were lost to follow-up. At the time of laparoscopic confirmation of endometriosis, a sealed envelope was opened and treatment was allocated randomly by a computer-generated randomization sequence to either laser treatment or expectant management. The patients who had laser treatment had vaporization of all visible endometriotic implants, adhesiolysis and uterine nerve transection with the CO_2 laser or the potassium titanyl phosphate (KTP/532) laser.

The patients in the 'no treatment' arm had only a diagnostic laparoscopy, although it was necessary to remove the serosanguinous fluid from the pouch of Douglas in order to perform a thorough inspection of the pelvic peritoneum. The patients were not informed whether they had laser treatment or no treatment (expectant management), and all patients had the same three portal incisions. Patients were followed up at 3 and 6 months after surgery by an independent observer – a research nurse, who was also unaware as to which treatment had been allocated. At 6 months follow-up the randomization code was broken and if the patient had received expectant management and had no treatment and was still in pain, then laser laparoscopy was offered to them almost immediately.

Results

The results were interesting because at three months after surgery, 18 out of 32 (56%) in the laser-treated group reported that their pain was better or improved compared with 15 of 34 (48%) in the expectant group. This difference was not statistically significant and the results of laser surgery were much lower than in our previous retrospective study.[20] Equally, we were very surprised to find that almost 50% of patients who had had a diagnostic laparoscopy alone appeared to be better or improved.

To our intense relief, at the six month follow-up, 20 of 32 (62.5%) in the laser group were better and the number in the control group had dropped to 7 of 31 (22.6%), which was a statistically significant difference. At three months, the median decrease in pain score was 2.6 for the laser group and 1.2 for the expectant group; this was not significant ($P = 0.9$, Mann-Whitney U-test). When the decrease in pain score from baseline to 6 months is analysed, the median decrease was 2.85 for the laser group and 0.05 for the expectant group. This difference was significant ($P = 0.01$, Mann-Whitney U-test). One of the problems of this study was that some of the very minimal changes in the peritoneum were interpreted as endometriosis merely by visual inspection with the laparoscope and no biopsy was permitted because that would, in itself, have acted as a cytoreduction of the implants. It is quite possible that some of these very subtle changes are not endometriosis at all, but merely represent post-inflammatory changes or even Walthard rests. If Stage I patients were excluded from the evaluation, then 73.7% of patients achieved pain relief which was similar to the number that reported pain relief in our retrospective study.[20]

Discussion

There are several interesting features in this study, which is the first one in the world to have been conducted in endoscopic laser surgery (although such randomized, prospective, double-blind studies are mandatory for the development of any new drug before it receives the approval of the statutory regulatory agencies). First, we were not entirely sure why the placebo response was so high at three months and yet dropped at six months. Indeed, when patients who claimed they were better at six months and then realized they had not had laser treatment often requested this treatment. This placebo response has also been reported by other investigators, notably Fedele et al.[28] We are not entirely sure whether the removal of peritoneal fluid in the pelvis, which contains high concentrations of pain-mediating substances, particularly prostaglandin F (PGF), is responsible for this alleviation of pain and that it may take 3 months of retrograde menstruation before new implants secrete sufficient amounts of PGF to create the same degree of pain.

Another possible explanation is a phenomenon well known among psychologists called 'pain memory', where the body anticipates pain and the mere reassurance of a laparoscopy and the expectation that one has had treatment for the disease gives relief of symptoms. Certainly, such relief is relatively short-lived and after six months the symptoms had not been relieved in the majority of patients who had not received laser treatment and yet even then, one fifth (22.6%) still maintained that pain was much less than before.

Advantages and disadvantages of the carbon dioxide laser

The carbon dioxide (CO_2) laser provides very precise vaporization of tissue layer by layer so that the surgeon can see when normal tissue is reached and all the abnormal tissue vaporized. Power output can be varied from 4 W to 100 W. Spot sizes can be selected from 2 mm to 10 mm. Average power densities can therefore be varied from 10 W/cm^2 to 1 500 000 W/cm^2. In practice, we usually use 10 W with a spot size of 0.45–0.50 nm in TEM ∞ mode. Greater average power densities improve surgical precision and speed but at the expense of reduced haemostasis.

The CO_2 laser has been used for endoscopic work for a number of years, and as a result maintenance services by a number of companies have now become well established. However, in the endoscopic field there has been a significant trend away from the CO_2 laser towards flexible fibre systems for a number of reasons:

1. Because of its long wavelength, the CO_2 laser beam cannot be passed down a standard flexible fibre. As a result, an articulated arm must be used which tends to be cumbersome and the accurate alignment of the mirrors requires constant maintenance to ensure effective transmission of the beam. For this reason, the laser generator cannot be easily moved to different locations in the hospital although, to some extent, sealed tube systems and carbon fibre arms are more robust.
2. Although some degree of haemostasis of smaller blood vessels may be achieved by defocusing the beam, it is difficult to stop haemorrhage from larger vessels. Therefore, the operator must have instant access to haemostatic clips, sutures or bipolar diathermy to stem the blood flow if anything larger than a capillary vessel is accidentally severed. This, combined with greater charring and smoke generation necessitating pressurized irrigation systems and smoke evacuation equipment, makes it a difficult laser to use and requires a large amount of teamwork from the operating theatre personnel.
3. The long focal length means that the beam retains effective power and can easily damage distal tissue after severing an adhesion. This is not a great problem if the beam hits a safe area of the pelvic sidewall or the adhesion can be pulled over the fluid-filled cul de sac as the laser energy will be absorbed. When performing a complicated enterolysis procedure this is not always possible and it is necessary to employ a backstop on the end of the probe or to use another non-reflective instrument.

Ovarian endometriomas (chocolate cysts) and treatment

There is considerable controversy over the pathogenesis of ovarian endometriomas and some authorities consider that there are three distinct forms of endometriosis: (1) peritoneal; (2) deep infiltrating disease; and (3) ovarian endometriomas.[29] As long ago as 1957, Hughesdon, a gynaecological pathologist at University College Hospital in London, suggested that bleeding from endometriotic implants on the posterior surface of the ovary caused the ovary to adhere to the peritoneum of the ovarian fossa. Therefore, because subsequent bleeding into the space enclosed by the adhesions prevents the escape of blood this results in invagination of the ovarian cortex as the endometrioma enlarges.[30] The majority of ovarian endometriomas would appear to fit into this category, since they are densely adhered to the peritoneum of the broad ligament close to the ureter and have to be freed by laparoscopic blunt dissection with a strong stainless steel probe and sometimes laparoscopic scissors. The ovary is gradually levered upwards away from the ovarian fossa taking care not to injure the ureter and during this process the endometrioma invariably ruptures. The haemosiderin-laden fluid is then aspirated and irrigated until the effluent runs clear and the whole of the inside of the endometrioma is photocoagulated with the emerald green KTP/532 laser which penetrates only a few millimetres and thus causes minimal damage to developing follicles under the surface (Fig. 7.2). If a KTP/532 laser is not available then superficial coagulation can be achieved by using a 'Bicap' bipolar endocoagulator (Cory Brothers, Horsham, UK) which attaches to the suction and irrigation equipment and is relatively simple and safe to use. The bipolar effect is achieved by the current passing between the peaks of adjacent ridges. The device is reusable but needs to be replaced after 8–10 applications.

An alternative technique is to initially aspirate the endometrioma at the first diagnostic laparoscopy procedure or under ultrasound control and then give the patient gonadatrophin-releasing hormone (GnRH) analogues for 3 months, after which time the shrunken endometrioma will have a relatively avascular capsule that can be vaporized effectively with the CO_2 laser. This particular laser will cause little damage to the developing follicles under the fibrous surface of the capsule, but would not work in the presence of the haemosiderin-laden fluid of the chocolate cyst.[11]

Some laparoscopic surgeons advocate stripping out the ovarian cyst capsule by traction and countertraction. In the case of a true endometrioma this merely results in stripping out the ovarian cortex and results in profuse bleeding. This requires bipolar coagulation to

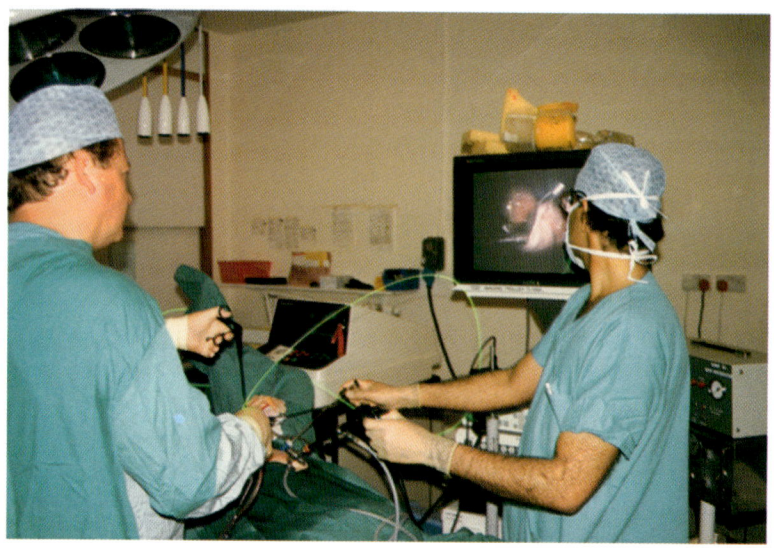

Figure 7.2
The KTP/532 laser being used to photocoagulate the interior of an ovarian endometrioma

control and the inevitable build up of heat results in damage to the developing oocytes beneath the surface. It is important to realize that not all 'chocolate cysts' are endometriomas and the chocolate-coloured material merely represents haemosiderin and is a reflection of internal bleeding into the cyst. In most of these situations the ovary is not adherent to the posterior leaf of the broad ligament. It is suspended free from the mesovarium and often represents a benign cyst-adenoma with internal haemorrhage or a haemorrhagic corpus luteum cyst, or occasionally an endometrioma that has arisen from coelomic metaplasia of invaginated epithelial inclusions.[29]

In whatever way the endometrioma is dealt with by laparoscopic surgery, it is important to be certain at the end of the procedure that there is reasonable haemostasis. If this is not possible, the ovary can be packed with Surgicel gauze (Ethicon Endosurgery, Edinburgh, UK), but on no account should there be any arterial bleeding at the end of the procedure. Sometimes, it is tempting to try and restore ovarian anatomy with laparoscopic sutures, but this should be resisted because sutures often result in tissue ischaemia, which is the main initiating factor in adhesion formation.[31]

Results

Photocoagulation of the endometrioma capsule with the KTP/532 laser is associated with a low recurrence rate.[32] Daniell and colleagues from Nashville have reported significant relief of pain and a pregnancy rate of 37.5% in 32 patients trying for conception.[33]

At the 1992 International Society for Gynaecological Endoscopy meeting in Washington, we reported our results on our first 102 patients with large endometriomas (between 3 cm–18 cm). We had been surprised to find that 80% of the patients had significant subjective improvement in pain and 57% of those trying to conceive became pregnant.[26] Most of the pregnancies occurred within the first few cycles and if they were to achieve a pregnancy it was most likely within the first 9 months. More recently, we reported a further 165 women who presented with large endometriomas exceeding 3 cm in diameter.[34] In this study, we used either the CO_2 or the KTP laser and found pain resolution in 74% of the women and a pregnancy rate of 45%. We noted that there was a higher recurrence rate (30%) in those treated with the CO_2 laser compared with only 12.5% in those who had been treated with the KTP laser. The slightly lower pregnancy rate than in the first series probably reflects the fact that this latter group included many patients referred from other centres who had already had previous laparotomies.

As Guildford hospital is a tertiary referral centre for women with severe endometriosis we see a large number of patients who have endometriotic cysts. Many of these patients have been operated on by gynaecological surgeons elsewhere in the UK, or from other parts of the world. We have been surprised by the variety of approaches to the management of endometriotic cysts, and in order to establish current clinical practice amongst gynaecological surgeons in the UK we carried out an anonymous postal survey in 2002.[35]

The participants were specialist gynaecologists (eligible to hold a certificate of completion of specialist training) who were Members or Fellows of the Royal College of Obstetricians and Gynaecologists of the United Kingdom during September 2000. An anonymous, self-administered, structured questionnaire was posted to 1240 gynaecologists. The postal questionnaire was returned by 651 consultants (52.5% response rate). This response rate is similar to a survey carried out by members of the British Society for Gynaecological Endoscopy on the prevalence of laparoscopic uterine nerve ablation in gynaecological practice.[36] It must be remembered that a significant proportion of obstetricians and gynaecologists in the UK pursue additional specialties, so it would appear that the majority of those concerned with gynaecological surgery did respond to the questionnaire. The survey indicated that 487 (74.8%) managed patients surgically and 179 (36.8%) treated them with a preoperative GnRH analogue. We were interested to find that even in the year 2000, a laparotomy was performed by 206 (42.3%) and the remaining 239 (49.1%) performed a laparoscopy in order to treat endometrioma.

We were disappointed by the very high percentage of surgeons who were still performing laparotomy. At our centre, we have not had to revert to a laparotomy in the past 16 years. We are convinced that ovarian endometriomas and severe endometriosis of the rectovaginal septum are easier to deal with at laparoscopy, once the surgeon has acquired the necessary skills and experience. Even when microsurgical techniques have been used at laparotomy, we see far more adhesion formation than patients who have been treated previously by laparoscopic surgery. The results of this survey showed that there is currently an equal preference for open versus endoscopic surgery. However, we feel very strongly that laparotomy should no longer be the surgical technique of first choice and if surgeons are unable to perform laparoscopic surgery they should refer patients to tertiary referral centres that have the necessary skills and equipment.

In our survey,[35] gynaecologists who performed a laparotomy usually performed an ovarian cystectomy (195; 94.7%), whereas those who performed a laparoscopy were equally divided between fenestration and ablation of the capsule (146; 61.1%) and stripping or excision of the cyst lining (127; 53.1%). The optimal technique for dealing with the endometrioma, once access has been gained, remains controversial. Our initial results with fenestration and ablation using the KTP laser showing an 80% subjective improvement in pain and 57% pregnancy rate were impressive.[26] However, this study was retrospective and attracts all the criticisms of such studies, except that it is very difficult to argue with the pregnancy rate because as Beretta et al[37] point out, a clinically confirmed pregnancy is an objective outcome. The numbers in each group were relatively small (32) and the time to pain recurrence in the cystectomy group was 19 months compared with 9.5 months in those having drainage and coagulation. Marginally better results were also seen in the pregnancy rate of 66.7% in the cystectomy group and 23.5% in those treated by drainage and coagulation. Unfortunately, this poor pregnancy rate compared to other studies using the KTP laser[26,32–34] (pregnancy rates of 45–57%) suggests that although this group was skilled at laparoscopic ovarian cystectomy, they were using a poor technique for drainage and coagulation in order to arrive at such a low pregnancy rate as 23.5%. A similar criticism can be applied to a retrospective study by Saleh and Tulandi.[38] In this study they showed that reoperation rates were much higher at 42 months in the fenestration and ablation group (57.8%) compared with the excision group (23.6%). Also, they showed that the reoperation rate with fenestration and ablation was independent of cyst size, but reoperation was much more likely after excision of larger cysts.

In our survey,[35] both the open (125; 60.7%) and the endoscopic surgeons (155; 64.9%) reported that they treated coexisting rectovaginal disease. This is important because ovarian endometriosis is a marker for more extensive pelvic and intestinal disease, which should be treated at the same time if the patient is to benefit from the operation.[39]

Deeply infiltrating endometriosis

Deep endometriosis is almost invariably located in the fibromuscular tissue of the pelvic sidewall, the rectovaginal septum, the uterosacral ligaments or sometimes in the uterovesical fold. When these lesions are excised or vaporized with the CO_2 laser, they are usually found to infiltrate over 5 mm in depth and this usually correlates with the severity of pain.[40]

In some women, however, no endometriosis can be seen laparoscopically but the induration can be clearly felt by a combination of rectal and vaginal examination. These lesions are spherical endometriotic nodules in the rectovaginal septum and can be clearly felt as painful nodules at that site and colposcopic examination of the vagina sometimes reveals dark-blue domed cysts, about 3–4 mm in diameter in the posterior vaginal fornix. These are the most severe lesions and have a tendency to spread laterally up and around the uterine artery and sometimes cause sclerosis around the ureter although, interestingly, never appear to invade the layers of the ureteric wall. The behaviour of this type of deep infiltrating disease, which is virtually unresponsive to drug therapy, is such that it can be considered an indirect argument for the hypothesis that deep endometriosis has escaped from the inhibitory influence of peritoneal fluid and is mainly under the control of the peripheral circulation.[40]

Possible environmental aetiological factors

Koninckx et al have suggested that dioxin and polychlorinated biphenyl pollution is a possible co-factor in the cause and development of deep infiltrating endometriosis.[41] This is resulting in a steadily increasing proportion of hysterectomies performed for this disease from 10% in 1965 to over 18% in 1984.[42] Using epidemiological data reported by the World Health Organization, Koninckx et al. link the highest concentrations of dioxin in breast milk in Belgium,[43] which appears to have the highest incidence of endometriosis in the world and much of this is of the deeply infiltrating type.[44] The highest concentration of cases is in the industrial corridor running along the south of the country (J Donnez, Personal communication).[45]

Dioxin has immunosuppressive activities and is a potent inhibitor of T lymphocyte function.[46–48] A group of rhesus monkeys which were chronically exposed to dioxin for a period of 4 years and followed by serial laparoscopies were found to develop endometriosis 7 years after the termination of dioxin exposure and in the majority of these cases it was of the deeply infiltrating variety.[49]

Dioxin is a potentially harmful by-product of the chlorine-bleaching process used in the wood pulp industry, which includes the manufacture of feminine hygiene products, such as tampons. It is of some concern that young girls are increasingly being encouraged to use tampons and therefore may be exposing the tissues of the rectovaginal septum and posterior fornix to chronic exposure with a known immunosuppressant. It has been suggested that a woman may use as many as 11 000 tampons in her lifetime and this represents a worrying level of dioxin exposure, which could result in deeply infiltrating endometriosis and it could explain the increasing incidence of this condition in young women.

Surgical treatment

Laparoscopic inspection, ultrasonography or magnetic resonance imaging (MRI) are not sufficiently adequate to delineate deep endometriotic lesions. This can only be done satisfactorily during surgical excision with electrosurgery, an ultrasonic scalpel or vaporization with a CO_2 laser until normal tissue is seen and palpated. Before performing any operative laparoscopy any patient complaining of dyschezia and perimenstrual rectal bleeding should have a proctoscopy and sigmoidoscopy, preferably during menstruation and appropriate radiological investigations. If the lesion extends laterally an intravenous urogram is required, but if it is confined to the rectovaginal septum it is our practice to perform an air contrast barium enema, sometimes combined with a vaginogram which should be carefully examined in the lateral views by a radiologist experienced with the evaluation of this disease.

A thorough bowel preparation is mandatory in all women suspected of having deep endometriosis and patients should be warned that there is a real risk of perforating the bowel. If this does happen, a colorectal surgeon should be available to repair such a defect. However, if bowel prep has been satisfactory it should not be necessary to require a colostomy. Indeed, some of the perforations can be adequately repaired transanally, or even laparoscopically.[50,53]

In the past, it has been necessary to resort to laparotomy for these patients but with increased experience in laparoscopic surgery, many of them can be treated by laparoscopy using CO_2 laser or electrosurgical excision or sharp dissection with scissors. In addition, it is sometimes necessary to perform vaginal excision either from below or by laparoscopy once the plane of cleavage has been developed between the rectum and the vagina.[49–52] Inevitably with this kind of surgery, which is probably the most difficult type of laparoscopy and requires considerable skill and experience, each surgeon will use the method that is best in his hands. We use a high power super-pulse CO_2 laser to develop the plane of cleavage between the rectum and the vagina, with special instrumentation to separate these two structures from below and careful palpation in order to avoid damaging the rectum. Even in highly skilled hands some bowel damage is sometimes inevitable. Nezhat and colleagues reported a series of 174 women where there were nine bowel perforations and a further two patients required ureteric stents.[52] Nevertheless, moderate to complete pain relief was achieved in 162 of the women. If dissection has to be very close to the rectum it is a wise precaution to fill the pelvis with warm Ringer's lactate solution and insufflate the rectum with air or methylene blue to look for any unrecognized rectal lacerations or perforations.[49] A vaginal incision is often, but not routinely, required and when the vagina is opened, the procedure may be completed vaginally or laparoscopically. In addition, it is sometimes possible to vaporize the vaginal dark-blue domed cysts via a colposcope with a finger inserted in the rectum to ensure that vaporization does not damage the rectum.

To excise uterosacral nodules, the peritoneum is incised lateral to the uterosacral ligament. It is necessary to first identify the ureter and occasionally to dissect it out along its course. Once it is displaced laterally the uterosacral ligament is resected beginning posteriorly and working towards the uterus. Once the nodule has been freed from the underlying tissue the anterior part of the ligament is cut and most of these deep uterosacral implants can be treated without any need for a vaginal incision. Patients with full-thickness bowel or bladder lesions require more extensive surgery, which is probably better dealt with by laparotomy, although some surgeons using advanced laparoscopy have reported successful results employing transanal circular stapling devices,[49] and laparoscopic and transanal or transvaginal repair with or without the help of colorectal surgeons.[53,54]

Although this type of surgery is very difficult and time consuming the results justify the effort, particularly since many of these patients do not respond to medical therapy. Koninckx and Martin analysed their results in 250 women in whom deep endometriosis had been excised with the CO_2 laser and showed a cure rate of pelvic pain in 70% with a recurrence rate of less than 5% with a follow-up period up to 5 years.[40] These results should be interpreted with some degree of caution because inevitably there is a learning curve in this type of surgery. Inspection of the data revealed that the completeness of excision has steadily increased with experience and the results of recent years strongly suggest an almost total cure rate with a very low recurrence rate.

Donnez and Nisolle reported a consecutive series of 500 cases with rectovaginal septum adenomyotic nodules treated by excision with the CO_2 laser.[55] They followed 242 of these patients for more than two years and only 3.7% had recurrent dysmenorrhoea and only 1.2% had dyspareunia. In this series there were only four rectal perforations, two of which were repaired by colpotomy and two others required a laparotomy. Donnez believes that the rectovaginal nodule is histologically similar to an adenomyoma – he describes this as a circumscribed nodular aggregate of smooth muscle, endometrial glands and endometrial stroma. As in the 'adenomyoma' secretory changes are frequently absent in these rectovaginal nodules. Occasionally, the invasion of the muscle by very active glandular epithelium without any stroma, proves that the stroma is not mandatory for invasion with this particular type of pathology which is more akin to adenomyosis found in the myometrium. He has suggested that because ciliated cells are present, which co-express both vimentin and cytokeratin, these nodules arise from Müllerian tissue and the histological characteristics are completely different from those observed in peritoneal lesions.[57,58] We have been using a similar technique at our centre, which involves opening up the rectovaginal septum with the CO_2 laser and vaporizing the visually abnormal tissue until normal soft fatty tissue is reached. If there is a marked vaginal component, then the dark-blue domed cysts are vaporized with the CO_2 laser directed via a colposcope with a finger in the rectum to prevent perforation of the rectum (Fig. 7.3). If the preoperative investigations, particularly the air contrast barium enema viewed laterally, suggest that the endometriosis penetrates through all layers of the bowel wall, they are treated by anterior

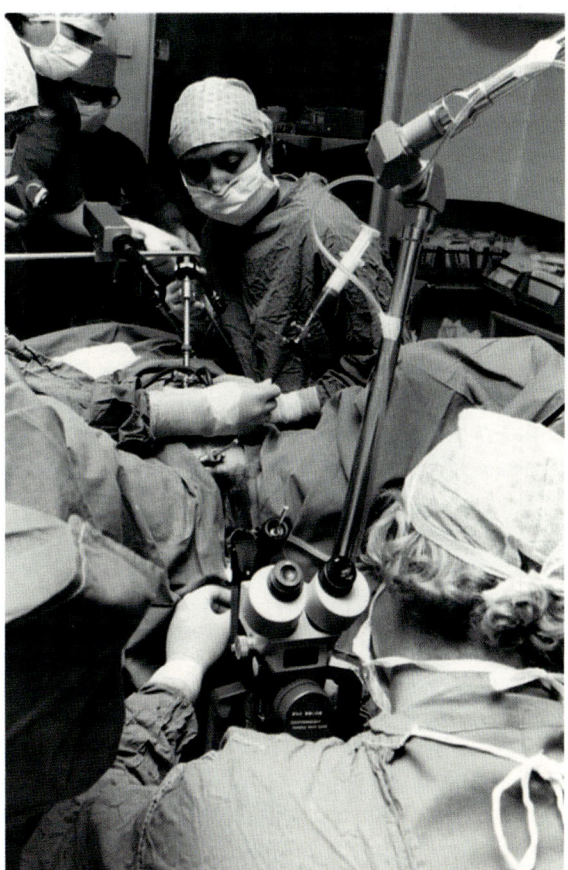

Figure 7.3

Vaporization of vaginal endometriosis (adenomysis) with the carbon dioxide (CO_2) laser via the colposcope after initial vaporization of deposits in the rectovaginal septum by CO_2 laser laparoscopic surgery

resection by a colorectal surgeon, although it is wise for the gynaecologist to be present in order to ensure as complete removal of deep infiltrating endometriosis as possible.

Since many of our patients referred for treatment of this condition come from all regions of the UK and many from overseas, it is very difficult to perform an adequate follow-up, and postal questionnaires are often unreliable. We therefore reviewed a cohort of consecutive patients with deep infiltrating endometriosis of the rectovaginal septum treated over a three month period (September to November 1999). There were 17 patients with a mean age of 34 (20–51 years): 10 had complained of rectal bleeding and had a barium enema and vaginogram and one was found to have a full-thickness lesion and was therefore treated by anterior resection; 12 patients (71%) had an arcus taurinus procedure that involves a radical excision of the uterosacral ligaments with vaporization of all abnormal tissue in the rectovaginal septum;[59,60] 3 patients had radical excision or vaporization of the uterosacral ligaments alone, which was performed with the CO_2 laser; and a further 3 patients had laser laparoscopy to the rectovaginal septum alone.

The procedure we employ is more rapid than other excisional techniques and the length of surgery was 32–80 minutes (mean 48 min). Severe dysmenorrhoea was present in 14 (82%), deep dyspareunia in 15 (88%), rectal pain (dyschezia) was present in 11 (64%) and rectal bleeding in 3 (18%). All patients were eventually contacted and satisfactory pain relief was reported in 92%. None of the patients in this small cohort have returned for repeat surgery and there were no complications from the laparoscopic surgery.

With the increasing numbers of referred patients with deep infiltrating endometriosis and the relatively few centres that are able to tackle this type of disease, we feel that CO_2 laser excision or vaporization is a relatively rapid procedure, allowing two or three cases to be performed on a morning operating list. We feel that the removal of as much abnormal tissue, with endometrial glands and stroma or fibromuscular hyperplasia, that can safely be achieved leads to excellent results allowing for satisfactory pain relief and the possibility of pregnancy. Although we appreciate that some laparoscopic surgeons have the necessary skill to perform reparative bowel surgery, we prefer to avoid bowel perforation if possible. In those few patients that have full-thickness lesions we feel that their treatment is the province of the colorectal surgeon.

We realize that a vaporization technique relies on the visual inspection and palpation of normal-looking tissue and does not rely on a histological report showing complete removal of the disease tissue. Nevertheless, although this approach is mandatory for cancer surgery, the two largest series looking at the correlation between symptoms and positive histology in this mysterious condition only found this to occur in about 50% of cases.[61,62]

Electrocoagulation of endometriosis

Electrocoagulation of endometriosis can only be used for superficial peritoneal disease and can be an alternative to the potassium titanyl phosphate (KTP) laser for coagulation of the capsule of an ovarian endometrioma. Bipolar electrosurgery, although excellent for achieving haemostasis in laparoscopic surgery, suffers from the basic physical problem in that it is difficult to assess the depth of penetration of the beam and there is always a risk that deeper deposits of endometriosis will remain untreated. Other electrosurgical coagulators, such as the argon beam coagulator, the helica thermocoagulator or the cold plasma coagulator, will only treat superficial peritoneal deposits and are not suitable and, indeed, are not designed for the treatment of deep infiltrating endometriosis.

Bipolar electrosurgery

In the bipolar system, the current from the electrosurgical generator flows through the active electrode, which is one of the blades of the forceps, through the intervening tissue to the other blade which acts as the inactive electrode, and thence back to the electrosurgical unit. This is an inherently safe system, because only the tissue grasped between the blades of the forceps is coagulated and ultimately desiccated, and no ground plate is required. The effect is therefore focused and although damage to adjacent tissue is minimized, it must be understood that there is a considerable build-up of heat in adjacent tissue.[63] Phipps devised a graph showing the extent of irreversible tissue damage that can occur to tissue, plotted against the distance from the bipolar forceps.[63] This is particularly important when using bipolar current to desiccate uterine arteries during laparoscopic hysterectomy and also deposits of endometriosis that are in close proximity to the ureter. The coagulated white area lateral to the forceps will be irreversibly damaged and it is important to realize that irreversible damage can occur at a temperature as low as 60°C.

Argon beam coagulator

Because of the way it has been advertised showing a bright blue light coming from the end of the generator and impinging on tissue some distance away, many people think the argon beam coagulator (ABC) is a laser. In fact, it is merely a way of delivering monopolar current via an electron channel, consisting of a flow of argon gas, which has the effect of blowing off the blood, char and debris from the target zone, thus allowing the unipolar current to directly impinge on a bleeding vessel. It is an excellent haemostatic energy source and is useful during vascular procedures, such as a myomectomy and a presacral neurectomy.[64] Surgeons also find it particularly useful for highly vascular procedures, such as partial hepatectomies.

The ABC produces less smoke than other similar energy sources, but it is vital to have an adequate suction system to siphon off the gas as there have been reports of deaths from argon gas embolism, both in animal studies,[65] and also in humans.[66] Death is due to a combination of high intraperitoneal pressures and open blood vessels. It can be avoided by using a high flow automatic insufflator that shuts off when the intraperitoneal pressure is greater than 20 mmHg, and just before firing the ABC a suction irrigation probe is placed close to the point of impact to aspirate the argon gas. This eliminates the accumulation of argon gas within the peritoneum and helps reduce the intraperitoneal pressure.

Although electrosurgical energy is invisible, when the electrons flow through the argon gas channel, there is an arcing effect that is visible and is similar to the glow seen with neon lights. This allows the surgeon to see the actual diameter of the beam when firing it laparoscopically and because there is a reduction in smoke with coagulation compared with electrosurgery and various lasers it allows excellent visibility of the tissue effects. The tip of the probe should be allowed to touch the planned impact site and then is backed away to a distance of 2–3 mm. After initial suction aspiration of the gas in the vicinity the device is then activated and the distance from the tip of the probe to the tissue is adjusted depending on the visible tissue effect. The 4 L/min plume of argon gas begins to flow just before the needle electrode is energized. This allows any excessive blood or irrigation fluids to be blown away from the impact site, thus allowing rapid haemostasis by direct coagulation of the exposed vessel. Since the spot size is 3 mm, fine cutting is difficult with the ABC, but it does allow superficial coagulation of endometriotic implants. However, it is not suitable for excisional techniques aimed to remove deep infiltrating endometriosis. Because of its excellent haemostatic properties, the ABC is an excellent device for presacral neurectomy, but care must be taken because accidents have been reported due to the electron channel of gas being deflected off the shiny surface of the peritoneum and causing serious injury to the pelvic sidewall vessels.

Helica thermal coagulator

The helica thermal coagulator (Helica Instruments, Broxburn, Lothian, UK) produces a similar effect to the argon beam coagulator but employs helium gas. When the foot switch is operated, a coronal-type flame issues from the end of the nozzle and has a high electron temperature but low molecular temperature, typically about 20°C, until the flame is brought close to the tissue surface where it is capacitively coupled or directly earthed. The coronal-type flame then changes to an arc discharge flame which has a higher molecular temperature, typically in the order of 800°C. The flame takes place in an atmosphere provided by the flowing helium gas which, being inert, minimizes oxidation of the tissue. The helica thermal coagulator is a power-controlled device and the voltage is reduced along the length of the flame, so only low electrical power is passed to the tissue. The power delivered to the surface can be controlled to within a few watts. The depth of penetration is easily controlled by the power setting and the distance of the probe from the tissue. The device is extremely versatile and easy to use and appears to be very safe, and is particularly effective for peritoneal surface endometriotic implants because it can cauterize soft tissue to a depth of one cell, allowing the diseased tissue to be removed layer by layer as with the CO_2 laser at rapid fluence. As with the argon beam coagulator, this device is only suitable for superficial peritoneal endometriosis because of its very limited depth of penetration, but is no use at all for dealing with deep infiltrating disease. It has the advantage that it is cheaper than a laser, but such considerations do not really apply considering its limited usefulness and surgeons should equip themselves with an energy source that can be used to deal with any type of endometriosis they find at the time of laparoscopic surgery.

Cold-plasma coagulator

The latest type of coagulator is the cold-plasma coagulator (CPC) (Soring, Quick Born, Germany) which has an even more superficial penetration than the argon beam coagulator or the helica thermal coagulator. It has an advantage in that it does not require an earthed plate and would appear to be extremely safe, although we await the results of clinical trials, which at the moment are being conducted in Russia.

Conclusion

There is really little to choose, in terms of clinical outcome, between the various surgical power sources. Operative laparoscopy is safe and effective, whether using sharp scissor dissection, the ultrasonic scalpel, electrosurgery or laser energy, provided that the surgeon is familiar with the physics of the modality used, and is also aware of complications that can occur with misuse, and takes every possible step to avoid them. The newer surgical modalities, such as the helica thermal coagulator, and the cold-plasma coagulator, require further evaluation and comparison with more established power sources, preferably in double-blind, prospective clinical trials. Currently, electrosurgery is by far the most popular and cheapest power source in endoscopic surgery. However, only the laser has been subjected to prospective, randomized clinical studies that have also been double-blind.

In the final analysis, the surgeon's own skill and experience, together with his or her preference of the technique employed, and careful patient selection play a more important role than the energy source in the clinical outcome of laparoscopic surgery.[67]

References

1. Einstein A. Zur quantentheorie der strahlung. Physio Z 1917;18:121–8.
2. Gordon JP, Townes CH, Zeigler HJ. The maser – new type of amplifier, frequency standard and spectrometer. Physiol Rev 1955;99:1264–74.
3. Schawlow AL, Townes CH. Infrared and optical lasers. Physiol Rev 1958;112:1940–8.
4. Maiman TH. Stimulated optical radiation in ruby. Nature 1960;187:493–7.
5. Patel GKN. Continuous-wave laser action on vibrational-rotational transitions of CO_2. Phys Rev 1964;136A:1187–93.
6. Bruhat M, Mage G, Manhes H. Use of CO_2 laser via laparoscopy. In: Kaplan I (ed) Laser surgery III. Proceedings of the 3rd Congress of the International Society for Laser Surgery. Tel Aviv: International Society for Laser Surgery;1979: 276.
7. Reich H, MacGregor TS, Vancaillie TA. CO_2 laser used through the operative channel of laser laparoscopes: in vitro study of power and power density losses. Obstet Gynecol 1991;77:40–7.
8. Adamson GD, Reich H, Trost D. CO_2-C-13 isotopic laser used through the operating channel of laser laparoscopes:a comparative study of power and energy density losses. Obstet Gynecol 1994; B83:717–24.
9. Reich H, Donnez J, Slatkine M, Schechter J. Suppression of thermal lensing in CO_2 laser laparoscopy with high flow rate abdominal insufflators. Gynaecol Endosc 1995;4:25–6.
10. Sutton CJG, Hodgson R. Endoscopic cutting with lasers. Minim Invasive Ther 1992;1:197–205.
11. Keckstein J. Laparoscopic treatment of polycystic ovarian syndrome. Baillière's Clin Gynaecol 1989;3:563–82.
12. Bellina JH, Hemmings R, Voros IJ, Ross LF. Carbon dioxide laser and electrosurgery wound study with an animal model. A comparison of tissue damage and healing patterns in peritoneal tissue. Am J Obstet Gynecol 148:327–31.
13. Allen JM, Stein OS, Shingleton HM. Regeneration of cervical epithelium after laser vaporisation. Obstet Gynecol 1983;62:700–4.
14. Baggish MS, Chong PP. Carbon dioxide laser microsurgery of the uterine tube. Obstet Gynecol 1981;58:111–16.
15. Bellina JH. Reconstructive microsurgery of the fallopian tube with the carbon dioxide laser. Procedure and preliminary results. Reproduction 1981;5:1–8.
16. Kelly RW. Laser surgery of the fallopian tube. In: William R Keye Jr. (ed) Laser surgery in gynecology and obstetrics, 2nd edn. Chicago: Year Book Medical Publishers, 1990:166–86.
17. Sutton C. Power sources in endoscopic surgery. Curr Opin Obstet Gynecol 1995;7:248–56.
18. Daniell JF, Brown DH. Carbon dioxide laser laparoscopy: initial experience in experimental animals and humans. Obstet Gynecol 1982;59: 761–4.
19. Sutton CJG. Initial experience with carbon dioxide laser laparoscopy. Lasers Med Sci 1986;1: 25–31.
20. Sutton CJG, Hill D. Laser laparoscopy in the treatment of endometriosis. A five year study. Br J Obstet Gynaecol 1990;97:181–5.
21. Feste JR. Laser laparoscopy: a new modality. J Reprod Med 1985;30:413–17.
22. Nezhat C, Winer W, Crowgey F, Nezhat F. Video laparoscopy of the treatment of endometriosis associated with infertility. Fertil Steril 1989;51: 237–40.
23. Davis GD. Management of endometriosis and its associated adhesions with the CO_2 laser laparoscope. Obstet Gynecol 1986;68:422–5.
24. Donnez J. Carbon dioxide laser laparoscopy in infertile women with endometriosis and women with adnexal adhesions. Fertil Steril 1987;48: 390–4.
25. Adamson GD, Lu J, Subak LL. Laparoscopic CO_2 laser vaporisation of endometriosis compared with traditional treatments. Fertil Steril 1988;50:704–10.
26. Sutton CJG. Endometriosis. Infertil Reprod Med Clin North Am 1995;6:591–613.
27. Sutton CJG, Ewen SP, Whitelaw N, Haines P. Prospective, randomised double-blind, controlled

trial of laser laparoscopy in the treatment of pelvic pain associated with minimal, mild and moderate endometriosis. Fertil Steril 1994;62: 696–700.
28. Fedele L, Bianchi S, Bocciolone L, Nola GD, Franchi D. Buserelin acetate in the treatment of pelvic pain associated with minimal and mild endometriosis: a controlled study. Fertil Steril 1993;59:516–21.
29. Donnez J, Nisolle M, Casanas-Roux F, Clerks F. Endometriosis: rationale for surgery. In: Brosen I, and Donnez J (eds) The current status of endometriosis. Carnforth, UK: Parthenon; 1993: 385–95.
30. Hughesdon PE. The structure of endometrial cysts of the ovary. J Obstet Gynaecol Br Emp 1957;44:69–84.
31. Raftery A. The effect of peritoneal trauma on peritoneal fibrinolytic activity and intraperitoneal adhesion formation. Eur Surg Res 1981; 13:397–401.
32. Marrs RP. The use of the KTP laser for laparoscopic removal of ovarian endometrioma. J Obstet Gynecol 1991;164:1622–6.
33. Daniell JF, Kurtz BR, Gurley LD. Laser laparoscopic management of large endometriomas. Fertil Steril 1991;55:692–5.
34. Sutton CJG, Ewen SP, Jacobs SA, Whitelaw N. Laser laparoscopic surgery in the treatment of ovarian endometriomas. J Am Assoc Gynecol Laparosc 1997;4:319–23.
35. Jones KD, Fan TC, Sutton CJG. The endometrioma: why is it so badly managed? Indicators from an anonymous survey. Hum Reprod 2002; 17:845–9.
36. Daniels J, Gray R, Kahn KS, Gupa JK. Laparoscopic uterine nerve ablation: a survey of gynaecological practice in the UK. Gynaecol Endosc 2000;9:157–60.
37. Beretta P, Franchi M, Gatzzi F, Busacca M, Zupi E, Bolis P. Randomised clinical trial of two laparoscopic treatments of endometriomas: cystectomy versus drainage and coagulation. Fertil Steril 1998;70:1176–80.
38. Saleh A, Tulandi T. Reoperation after laparoscopic treatment of ovarian endometriomas by excision and fenestration. Fertil Steril 1999;72: 322–4.
39. Redwine DB. Ovarian endometriosis: a marker for more extensive pelvic and intestinal disease. Fertil Steril 1999;72:310–15.
40. Koninckx PR, Martin DC. Treatment of deeply infiltrating endometriosis. In: Sutton CJG (ed) Gynaecologic surgery and endoscopy. Current opinion in obstetrics and gynaecology (Vol. 6). 1994:231–41.
41. Koninckx PR, Braet P, Kennedy S, Barlow DH. Dioxin pollution and endometriosis in Belgium. Hum Reprod 1994;9:1001–2.
42. National Center for Health Statistics: Hysterectomies in the United States. 1965–84. Hyattsville MD. National Center for Health Statistics, vital and health statistics. Data from the National Health Survey; 1987. Series 13, No 92, DHSS Publ. (PHS) 88–175.
43. World Health Organization (WHO). Level of PCBs, PCDDs and PCDFs in breast milk: Result of WHO co-ordinated interlaboratory quality control studies and analytical field studies. WHO Environmental Health Series: 1989.
44. Martin DC, Hubert GD, Van der Zwaag R, El Zeky FA. Laparoscopic appearances of peritoneal endometriosis. Fertil Steril 1989;51:63–7.
45. Donnez J. Personal communication.
46. Holsapple MP, Snyder NK, Wood SC, Morris DL. A review of 2,3,7,8-tetrachlorodibenzo-p-dioxin-induced changes in immunocompetence. Toxicology 1991;69:219–55.
47. Neubert R, Jacob-Muller U, Stahlmann R, Helge H, Neubert D. Polyhalogenated dibenzo-p-dioxins and dibenzofurans and the immune system. Arch Toxicol 65:213–19.
48. Rier SE, Martin DC, Bowman RE, Dmowsky WP, Becker JL. Endometriosis in Rhesus monkeys (*Macaca mulatta*) following chronic exposure to 2,3,7,8-tetrachlorodibenzo-p-dioxin. Fundam Appl Toxicol 1993;21:433–41.
49. Reich H, McGlynn F, Salvat J. Laparoscopic treatment of cul-de-sac obliteration secondary to retrocervical deep fibrotic endometriosis. J Reprod Med 1991;3:516–22.
50. Martin DC. Laparoscopic treatment of advanced endometriosis. In: Sutton CJG, Diamond M (eds) Endoscopic surgery for gynaecologists. London: WB Saunders, 1993:229–37.
51. Martin DC. Laparoscopic and vaginal colpotomy for the excision of infiltrating cul-de-sac endometriosis. J Reprod Med Obstet Gynaecol 1988;33:806–8.
52. Nezhat C, Nezhat F, Pennington E. Laparoscopic treatment of infiltrative rectosigmoid colon and

53. Redwine DB. Non-laser resection of endometriosis. In: Sutton CJG, Diamond M (eds) Endoscopic surgery for gynaecologists. London: WB Saunders, 1993: Ch 29, 220–8.
54. Redwine DB, Sharpe DR. Laparoscopic segmental resection of the sigmoid colon for endometriosis. J Laparoendoscop Surg 1991;1: 217–20.
55. Donnez J, Nisolle M, Smets M, Bassil S, Casanas-Roux F. Rectovaginal septum adenomyotic nodules; a series of 500 cases. Br J Obstet Gynaecol 1997;104:1014–18.
56. Zaloudek C, Norris HJ. Mesenchymal tumours of the uterus. In: Kurman R (ed) Blaustein's pathology of the female genital tract. Berlin: Springer, 1987:373.
57. Nisolle M, Paindavenie B, Bourdon A, Berliere M, Casanas-Roux F, Donnez J. Histologic study of peritoneal endometriosis in infertile women. Fertil Steril 1990;53:984–8.
58. Jones KD, Sutton CJG. The colposcopic approach to rectovaginal endometriotic nodules. Min Invasive Ther Allied Technol (in press).
59. Jones KD, Sutton CJG. Arcus Taurinus: the mother and father of all LUNAs. Gynaecol Endosc 2001;6:19–23.
60. Sutton CJG. Surgical management of pelvic pain in endometriosis. In: Maclean AB, Stones RW, Thornton S (eds) Pain in obstetrics and gynaecology 2002;154:164–83.
61. Damario MA, Horowitz IR, Rock JA. The role of uterosacral ligament resection in conservative operations for uterosacral ligament resection in conservative operations for recurrent endometriosis. J Gynecol Surg 1994;10: 57–61.
62. Chapron C, Dubuisson JB, Fritel X et al. Operative management of deep endometriosis infiltrating the utero-sacral ligaments. J Am Assoc Gynecol Laparosc 1999;1:31–7.
63. Phipps J. Thermometry studies with bipolar diathermy during hysterectomy. Gynaecol Endosc 1993;3:5–7.
64. Daniell JF. Laparoscopic use of the argon beam coagulator. In: Sutton CJG, Diamond M (eds) Endoscopic surgery for gynaecologists. London: WB Saunders, 1993:71–6.
65. Palmer M, Miller CW, van Way CW, Orton EC. Venous gas embolism associated with argon-enhanced coagulation of the liver. J Invest Surg 1993;6(5):391–9.
66. Anonymous. Fatal gas embolism caused by over pressurisation during laparoscopic use of argon enhanced coagulation. Health Devices 1994; 23(6):257–9.
67. Tulandi T, Bugnah M. Operative laparoscopy: surgical modalities. Fertil Steril 1995;63: 237–45.

8

Excision of endometriosis with the carbon dioxide laser
Robert B. Albee Jr.

Historical perspective

In the early 1950s endometriosis was considered to be a disease that was curable by conservative excisional surgery at laparotomy.[1] Recently, however, the most common treatments chosen have been non-aggressive laparoscopic thermal ablative techniques (such as laser vaporization, electrocoagulation, or endocoagulation), medical suppression, or removal of the reproductive organs with retention of endometriosis. The length and difficulty of endoscopic excisional procedures, inadequate reimbursement, fear of adhesion formation, and the misconception that new disease was a common sequelae to all methods of surgical treatment led many gynecologic surgeons to abandon excision.

If the ultimate desire is to remove the disease from the body, thermal ablative techniques may be adequate only for superficial lesions, because they typically leave the deep disease in situ. For this reason, many experts treat endometriosis by excision.[2-4] Medical treatment does not cure or remove endometriosis.[5-12] Even after removal of the uterus, tubes, and ovaries 10–31% of patients require reoperation for recurring symptoms.[13] Finally, adhesion formation can be a consequence of leaving a biologically active disease in the body. Adhesions forming as a response to excision of all disease occur in the immediate postoperative period, occur only once and are not continuously formed unless there are other sources of peritoneal irritation, such as persistent endometriosis or infection. The sooner all endometriosis is removed, the sooner comes the end of the ongoing formation of new adhesions. Today's techniques for ovum recovery and assisted reproduction have rendered obsolete the concerns of adhesion-induced infertility after excision. Furthermore, it is much easier for a mother to care for a newborn when her pain from endometriosis has been relieved. Patients choosing pregnancy before aggressive treatment of their endometriosis often must face the pain of their disease at a time when the demands of an infant are significant.

Introduction of the carbon dioxide laser into laparoscopy

The carbon dioxide (CO_2) laser was the first laser used at laparoscopic surgery. Its early use was plagued by ineffective beam alignment systems and the accumulation of laser plume, requiring evacuation and frequent re-establishment of the pneumoperitoneum. However, newer laser arms are far more reliable in maintaining accurate alignment, high flow insufflators re-establish the pneumoperitoneum rapidly with resultant rapid smoke evacuation, and the introduction of direct couplers has greatly enhanced the ease with which the CO_2 laser is used at laparoscopic surgery.

Carbon dioxide laser physics

The term 'laser' is an acronym for 'light amplification by stimulated emission of radiation'. The CO_2 laser is an invisible laser beam of infrared light, with a wavelength of 10 600 nm. The beam is generated by exciting CO_2 molecules in an optic resonator. The laser output is an invisible monochromatic, coherent, and collimated emission delivered as a noncontact-free beam. Water is the target chromophore for the CO_2 laser. The CO_2 laser energy is almost completely absorbed by water. When delivered to living cells and provided sufficient energy, instantaneous boiling of intracellular water occurs, resulting in an explosion (i.e. vaporization of tissue), with lateral thermal spread often less than 100 µm.

By adjusting the power density (PD), the CO_2 laser can also be used for cutting (similar to a knife). The factors affecting PD include power setting, spot size, degree of focus of the beam.

The PD can be calculated by a simple formula, as follows: PD = Power (in watts [W]) × 100/spot size (spot diameter in cm²). Defocusing the beam increases the spot size, decreasing the power density. The average PD required for vaporization is 700–1000 W/cm². For cutting, vaporization requires a higher PD of as much as 1000–1200 W/cm². The CO_2 laser beam can be delivered in an intermittent or continuous mode.

Advantages and disadvantages of the carbon dioxide laser

Advantages of the CO_2 laser include the following:

- The energy is absorbed by water; therefore moist surfaces have some resistance to damage from scatter.
- Power density (PD) and shutter speeds can be adjusted flexibly.
- There is a short depth of tissue absorption.
- A highly focused beam allows minimal lateral tissue damage which results in rapid healing and a reduced potential for injury to adjacent structures.
- The noncontact energy source allows continuous visual monitoring of the tissue at the point of impact.

Disadvantages of the CO_2 laser include the following:

- There is minimal coagulation effect.
- The laser plume requires evacuation.
- The equipment is expensive, heavy, difficult to transport, and takes up a moderate amount of space.
- 'Thermal blooming' occurs when gases inside the scope are heated diffusing the laser beam and altering the power density. This problem has been reduced by using CO_2 isotopes.
- The Lumenis, UltraPulse 'L' series uses a $C_{13}O_2$ isotope that lases at a wavelength of 11.1 µm which does not suffer from the absorption issues in the CO_2 insufflated laparoscopic environment as the standard $C_{12}O_2$ 10.6 µm laser.

For many experts, the CO_2 laser has become the preferred energy source for excising endometriosis. Continuous plume evacuation has greatly reduced the time spent evacuating and recreating the pneumoperitoneum. Laser beam alignment problems no longer exist. The focused laser is so exact that there is greatly reduced danger to adjacent structures when compared to electrical sources or other contact sources. Most importantly, any difficult dissection is aided when you never lose visual contact with the tissue at the time energy is being delivered. Delicate dissections through distorted planes can be performed using the CO_2 laser beam while leaving a very narrow zone of lateral tissue damage.

EXCISION OF ENDOMETRIOSIS WITH THE CARBON DIOXIDE LASER

Equipment

An acceptable laser should have the capability of providing at least 25 W in a rapid pulse mode, and a minimum of 40 W in a continuous mode, such as a Lumenis UltraPulse 5000L. Other considerations are the alignment mechanism and ease of attachment to a laparoscope. A good quality camera and monitor are vital. A high flow carbon dioxide insufflator capable of delivering a volume of at least 30 l/min is very helpful. A video printer makes it easy to illustrate to others the specifics of what has been found and how it has been treated, allowing others to appreciate the surgery accomplished (Fig. 8.1).

Room and patient set-up

Proper arrangement of equipment in the operating room makes surgery more efficient. The laser generator can be positioned on the side of the operating table opposite the surgeon and out of the way of the assistant. A mobile cart with the television monitor, light source, camera box, and insufflator can be positioned on the side of the table opposite the surgeon as well. The assistant can then stand between the mobile cart and the laser generator. A second video monitor can be positioned next to the surgeon for the assistant to observe during surgery. An electrosurgical generator can be positioned behind the surgeon (Fig. 8.2). The scrub nurse and his or her tray can stand between the patient's legs. Other necessary equipment includes a suction-irrigator and a simple but sufficient selection of laparoscopic tools, such as atraumatic graspers. (Fig. 8.3) A suction-irrigator allows continuous suction while using the central channel for instrumentation, such as a small bipolar, or grasper.

The anesthesia personnel and equipment occupy their traditional spot at the head of the table. After the induction of general anesthesia, the patient is placed in the dorsal semi-lithotomy position with her legs in protective stirrups. A warming system applied to the upper torso can help avoid hypothermia, especially during a long surgery. Both arms can be placed down at the patient's side using ulnar nerve gel protection. Standard laparoscopy drapes work well. An intrauterine manipulator is a must for proper exposure of the deep pelvis during surgery. Each patient is bowel prepped since intestinal endometriosis is difficult to predict with absolute certainty.

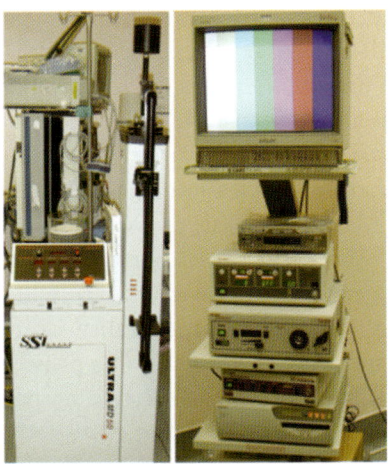

Figure 8.1
Left: the Lumenis UltraPulse 5000L laser used by the author. Right: a video cart with a video monitor on top with video cassette recorder, insufflator, light source, camera box and printer below

Basic surgical principles

Although no two surgeries will be the same, there are important basics that can be applied to each surgery. Visualize thoroughly the upper and lower abdomen as well as the pelvis. This

SURGICAL MANAGEMENT OF ENDOMETRIOSIS

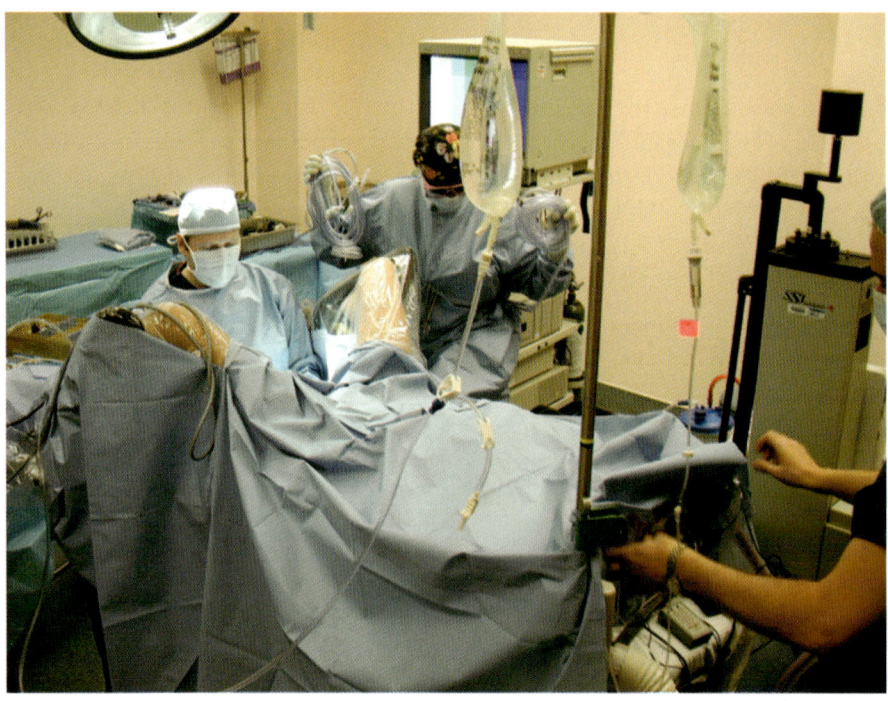

Figure 8.2
The patient is placed in dorsal semi-lithotomy position with a warming system to maintain body heat. The patient's arms are tucked by her sides and protected with foam

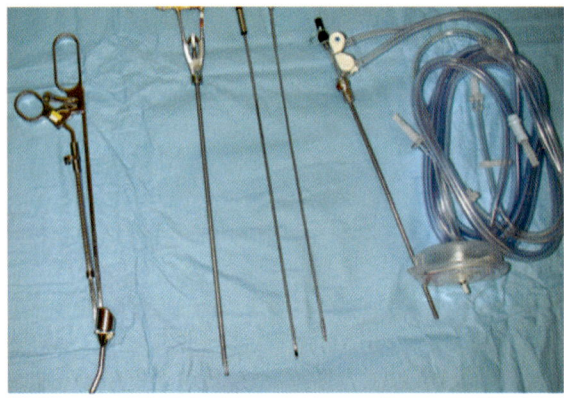

Figure 8.3
The equipment for advanced laser excision of endometriosis can be quite simple, consisting of an intrauterine manipulator on the left, various types of atraumatic graspers, and a suction-irrigator on the right

should include the diaphragms, liver, gall bladder, small and large intestine, stomach, appendix, and ileocecal valve. Develop an initial plan for the treatment of all the disease found. If possible before excising, restore all areas of distorted anatomy back to normal. Before excising lesions, circumscribe all areas of endometriosis or any other type of peritoneal abnormality with a peritoneal incision so it will not be forgotten later. Any abnormality of the peritoneum must be considered to be possible endometriosis until proven otherwise by pathologic evaluation.[14]

Commonly during surgery the laser seems to be less and less effective on the tissue. Here are the most common problems and their solutions:

1. Too much plume in the abdomen. Suction out all plume, using constant suction

through the suction-irrigator, and add a 'Paul filter' to one of the outflow valves on the port sleeves.
2. A loose connection between the scope and the coupler or laser articulating arm. Have the circulating nurse re-tighten all connections.
3. Water or debris has accumulated inside the scope. Remove the scope and clean the channel with a soft brush. We keep a sterile one on the field at all times.
4. Saline or fat is dripping on to the scope lens from the anterior abdominal wall. Suction out all excess saline and fat.
5. Saline is accumulating on the tissue by running down from the abdominal gutters. Take the patient out of the Trendelenburg position and suction out all accumulated saline and blood.

During excision, it is necessary to identify and isolate the visceral structures of concern proximal to the area to be worked on. This may require lysis of adhesions, dissection of the retroperitoneal or rectovaginal spaces, ureterolysis, and manipulation or insufflation of the colon or bladder. Once a lesion is isolated from surrounding structures, it is undermined and removed. Two bipolar instruments are used to control vessels that the laser does not coagulate. Most of the time, the small 3 mm bipolar passed through the suction-irrigator is all that is needed to control bleeding. When a larger instrument is needed, the suction irrigator is replaced with an instrument, such as a Gyrus 5 mm bipolar dissecting forceps. Each specimen is labeled and sent to pathology. The information gained from the pathology reports has proven vital in many situations, is very reassuring to the patient, and is the foundation for scientific understanding of the disease.

Laparoscopic excision with the carbon dioxide laser

Some general principles concerning excision with the CO_2 laser apply to most surgical situations. Each area of interest is circumscribed first with 12 W rapid pulse. The initial circumscribing laser incision passes just through the peritoneum. As the dissection continues beneath the peritoneum, the power is increased to 15–20 W pulsed unless surgery is occurring directly over a dangerous area. One edge of the peritoneum beside the lesion is then elevated with traction to help distinguish the site of the attachment of the endometriosis and associated scarring to normal tissue. Backstopping is performed whenever appropriate using the suction-irrigator in most cases. Staying in normal tissue immediately adjacent to the abnormal, the laser beam works around and underneath the involved area. Abnormal tissue is characterized by increased density, change in color, abnormal vascularity, and the presence of scar. When the specimen is totally free, it is removed through one of the port sheaths.

As experience increases, it becomes easier to know when to use blunt dissection and when to excise sharply using the laser. Hydrodissection is not particularly helpful in many cases because dense retroperitoneal fibrosis will not yield to it, and hydrodissection can be a hindrance since if the tissues are totally wet, the laser energy will be absorbed by the saline.

Simple excision without anatomic distortion

Superficial disease (Fig. 8.4) provides a good opportunity to get experience using laser excision. Low power can be used to circumscribe lesions (Fig. 8.5). After the area has been outlined, the dissection can be extended directly through the peritoneum. The edge of

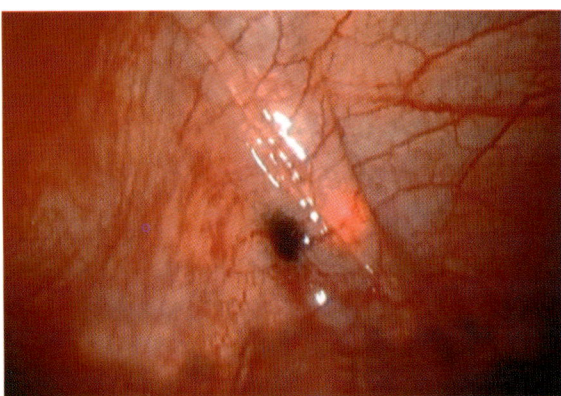

Figure 8.4
A black 'powder burn' lesion with no associated scarring or neovascularity is seen over the right uterosacral ligament. The depth of invasion is not obvious by inspection of the surface

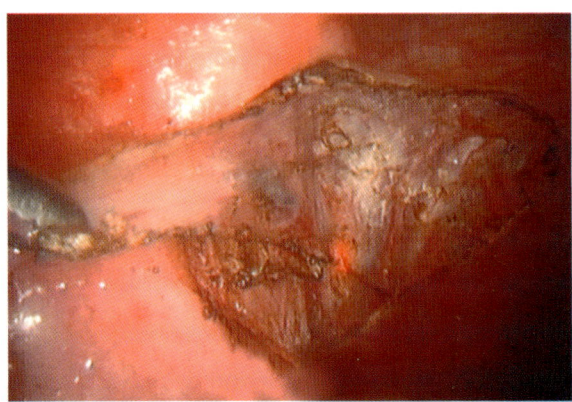

Figure 8.6
The abnormal peritoneum is grasped and pulled under strong traction while the laser separates the retroperitoneal tendrils from the underlying structures. Note that the bottom side of the black lesion is visible in the peritoneum being resected, ensuring complete removal of this lesion

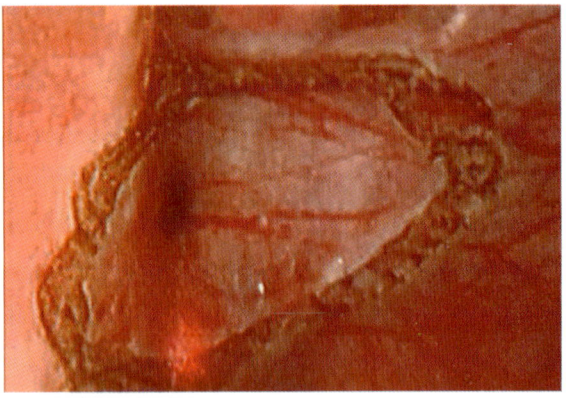

Figure 8.5
The lesion has been circumscribed with a low power laser incision carried just through the peritoneum

the peritoneum can then be grasped and upward traction applied (Fig. 8.6). This traction will help to distinguish the site of the attachment of the endometriosis/scarring to underlying normal tissue. Dissection can continue using the blunt tip of the suction-irrigator or can be done sharply using the laser. The undersurface of the lesion can be examined as it is separated (Fig. 8.6). Once complete excision has been accomplished the specimen can be removed through one of the ports and sent to pathology for evaluation. Examination of the excision site helps ensure that none of the lesion has been left behind. Often, the site is clean and blood-free. As skill develops, delicate dissection can be performed over veins leaving them intact. Smooth reperitonealization can be expected without adhesion formation in the majority of these locations (Fig. 8.7).

It is common to see superficial disease mixed together with surface scarring, foreign body reaction, fibrosis, and other changes that are secondary to prior thermal ablative treatments (Fig. 8.8). These changes make it difficult to know whether or not underlying endometriosis is present. Therefore, it is important to remove all abnormal peritoneum. Only with excision, is it possible to tell how deeply the changes penetrate below the surface (Fig. 8.9). It is easy, however, to examine the base of the area left after excision and know if any disease remains (Fig. 8.10). One of the remarkable properties of excision is that no matter how superficially or how

EXCISION OF ENDOMETRIOSIS WITH THE CARBON DIOXIDE LASER

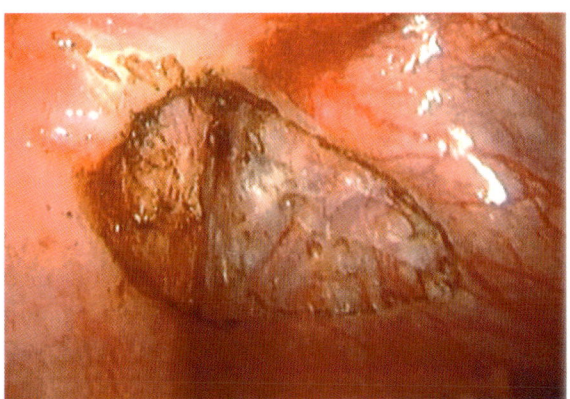

Figure 8.7
The resected area is clean and free of bleeding, carbon, or other debris. Underlying deeper veins have been protected

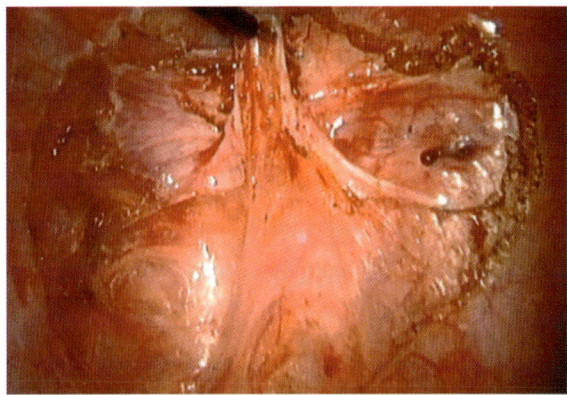

Figure 8.9
The abnormal peritoneum is placed on upward traction and the laser is severing the retroperitoneal tissue allowing complete removal of the lesions without damage to underlying vital structures

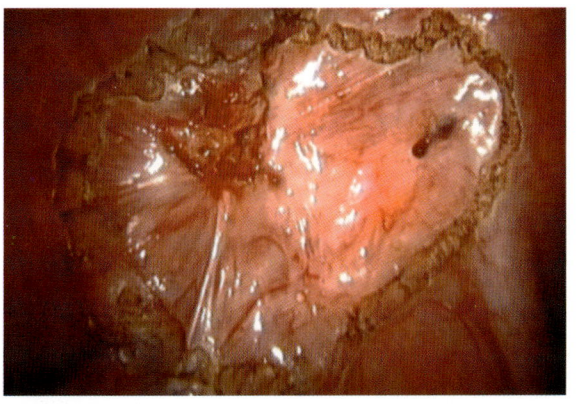

Figure 8.8
This is a hemorrhagic lesion of the left pelvic sidewall with some associated scarring and adjacent clear papules and whitish fibrosis in a patient with previous attempts at thermal ablation. The excision process is again initiated with a laser incision circumscribing the abnormal peritoneum to be removed along with every abnormality on its surface

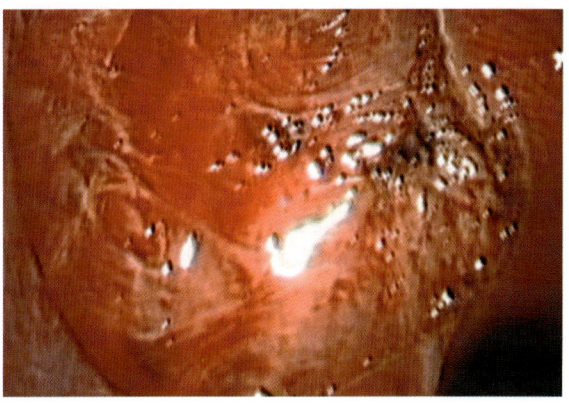

Figure 8.10
The excision process is complete. No macroscopic or microscopic endometriosis is present since the excision process has extended to healthy normal tissue. A small bleeder will be controlled with bipolar coagulation

Deep excision without anatomic distortion

deeply the endometriosis has invaded, the resulting surgical defect is largely the same in all patients. For this reason, excision sites will heal remarkably well with fresh peritoneum within a few weeks.

Irregular surface contour, clear papules, red implants, and whitish fibrosis are commonly associated with superficial disease, but some apparently 'superficial' disease is much more widespread than noted on initial casual observation (Fig. 8.11). Although not commonly available in the operating room, 'digital embossing' can be used to show the subtle changes which every surgeon needs to look for (Fig. 8.12). It is not uncommon for undiscernible deep disease to be present. Techniques that can be used to put pressure and/or tension on a lesion and demonstrate its morphology include movement of a manipulator inside the rectum or vagina, movement of the uterus, filling the bladder with saline, and using additional instruments to squeeze or bump it. Thermal ablative techniques will totally ignore such deep disease because once the surface is treated the deeper tissues are typically not evaluated further.

Excision of deep endometriosis can vary considerably depending on the anatomic area involved. Knowledge of the local anatomy is imperative. Neovascularity and vascular engorgement should be expected. A rectal manipulator helps identify the colon wall and provide countertraction when working on a rectal lesion (Fig. 8.13). The principle of traction and countertraction are just as important in laparoscopic surgery as they are in conventional surgery and it is essential to have two intraabdominal sources of traction to fulfill this principle. A small grasper can be used through the suction-irrigator (placed through the left lower quadrant 5 mm port) and an atraumatic grasper through the right lower quadrant port.

It is imperative to determine the depth of invasion of the lesion into adjacent viscera. Excision is the only technique that allows this

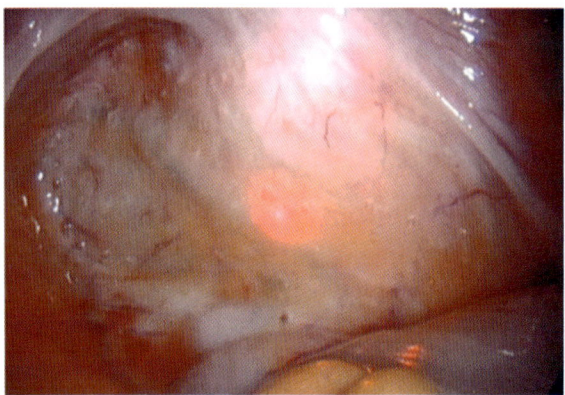

Figure 8.11
In the cul de sac, are clear papules, red and white lesions, and an irregular surface texture

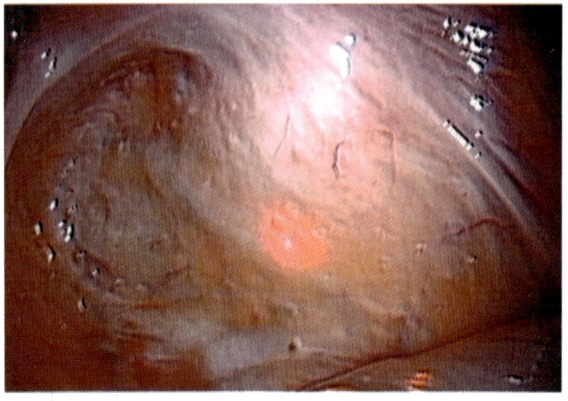

Figure 8.12
'Digital embossing' allows more precise delineation of subtle peritoneal lesions and can make them more apparent, although deeper nodules may remain undetectable

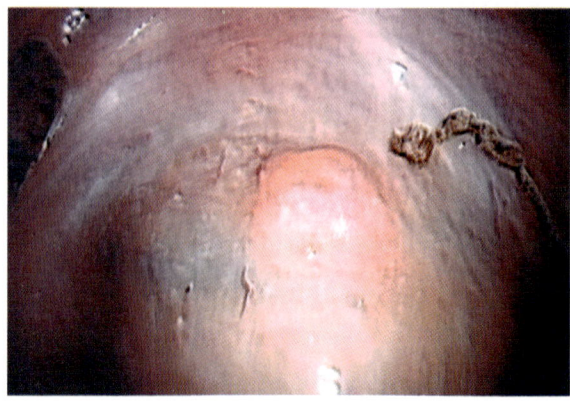

Figure 8.13
When a rectal probe is inserted, a small nodule high in the central cul de sac is identified. Laser excision of the abnormal cul de sac peritoneum has begun in the vicinity of the right uterosacral ligament

type of evaluation to be made. If extensive excision is performed but some deeply invasive disease is left behind, the surgery will not be totally successful. Persistent disease inevitably causes problems, and repeat surgeries may be more difficult than initial surgeries.

After a deeper lesion is circumscribed, it is isolated from surrounding normal tissue and vital structures using blunt and sharp dissection (Fig. 8.14). In the area anterior to the rectum and without much lateral involvement, blood vessels are small and a small bipolar coagulator is sufficient to control vessels. If the dissection extends into the pararectal space larger arterioles will be encountered which require the larger bipolar coagulator. Occlusive pressure provided by lateral displacement of the rectal manipulator or direct clamping of the vessel using the small grasper provide time to insert the bipolar coagulator when brisk bleeding is encountered. It is important to learn how to clean blood from the lens of the laparoscope using a stream of saline from the suction-irrigator.

After excision is complete, the site should be clean and dry. Underlying vascular structures can remain intact (Fig. 8.15). The viscera adjacent to areas of excision should always be evaluated after the excision is complete. The retrocervical space can be surprisingly large, and many lesions dissect off the surface of the colon nicely. At the completion of this type of dissection an atraumatic clamp can be used to cross and occlude the colon at the pelvic brim. The pelvis is then flooded with saline and the colon is filled with air. The absence of a stream of bubbles from a leak point confirms the integrity of the bowel wall.

Deep excision with anatomic distortion and organ involvement

Deep excision with anatomic distortion presents the greatest challenge since it may require resection of bowel, bladder, or ureter as well as reconstructive ovarian surgery. Each challenge is unique and a thoughtful perspective plus experience will be needed to understand the anatomic

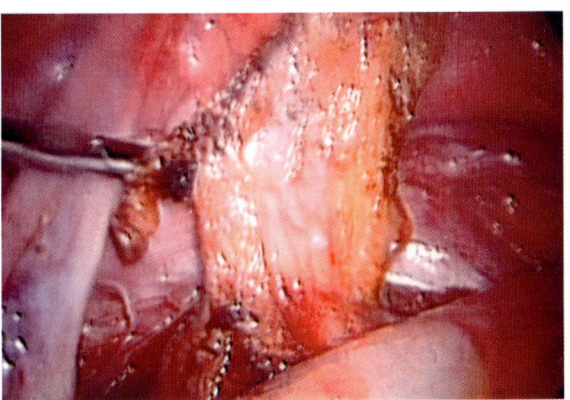

Figure 8.14
A lesion of endometriosis is being dissected off of the anterior rectal wall. The basic surgical principles of traction and countertraction are supplied by two atraumatic graspers (one is out of the frame at top) and by a rectal probe pushing posteriorly. On the anterior bowel wall vessels are small, while in the pararectal gutters, larger vessels will be found

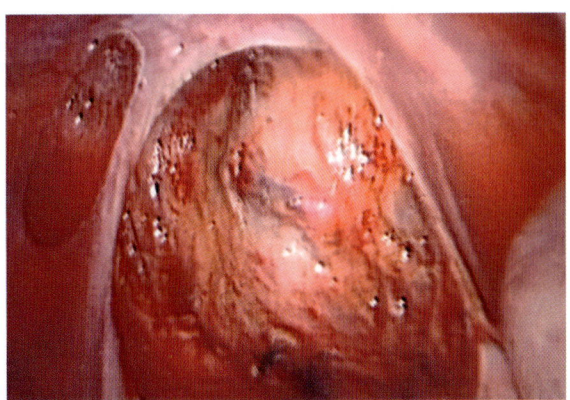

Figure 8.15
After excision of a small rectal nodule the site is clean and dry. The central bulge is the rectal wall, and the dissection is bordered by the intact uterosacral ligaments. Bowel wall integrity can be checked by underwater air pressure examination with air insufflated transanally

SURGICAL MANAGEMENT OF ENDOMETRIOSIS

changes that have occurred over time due to the disease and the effects of previous surgery.

In these situations it may be impossible to start out circumscribing the areas of planned excision. The first step is often to dissect out vital structures and evaluate them for the presence or absence of endometriosis, and then attempt to restore normal anatomy. The ability to do a retroperitoneal dissection to isolate the ureter and to protect the iliac and hypogastric vessels is essential to safe treatment of advanced stage endometriosis when there is significant sidewall distortion. Similarly, the gynecologic surgeon desiring to be proficient in excising endometriosis must master the ability to explore and dissect out the rectovaginal septum when there is an obliterated cul de sac or deep disease in the uterosacral ligaments.

Excision provides the most accurate diagnosis of the location of endometriosis and of the extent of invasion. Treatment of deep endometriosis may require a multi-organ approach. Patient care centers wishing to treat this problem should have a surgeon or surgeons who are able to treat any manifestation of the disease in any location inside the abdomen.

Ovarian endometriomas

One type of deep excision commonly associated with anatomic distortion is the ovarian endometrioma. It is often densely adherent to the adjacent uterosacral ligament, pelvic sidewall, uterus, and intestine (Fig. 8.16).

The bowel must first be restored to its normal position by dissecting it from the ovary, pelvic sidewall, and uterosacral ligament. This allows the surgeon to access the retroperitoneal space to isolate the ureter and follow its course. The start of a retrocervical dissection is also necessary to reduce the attachment of the lower sigmoid to the posterior cervix (Fig. 8.17).

The CO_2 laser is an excellent tool for these types of dissections because used at low power,

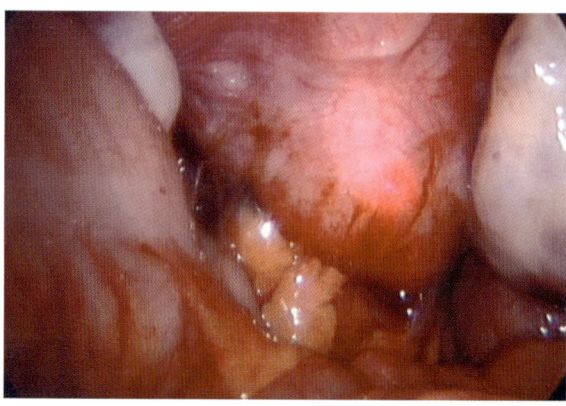

Figure 8.16
Complete obliteration of the cul de sac in Stage IV endometriosis is seen, with the ovaries bilaterally adherent to their respective sidewalls and uterosacral ligaments. Surgery begins by freeing the ovaries from their adhesive attachments

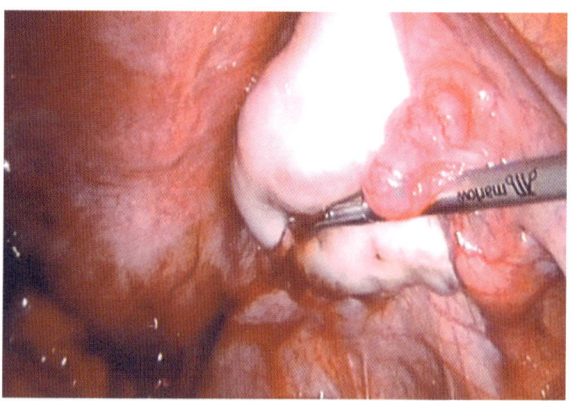

Figure 8.17
The right ovary has been partially freed from the posterior cervix but is still adherent to the right broad ligament over the region of the right ureter which can be seen in the right lower frame

a plane between two densely fused surfaces can be identified by gently feathering the surface with the laser and then using blunt dissection. There is no need for additional instruments that may obstruct vision. The pinpoint control of the laser beam minimizes bleeding by not entering adjacent tissues. In some of these situations, too much blunt dissection results in tearing one surface off the other without getting into the proper plane. Too much sharp dissection can create multiple wounds into the surfaces resulting in a macerated appearance, which is more likely to create bothersome bleeding.

It is important to totally separate the ovary from the sidewall. This allows the surgeon to determine if there is disease on the sidewall which must be excised. It also gives full access to the ovary so that the endometrioma can be excised (Fig. 8.18). During this part of the dissection the surgeon should try to keep the capsule of the ovary intact. This helps to avoid leaving a remnant on the sidewall. At this point, the endometrioma can be excised from the ovary. This can be accomplished in the same way that excision is performed elsewhere. Continuous energy at high power is best for ovarian dissection. Although it does create more smoke, it reduces bleeding. The depth of the endometrioma must be determined as the dissection progresses, but preserving a thin layer of any surrounding normal ovarian capsule is of great importance in order to create a defect in the ovary which involutes well and leaves little raw surface area on which adhesions might form.

The laser can then be used as an ablative tool on the raw surface of the stromal crater that has been created. This creates a surface contraction that helps to involute the ovary (Fig. 8.19). Bleeding becomes more of a problem deep in the stroma closer to the uteroovarian ligament, and coagulation may be required.

Once the ovary is fully involuted a choice must be made regarding the use of anti-adhesives. A well-involuted ovary with edges that reapproximate well may heal with few if any adhesions. On the other hand, a gap in the stroma is best covered (Fig. 8.20). In patients who require ovarian cystectomy, three months of ovarian suppression can be very helpful. If a freshly bivalved ovary attempts to ovulate before complete healing, there is a significant chance of stromal hemorrhage causing cyst formation and significant pain. Even if no hemorrhage occurs, postoperative ovarian activity is likely to be more painful until healing is complete.

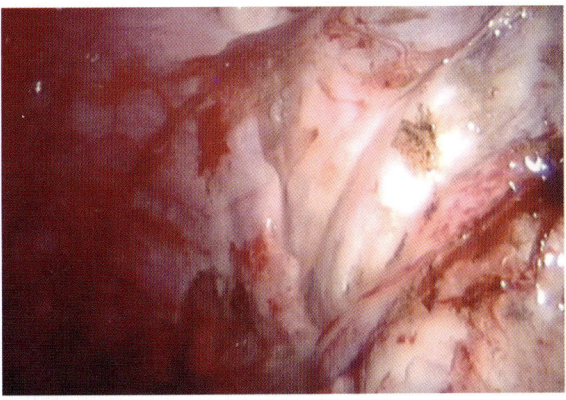

Figure 8.18

If an ovary is adherent to its sidewall, it must be freed up, after which the surface abnormality and underlying cyst can be excised. Continuous energy at high power reduces bleeding, although creates more smoke

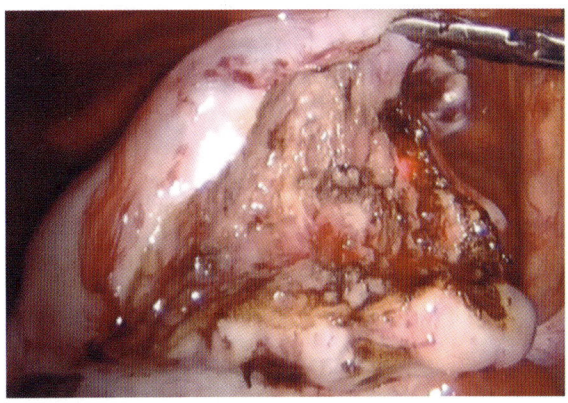

Figure 8.19

Leaving as much of a margin of normal ovarian tissue and cortex around the area excised may help reduce the chance of postoperative adhesions. Once the cyst has been dissected out, the cavity can be vaporized lightly to induce some contraction of the stroma to help involute and close the defect without suture

SURGICAL MANAGEMENT OF ENDOMETRIOSIS

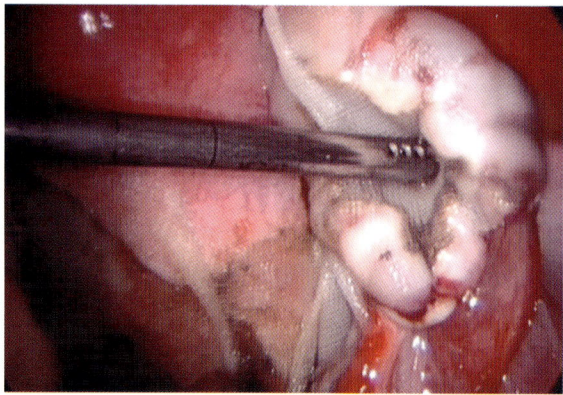

Figure 8.20

The involuted ovary can be wrapped with INTERCEED, if there is a gap in the stroma

Philippe Koninckx recommends certain patients with ovarian endometriosis be treated using a two-stage procedure. Using this approach, the first laparoscopy is performed without a bowel preparation. At the time of laparoscopy, after carefully evaluating the abdomen and pelvis, a large window is made in the cyst wall, followed by irrigation of the cyst. The cyst wall may be treated using thermal ablation techniques, but adhesions are not lysed and other areas of endometriosis are not treated at this time. Postoperatively, three months of LH-RH agonist treatment is given to reduce the size of the cyst. The decision is then made regarding a second laparoscopy to treat the remaining disease. This decision is made based on patient comfort, cyst size, and tolerance to the agonist. The advantages to this approach are that the first case can be scheduled without a bowel prep as a day surgery. Additionally, a much more specific plan can be made prior to the second surgery with regard to organ preservation, adhesiolysis, length of stay, possible additional procedures which may be required, and general surgical or urological surgical assistance.

Vaginal involvement

When endometriosis invades deep into the floor of the pelvis, there may be involvement of the retrocervical space down to the level of the rectovaginal septum or even further. The upper rectum and the posterior vaginal wall may also be involved. The CO_2 laser is a wonderful tool for excision in this lower pelvic space where everything funnels posteriorly due to the fact that the energy is delivered in a beam and requires no direct contact with the tissue. Using most of the other techniques, the instrument carrying energy must be placed on the intended point of dissection which obscures vision to some extent. Often, the initial views of the lesion are obscured by overlying adhesions and distorted anatomy (Fig. 8.21). Once the floor of the pelvis has been exposed, it is possible to outline the lesion and the intended dissection. It is helpful to begin this type of dissection around the lateral margins and extend the surgical plane into the pararectal space if necessary (Fig. 8.22). When accomplished on both sides, the lesion is outlined laterally but still attached anteriorly and posteriorly (Fig. 8.23). It may not be possible to tell initially the extent of invasion into the

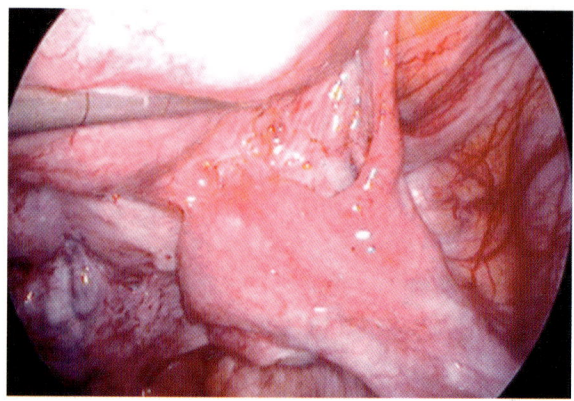

Figure 8.21

Invasive endometriosis of the cul de sac and pelvic floor is partially hidden beneath the adherent right tube and ovary

EXCISION OF ENDOMETRIOSIS WITH THE CARBON DIOXIDE LASER

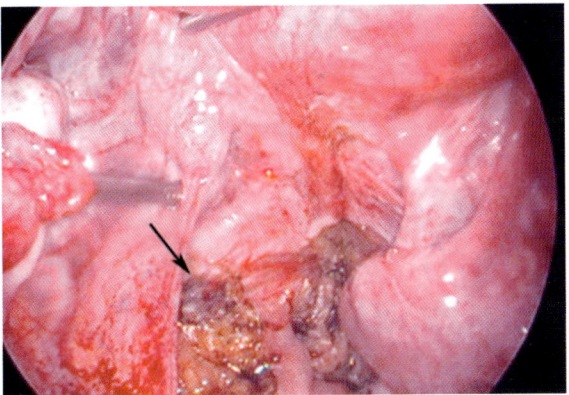

Figure 8.22
Since there are no instruments to impede the surgeon's view during laser surgery, the dissection of the ovary from the pelvic floor can be straightforward and less risky. After the right tube and ovary are freed, the pelvic floor is exposed. A nodular lesion is seen as a bluish area (→)

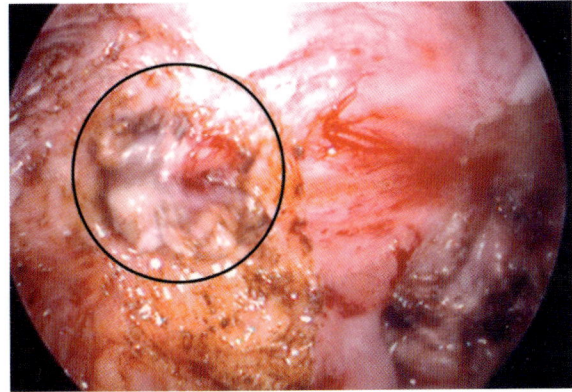

Figure 8.23
After further dissection, the nodule is seen still attached to the underlying posterior vaginal wall (circle) and to the bowel

bowel or vaginal wall. Dissection must be continued cautiously using the rectal manipulator and vaginal probes for assistance. The ideal dissection leaves the deepest point of invasion until the end (Fig. 8.24). Once isolated at this point, the extent of the lesion is fully understood and appropriate plans made for the nature of the

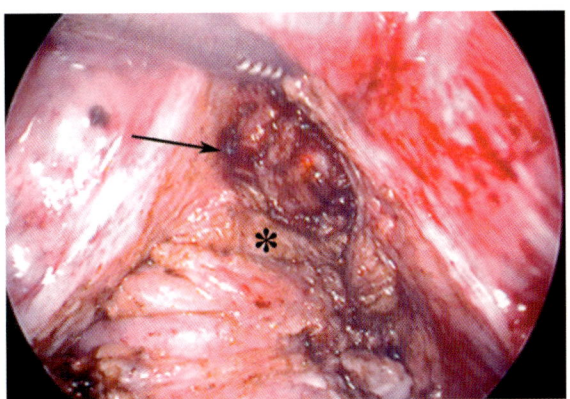

Figure 8.24
The lesion (→) has been dissected off the bowel wall (∗) and remains attached only to the posterior vaginal wall

surgery required to remove it. Finally, the involved tissue is resected with the lesion in situ. Resultant defects of bowel or vagina can then be repaired (Figs 8.25, 8.26).

Nodule in the anterior cul de sac
Endometriosis in the anterior cul de sac often appears to be more deeply invasive into the bladder than it actually is. The bladder may

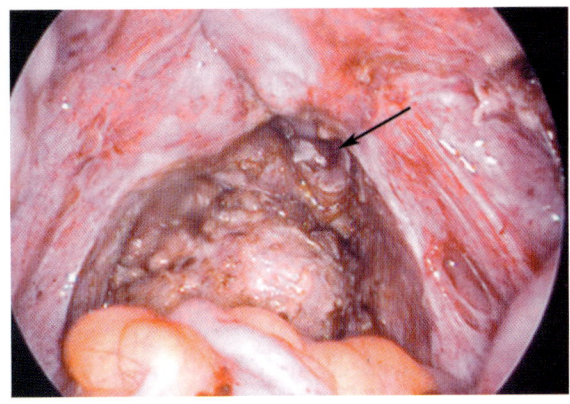

Figure 8.25
The nodule has been removed by creating a small opening into the vagina (→). All invasive endometriosis has been removed without damage to the adjacent rectum. This patient conceived 9 months following surgery

SURGICAL MANAGEMENT OF ENDOMETRIOSIS

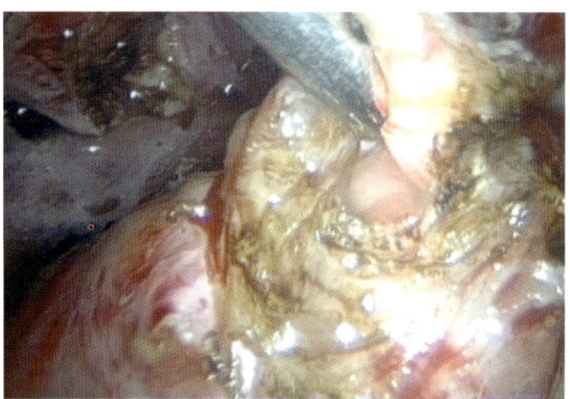

Figure 8.26

A similar case is shown where entry into the lumen of the bowel was eventually required to completely excise rectal endometriosis

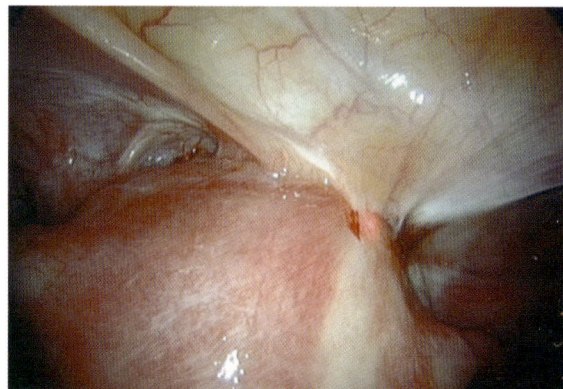

Figure 8.27

The uterus is in the left lower part of the frame and the bladder peritoneum is adherent across the anterior fundus, exhibiting a 'rolling' morphology

totally cover up the lesion and be found adhered to the anterior surface of the uterus above it (Fig. 8.27). It is usually more common that the lesion invades the myometrium rather than the bladder detrusor muscle. Occasionally, the bladder muscularis is invaded, and it is important to be prepared to resect the entire lesion if it is found to be penetrating. As in all nodular disease, the lesion must be isolated from all adjacent tissues leaving the point of greatest penetration as the final stage. This is another area where it is helpful to develop the lateral margins first so that separation is obtained between the bladder and the uterus along the lateral margins of the nodule. Then, as the dissection is advanced both anteriorly and posteriorly, it is possible to identify the margins of the nodule and the degree of invasion of surrounding structures. Nodules that penetrate the myometrium can then be resected off. This may leave a raw surface area much like a myomectomy which can then be covered or sutured closed (Fig. 8.28). Pathology on such specimen may reveal uterine muscle surrounding portions of the endometriosis or adenomyoma. The urinary bladder can be filled with contrast material to demonstrate its integrity.

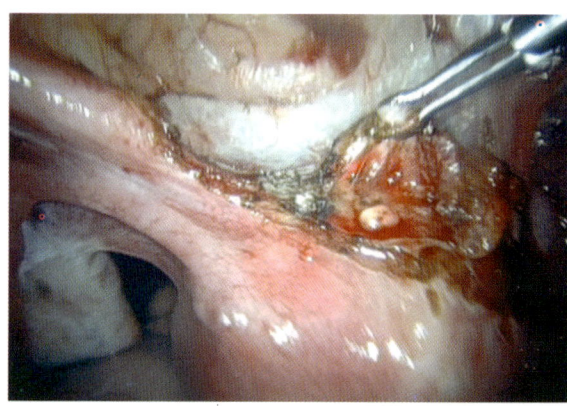

Figure 8.28

The lesion has been dissected off the region of the bladder and is seen to mainly involve the anterior uterine fundus

Invasive lesions of the colonic wall

Invasive lesions of the bowel wall may be surprisingly subtle in their appearance (Fig. 8.29). Sometimes, all that is seen is superficial scarring or thickened serosa. The rectal manipulator is very helpful in quickly demonstrating the presence of an unexpected deeper nodule. By passing the manipulator through the underlying bowel lumen, nodules are more easily seen as

EXCISION OF ENDOMETRIOSIS WITH THE CARBON DIOXIDE LASER

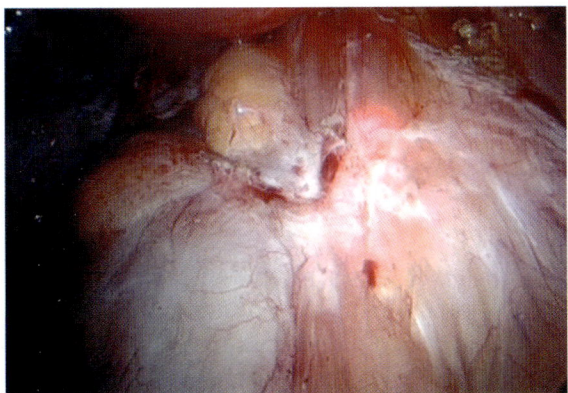

Figure 8.29

A nodule of endometriosis of the bowel may have a visually innocuous morphology

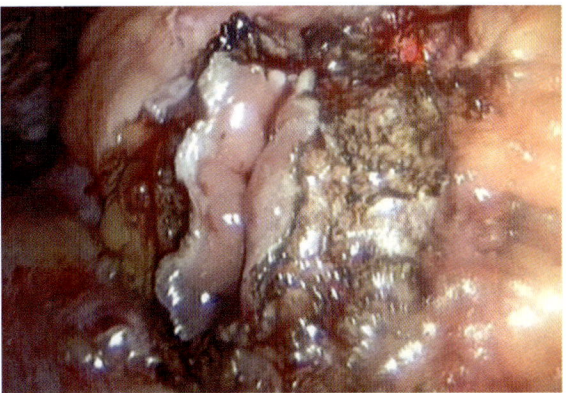

Figure 8.31

Full-thickness penetration into the bowel lumen is sometimes necessary for complete treatment of nodular intestinal endometriosis

raised areas that pass over the manipulator in a bumpy fashion. Direct contact with the suction-irrigator may reveal the more dense tissue of the nodule compared to the softer normal bowel wall. After circumscribing the lesion, dissection can be carried out circumferentially using mainly sharp/laser dissection (Fig. 8.30). Attempts to dissect the lesion off the serosa of the intestine meet with dense resistance and increased vascularity. As the dissection is carried around the lesion deeper into the bowel wall, the mucosa is ultimately encountered (Fig. 8.31). Often, there are no obvious longitudinal or transverse muscle fibers to be seen. In the bowel wall, endometriosis seems to replace rather than to infiltrate the muscularis. Once the lumen of the bowel is encountered, it is usually easier to remove the remainder of the lesion minimizing the size of the bowel wall fenestration. If the lesion size is small enough, the fenestration may be closed with a standard double layer closure (Fig. 8.32). The bowel wall integrity can then be tested.

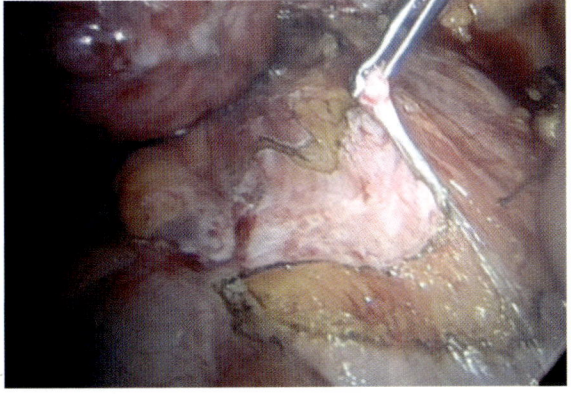

Figure 8.30

The laser is used to begin circumscribing the nodule

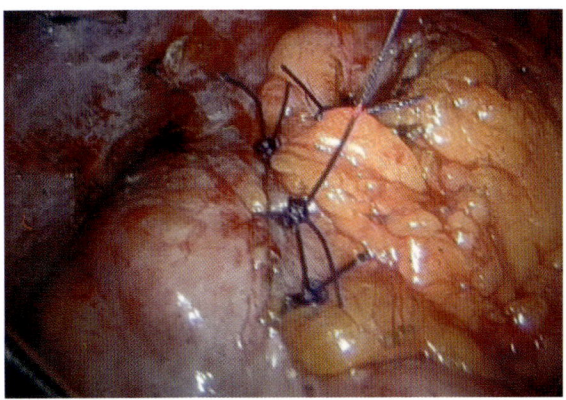

Figure 8.32

The rectal defect has been closed with interrupted sutures and integrity of the bowel wall is proven with an underwater air pressure examination

Summary

Surgical excision is the cornerstone of the treatment of endometriosis by experts in the disease. It can be performed using a number of different energy sources. Variation in types of energy used need not influence the most important outcome, which is the safe removal of all disease. On the other hand, the energy used may impact the amount of bleeding that occurs, the ease of accomplishing the desired result, the amount of time required to do the surgery, the equipment needed to perform the operation, the amount of adhesions that form, and the amount of time necessary to heal.

The carbon dioxide laser is a useful tool for the surgeon who wants to be prepared to laparoscopically excise endometriosis in all locations. The CO_2 laser has proven itself in virtually all situations. It leaves a very minimal zone of injury lateral at the point of incision. It offers the best visualization of tissue during dissection because the energy is applied through a beam which can be continuously monitored without touching the tissue. Healing is remarkably rapid after laser excision, because there is a minimum of devitalized tissue left behind. It can be used for bladder resection and repair, rectum, colon, and small bowel resection and repair, ureteral resection and repair, partial vaginectomy, excision of nodules in the rectovaginal septum as well as in many other situations.

Since 1990, I have treated over 1000 patients exclusively by excising all disease with the CO_2 laser. These patients form the basis of an ongoing prospective observational study. Data is collected by questionnaire annually and personal interviews at the time of follow-up. In this group of patients, the rate of endometriosis 'recurrence' documented by 'observation' at the time of surgery is 13%. The rate of recurrence documented by pathologic evaluation is 9%. Endometriosis is a curable disease.

References

1. Meigs JV. Etiologic role of marriage age and parity; conservative treatment. Obstet Gynecol 1953; 2:46–53.
2. Koninckx PR, Martin D. Treatment of deeply infiltrating endometriosis. Curr Opin Obstet Gynecol 1994;6:231–41.
3. Redwine DB. Conservative laparoscopic excision of endometriosis by sharp dissection: life table analysis of reoperation and persistent or recurrent disease. Fertil Steril 1991;56:628–34.
4. Vercellini P, Chapron C, DeGiorgio O, Consonni D, Frontino G, Crosignoni PG. Coagulation or excision of ovarian endometriomas? Am J Obstet Gynecol 2003;188:606–10.
5. Nisolle-Pochet M, Casanas-Roux F, Donnez J. Histologic study of ovarian endometriosis after hormonal therapy. Fertil Steril 1988;49:423–6.
6. Parazzini F, Fedele L, Busacca M, Falsetti L, Pellegrini S, Venturini PL, Stella M. Post surgical medical treatment of advanced endometriosis: Result of a randomized clinical trial. Am J Obstet Gynecol 1994;171:1205–7.
7. Fedele L, Bianchi S, Zanconato G, Tozzi L, Raffaelli R. Gonadotropin-releasing hormone agonist treatment for endometriosis of the rectovaginal septum. Am J Obstet Gynecol 2000; 183:1462–7.
8. Shaw RW. Endometriosis: Current evaluation of management and rationale for medical therapy. In: Brosens IA, Donnez J (eds) The current status of endometriosis. London: Parthenon, 1993: 371–83.
9. Fedele L, Bianchi S, Bocciolone L, Dinola G, Franchi D. Buserelin acetate in the treatment of pelvic pain associated with minimal and mild endometriosis – A controlled study. Fertil Steril 1993;59:516–21.
10. Fedele L, Arcaini L, Bianchi S, Baglioni A, Vercellini P. Comparison of cyproterone acetate and danazol in the treatment of pelvic pain associated with endometriosis. Obstet Gynecol 1989; 73:1000–4.
11. Fedele L, Bianchi S, Arcaini L, Vercellini P, Candiani GB. Buserelin versus danazol in the treatment of endometriosis-associated infertility. Am J Obstet Gynecol 1989;161:871–6.
12. Redwine DB, Elstein M, Shaw R, Barlow DH, Kellerman LA. Nafarelin versus danazol versus surgery. Fertil Steril 1992;58:455–6.
13. Namnoum AB, Hickman TN, Goodman SB, Gehlback DL, Rock JA. Incidence of symptom recurrence after hysterectomy for endometriosis. Fertil Steril 1995;64:898–902.
14. Redwine DB. Age related evolution in color appearance of endometriosis. Fertil Steril 1987;48:1062–3.

9

Fiber laser excision of endometriosis

Thomas L Lyons

Management of endometriosis has always been based on symptomatic relief.[1,2] Despite the fact that the disease seems to be endemic and that voluminous research has been performed in order to find a non-invasive cure, management remains centered around the use of surgical extirpation with medical placation.[3] Although extensive efforts have been made in attempts at improving fecundity rates, results remain marginal.[4,5] Neither medical therapy nor surgery alone or in combination produces significant improvement in pregnancy rates. However, for relief of pain both medical and surgical therapies have been employed with success although cure rates are not available. For invasive rectovaginal disease and large endometriomas, surgical therapy appears to be the only solution as medical therapy has demonstrated no efficacy in these areas.[6,7]

Surgical therapy revolves around three basic techniques:

1. Vaporization – laser, electrosurgical
2. Coagulation/ablation – laser, electrosurgical
3. Excision – laser, electrosurgery, scissors, harmonic scalpel.

Of these techniques, excision is by far the most appropriate. If the surgeon has significant expertise in the recognition of endometriosis occasionally vaporization or coagulation of superficial disease can be used, but in most cases excision is the wiser choice. Excision offers the advantages of pathologic confirmation and adequate removal of the lesion. Because endometriosis may extend several centimeters into the tissue and because epithelial cancers can mimic this disease it is always wise to have a histologic confirmation of the diagnosis.[8]

Laparoscopy has been defined as the gold standard in surgical treatment of endometriosis for several reasons:[9]

- Minimally invasive approach
- Superior visualization with 4–10 × power magnification
- Superior access – posterior pelvis and cul de sac
- Microsurgical accuracy of excision
- Decreased risk of scarring
- Ability to repeat the surgery without compromising results.

The surgical approach to endometriosis should be aggressive and according to the patient's symptomatology. All patients should be bowel prepped and counseled appropriately preoperatively. Although staged procedures are used by some surgeons, a single stage approach is preferable if the clinical picture warrants this type of surgery. Pain mapping on pelvic examination should be performed preoperatively using a systematic regimen with particular attention to the cul de sac, each uterosacral ligament, and uterus as separate areas of palpation. Operative pain mapping by patient-assisted laparoscopy[10] may sometimes be helpful if the patient's history is vague and pelvic examination does not reproduce symptoms. Ovarian conservation is possible in a large percentage of patients and, despite using an aggressive surgical approach, hysterectomy is rarely necessary unless coexisting uterine symptoms or disease is present.[11]

Rectovaginal disease is present in less than 10% of patients with endometriosis but may be present in a higher proportion, particularly in patients with a combination of dyspareunia, dyschezia, or cyclic rectal bleeding. Anterior full-thickness disk resection of the rectosigmoid colon may be indicated and should be performed when the disease process involves this area.[12] While a 1–3% rate of complications following full-thickness bowel resection has been reported in the general surgical literature,[13] it should be remembered that patients with endometriosis are young and healthy compared to most general surgery patients, and the rate of complications following bowel surgery is much lower in these patients. Rectovaginal disease can be treated laparoscopically with or without bowel resection.[14–17] General surgery consultation should be available in these cases. Segmental resection of the rectosigmoid colon is rarely indicated but may be accomplished at laparotomy,[18–20] or laparoscopy,[21–23] by a multidisciplinary team.

Urologic involvement is not common but must be considered. In presumed Stage III–IV disease this author prefers a preoperative intravenous pyelogram (IVP) for documentation of ureteral patency. Retroperitoneal fibrosis has been reported postoperatively and in extensive sidewall dissections consideration of ureteral wrapping with INTERCEED, Spraygel, other adhesion barriers (see below), or omental graft may be indicated.[24]

Methods

Equipment

We prefer the Contact neodymium-yttrium-aluminum garnet (Nd:YAG) laser for excision of endometriosis but the technique may be accomplished using other modalities. Lasers in general can offer some advantages to the operator in this often demanding dissection process. The types of fiber lasers currently available for use are Nd:YAG, potassium titanyl phosphate (KTP), argon, homium, and a series of tunable dye or diode lasers.[25,26] The advantages of these types of lasers predominately revolve around the ease of access. The laser fiber is easily passed through the working channel of the operating laparoscope or through secondary laparoscopic portals. The small diameter of these fibers and the inherent flexibility can aid in the ease of use of the tool to accomplish the dissection.

The Contact Nd:YAG laser (Surgical Laser Technologies, Oaks, PA) uses a patented process of optically coating a synthetic sapphire tip of varying shape and size which prevents the YAG energy from exiting the tip. This creates superheating of the tip thus creating an efficient, accurate endothermy device. So-called sharpened fibers have a similar action but do not function, in our opinion, as effectively as the thermal area is limited to the tip alone. This area is only 1–2 mm in length and therefore limits the ability to use the coagulating effects of the broad sides (1–2 cm in length). The Contact laser scalpel shape we favor is a cone-shaped tip which has a point of 400–600 μm in diameter (Fig. 9.1). This focused tip is a highly efficient cutting device and the side of the shaft can be used to coagulate and seal vessels up to 2 mm in diameter. The absence of a need to 'back stop' the contact laser facilitates the dissection of the retroperitoneal spaces, and the discrete nature of the tool allows the operator to work at point blank range with ureter, bowel, and other structures where limitation of energy transfer is critical. This lack of energy spread allows penetration depths of 100–300 μm enhancing dissection planes without tissue distortion.

Carbon dioxide (CO_2) lasers are highly effective cutting devices and are efficient at vaporizing lesions but because this laser uses an invisible beam of laser energy care must be taken to not allow penetration of the energy to unwanted depths. This is particularly true over vital structures including ureter, bowel and vasculature. In order to prevent this accident, irrigant is forced under the tissues in a technique called hydrodissection or aquadissection as a backstop for the CO_2 beam. However, this technique is unnecessary when using fiber lasers and can distort the surgical planes making accurate and discrete dissection more difficult.

When using the laser as a cutting tool we find the BiCoag dissecting forceps indispensable (Gyrus Medical, Cardiff, Wales) as our choice for control of larger vascular pedicles and for surface fulguration of microscopic bleeding. These forceps enable the physician to grasp, dissect, and seal vessels, without changing instrumentation, thus making the procedure move at an improved pace while maintaining excellent hemostasis. The combination of the Contact Nd:YAG laser scalpel and the bipolar dissecting forceps improves efficiency, even in the most challenging cases, and thereby decreases both clinical and economic morbidity.[27]

Technique

The open (Hasson) technique is used to enter the abdomen. This primary trocar can be placed in several ways other than the open technique but we choose this technique because of the incidence of multiple prior procedures in this group of patients and the incidence of de novo adhesions with endometriosis alone. This first trocar is of 10/12 mm diameter, while other trocars are 5 mm (Fig. 9.2). Generally, three 5 mm trocars are used allowing the operator to triangulate most pathology in the pelvis and to best take advantage of help from the surgical assistant. A good uterine manipulator is very helpful in these dissections and is manned by the scrub nurse who is stationed between the patient's legs. Good Trendelenburg is optimal at 27–30 degrees and will allow the bowel to mobilize out of the pelvis. Pneumoperitoneum at 14 mmHg is maintained throughout the procedure. In some cases,

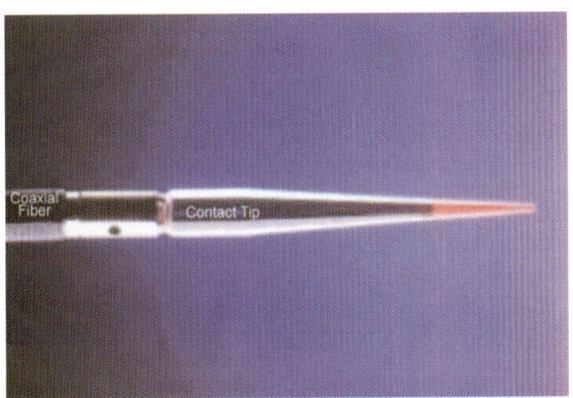

Figure 9.1
The Contact Nd:YAG laser scalpel

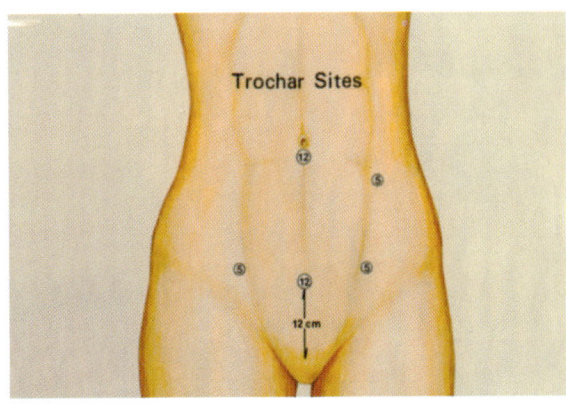

Figure 9.2
Trocar sites

where the patient is obese, 17 mm of pressure may be necessary for exposure.

The case is begun with restoration of normal anatomic relationships, beginning with adhesiolysis until all endometriotic disease can be visualized. The ureters are then identified for protection using one of two approaches. The medial approach is used if the peritoneal surfaces medially are available and the track of the ureter can be identified along its course through the pelvis. An incision will then be made alongside the ureter which will be dissected the length of the pelvis until reaching the tunnel in the cardinal ligament. Also, at this time the rectosigmoid colon is identified and separated from the uterosacral ligaments and vaginal cul de sac. Now all areas of abnormal peritoneum are circumscribed using the laser scalpel followed by excision to the level of normal tissue (Figs 9.3–9.7).

If the medial peritoneal surfaces are obscured due to disease or scarring then the lateral approach to the retroperitoneal space is used. An incision is made in the peritoneum of the avascular triangle perpendicular to the round ligament and parallel with the tube and is extended from the round ligament to the pelvic brim or the iliac vasculature. Then using blunt

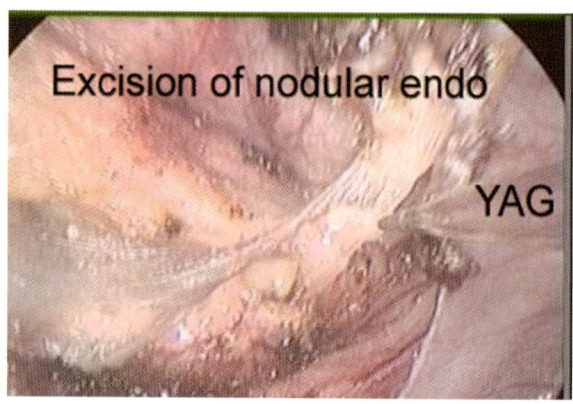

Figure 9.4

Nodular disease of the pelvic sidewall/uterosacral area is seen extending more deeply into the tisssues. Here the entirity of the lesion is dissected using the contact Nd: YAG laser scalpel. Note: absolute hemostasis

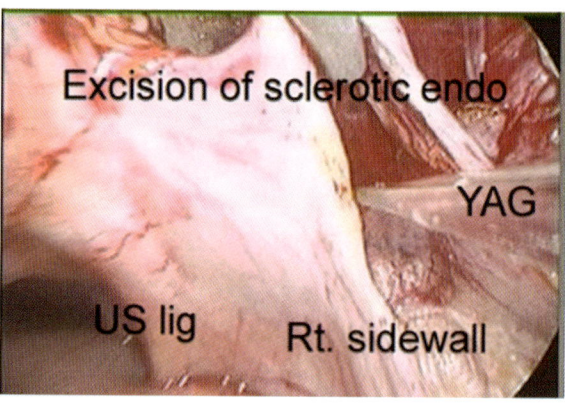

Figure 9.5

Endometriosis has caused thickening of the peritoneum of the right broad ligament. The Nd:YAG laser (YAG) has created an incision through normal peritoneum adjacent to the thickened peritoneum which is being held on traction by the grasper at the top middle of the frame. Retroperitoneal dissection allows the ureter to be kept out of harm's way

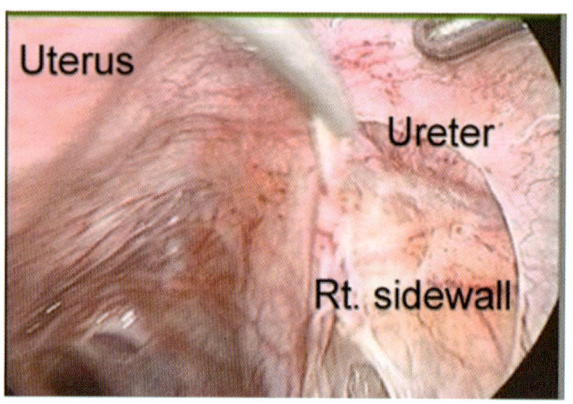

Figure 9.3

Skinning excision of endometriosis of the sidewall

dissection the broad ligament vasculature and the ureters are identified and separated from the overlying diseased peritoneum. The remainder of the dissection is the same but this technique gives access to the hypogastric arteries and their

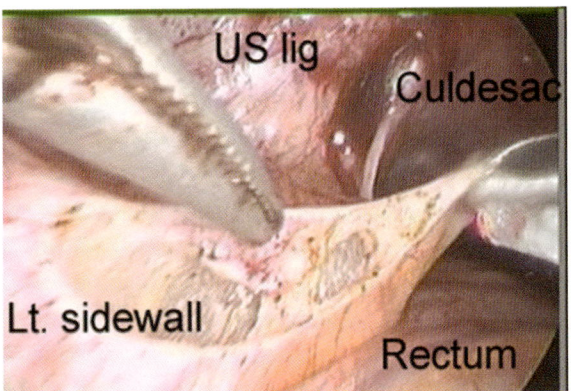

Figure 9.6
Superficial endometriosis over the left ureter proximal to the left uterosacral ligament (US lig) has been partially isolated with a peritoneal incision. The peritoneal incision is held on stretch bhy the grasper at the right of the frame, while a second grasper points at the small lesion

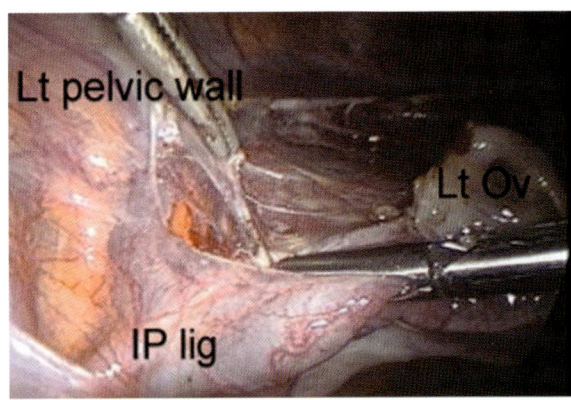

Figure 9.8
Retroperitoneal dissection through the left avascular triangle has begun just lateral to the left infundibulopelvic ligament (IP lig). This approach is useful when an adherent ovary and retroperitoneal fibrosis makes dissection through the broad ligament peritoneum problematic

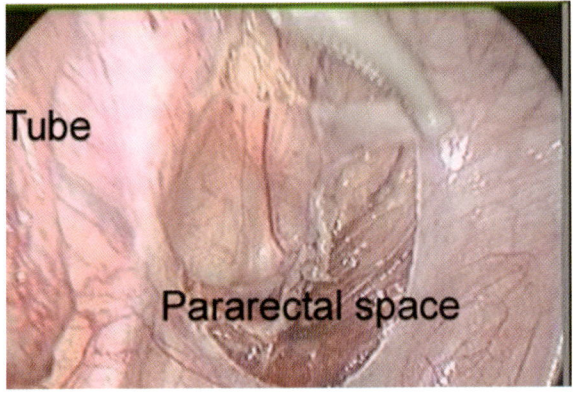

Figure 9.7
Endometriosis of the base of the left uterosacral ligament has been circumscribed with a peritoneal incision which immediately exposes the sizable lateral rectal vessels traversing the pararectal space. The left fallopian tube is seen at the extreme of the frame

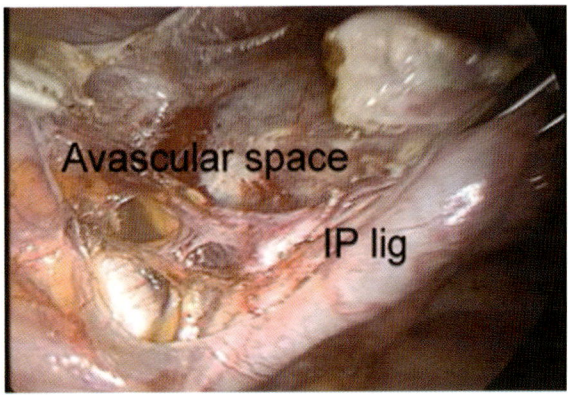

Figure 9.9
The left avascular triangle has been opened widely and the retroperitoneal dissection has been carried posteriorly, allowing the surgeon views of the left common iliac artery, internal iliac vessels, the ureter, and the posterior leaf of the broad ligament

tributaries and allows aggressive resection of all diseased tissue (Figs 9.8, 9.9).

Areas of endometriosis involving the ovaries are treated using ablation of surface lesions and drainage and removal of cysts. Endometriomas are drained and the interior surfaces are stripped and/or ablated. Removal of the cyst wall[28] decreases chances of recurrence of these endometriomas versus ablating their surfaces.[29]

Aggressive resection of cul de sac nodules, rectovaginal disease, and uterosacral/cervical disease is done using the Contact Nd:YAG laser scalpel. Bowel treatment is saved for the last part of the procedure along with removal of the appendix. Anterior disk resection of the rectum or rectosigmoid colon is accomplished by excising the lesion or nodule with the Nd:YAG laser scalpel and then the bowel is closed in two layers. The first layer is 3-0 Vicryl placed in a running fashion, followed by a layer of 3-0 silk placed in a running, locking fashion. Occasionally, full-thickness excision is not necessary and in these cases a reinforcing suture of running 3-0 silk will be used. Segmental resection of the bowel is rarely necessary but can be accomplished using the EEA circular stapler (Ethicon Endosurgery, Cincinnati, OH) to anastomose the bowel segments.

Copious irrigation is used of warmed Lactated Ringers solution in order to keep the tissues moist and to cleanse the area of debris and blood. This process clears the area for better visualization and potentially decreases postoperative adhesions. Adhesion barriers are used in all cases. INTERCEED has been used in the past as well as Adept (ML Laboratories, London, UK) for this purpose. Spraygel (Confluent Medical, Boston, MA) is a new barrier which has shown promise in Europe and can be used even when bowel surgery has been performed. This is a spray on application that certainly could be superior to INTERCEED given positive results in upcoming clinical trials. Postoperative adhesive disease remains a part of the puzzle that has not been completely solved and could contribute significantly to improving clinical outcomes.

Postoperatively, the patients may recover in an outpatient setting and are discharged uniformly within 23 hours. Liquids are encouraged immediately, and the patient is ambulated as soon as she is able in the extended recovery area. Most patients are able to return to normal activity within 7–10 days without compromise. Careful preoperative preparation of the patient for this postoperative scenario is imperative and can improve the overall course of the recovery period. Retroperitoneal fibrosis can occur following extensive lateral wall dissections and must be considered if the patient's postoperative course is abnormal. Avoidance of devascularization of the areas lateral to the ureter and the use of adhesion barriers in this area can help to mitigate this potential problem.

Recognition of injury during the procedure is the most important caveat during these types of procedures. Postoperative cystoscopy, sigmoidoscopy, and any other intraoperative maneuvers necessary to ensure that there has been no loss of integrity to bowel or urinary tract is reassuring and appropriate whenever extensive dissections involve these non-gynecologic structures.

Discussion

The greatest challenges for the gynecologist are to identify the endometriotic lesions, which may occur in many different colors or configurations,[30] and to biopsy and excise all of these suspicious areas to a depth that is sufficient to eliminate the disease. Invasive lesions that have been associated with pain must be recognized and removed in their entirety in order to obtain the clinical results desired. The surgeon must be cognizant that some of the old stereotypical notions regarding endometriosis and the patients who should be considered at risk for the disease are inaccurate. Therefore, at any age and at any parity, the patient presenting with pelvic pain must be evaluated with endometriosis primary in the differential diagnosis.

Sufficient literature has been generated to show that an excisional approach to endometriosis results in better clinical outcomes. In the area of symptom relief, pain is certainly less likely to recur if aggressive removal of disease has been performed.[31] The data are less conclusive when pregnancy rates are considered, but the relationship between endometriosis and pregnancy is difficult to define and the ameliorative effects of the pregnant state on endometriosis are now in question.[32, 33]

Medical therapy for endometriosis centers on the use of a pseudomenopausal state (GnRH agonists), which has been shown to be effective in symptom reduction and can be helpful as an adjuvant to good surgical therapy in producing higher successful pregnancy rates in some investigations.[34, 35] The decision now is not whether surgery is integral therapy but rather how can this excisional surgery best be performed.[36, 37] The use of the technology described (Contact Nd:YAG laser), combined with meticulous adherence to proven surgical principles (hemostasis, traction/countertraction, and reapproximation/restoration of anatomic planes), can provide the patient with a low morbidity, cost-effective approach to an extremely difficult gynecologic problem. The use of various energy sources for the purpose of cutting and/or coagulation is dependent on the operator's knowledge of the physics and properties of those energy sources. Lasers have been used effectively in this area with safety and accuracy and will continue to be a part of the regimen for the laparoscopic surgeon in the future.

References

1. Mettler L, Geisel H, Semm K. Treatment of female infertility due to obstruction by operative laparoscopy. Fertil Steril 1979;32:384–9.
2. Redwine DB. Treatment of endometriosis associated pain. In: Olive DL (ed) Endometriosis: Infertility and reproductive medical clinics of North America. Philadelphia: WB Saunders, 1992:697–720.
3. Martin DC. CO_2 laser laparoscopy for endometriosis associated with infertility. J Reprod Med 1986;31:1089–94.
4. Marcoux S, Maheux R, Berube S and the Canadian Collaborative Group on Endometriosis. Laparoscopic surgery in infertile women with minimal or mild endometriosis. N Engl J Med 1997;337:217–22.
5. Adamson GD, Pasta DJ. Surgical treatment of endometriosis-associated infertility: Meta-analysis compared with survival analysis. Am J Obstet Gynecol 1994;171:1488–505.
6. Gant NF. Infertility and endometriosis: Comparison of pregnancy outcomes with laparotomy versus laparoscopic techniques. Am J Obstet Gynecol 1992;166:1072–81.
7. Canis M, Pouly JL, Wattiez A, Manhes H, Mage G, Bruhat MA. Incidence of bilateral adnexal disease in severe endometriosis (r-AFS stage IV): Should a stage V be included in the AFS classification? Fertil Steril 1992;573:691–2.
8. Garry R. Endometriosis: an invasive disease. Gynecol Endosc 2001;10(2):79–82 (Editorial).
9. Gomel V. Operative laparoscopy: a time for acceptance. Fertil Steril 1989;52:1–1.
10. Demco LA. Mapping the source and character of pain due to endometriosis by patient assisted laparoscopy. J Am Assoc Gynecol Laparosc 1998;5:241–5.
11. Redwine DB. Conservative laparoscopic excision of endometriosis by sharp dissection: life table analysis of reoperation and persistent or recurrent disease. Fertil Steril 1991;56:628–34.
12. Martin DC, Hubert GD, Levy BS. Depth of infiltration of endometriosis. J Gynecol Surg 1989;5:55–60.
13. Tuson JR, Everett WG. A retrospective study of colostomies, leaks and strictures after colorectal anastomosis. Int J Colorectal Dis 1990;5:44–8.
14. Brosens IA. New principles in the treatment of endometriosis. Acta Obstet Gynecol Scand Suppl 1994;159:18–21.
15. Koninckx PR, Martin D. Treatment of deeply infiltrating endometriosis. Curr Opin Obstet Gynecol 1994;6(3):231–41.
16. Redwine DB. Laparoscopic en bloc resection for treatment of the obliterated cul de sac in endometriosis. J Reprod Med 1992;37:695–8.
17. Redwine DB, Wright J. Laparoscopic treatment of obliteration of the cul de sac in endometriosis: Long term followup. Fertil Steril 2001;76:358–65.
18. Coronado C, Franklin RR, Lotze EC, Bailey HR, Valdes CT. Surgical treatment of colorectal endometriosis. Fertil Steril 1990;53(3):411–16.
19. Gray LA. Endometriosis of the bowel: role of bowel resection in superficial excision and oophorectomy in treatment. Ann Surg 1973;177(5):580–587.
20. Magos A. Endometriosis: radical surgery. Ballière's Clin Obstet Gynecol 1993;7(4):849–64.
21. Redwine DB, Sharpe DR. Laparoscopic segmental resection of the sigmoid colon. J Laparoendosc Surg 1991;1:217–20.
22. Sharpe DR, Redwine DB. Laparoscopic segmental resection of the sigmoid and rectosigmoid colon for endometriosis. Surg Laparosc Endosc 1992;2:120–4.
23. Redwine DB, Koning M, Sharpe DR. Laparoscopically assisted transvaginal segmental bowel resection for endometriosis. Fertil Steril 1996;65:193–7.
24. Lyons TL. Laparoscopic resection of rectovaginal endometriosis using the Contact Nd:YAG laser and primary closure with suturing techniques. J Pelv Surg 1996;2(1):8–11.
25. Martin DC. CO_2 laser laparoscopy for endometriosis associated with fertility. J Reprod Med 1986;31:1089–96.

26. Daikuzono N, Joffe SN. Artificial sapphire probe for contact photocoagulation and tissue vaporization with the Nd:YAG laser. Med Instrument 1985;19:173–8.
27. Lyons TL, Winer W. An innovative bipolar device for laparoscopic use. J Am Assoc Laparosc. In press.
28. Reich H, McGlynn F. Treatment of ovarian endometriomas using laparoscopic surgical techniques. J Reprod Med 1986;31:577–84.
29. Fayez JA, Vogel MF. Comparison of different treatment methods of endometriomas by laparoscopy. Obstet Gynecol 1991;78:660–5.
30. Martin DC, Hubert GD, VanderZwaag R, El-Zeky FA. Laparoscopic appearances of peritoneal endometriosis. Fertil Steril 1989;51:63–7.
31. Garry R, Clayton R, Hawe J. The effect of endometriosis and its radical laparoscopic excision on quality of life indicators. Br J Obstet Gynaecol 2000;107(1):44–54.
32. McArthur JW, Ulfelder H. The effect of pregnancy on endometriosis. Obstet Gynecol Surv 1965;20:709–33.
33. Hanton EM, Malkasian GD, Dockerty MB, Pratt JH. Endometriosis: symptomatic during pregnancy. Am J Obstet Gynecol 1966;95:1165–6.
34. Winkel CA, Bray M. Treatment of women with endometriosis using excision alone, ablation alone or ablation in combination with leuprolide acetate. In: Proceedings of the 4th World Congress on Endometriosis, Yokohama, 1996: 55.
35. Parazzini F, Fedele, L, Busacca M et al. Postsurgical medical treatment of advanced endometriosis: results of a randomized clinical trial. Am J Obstet Gynecol 1994;171:1205–7.
36. Bateman BG, Kolp LA, Ntits S. Endoscopic versus laparotomy management of endometriomas. Fertil Steril 1995;62:690–5.
37. Canis M, Mage G, Manhes H, Pouly JL, Wattiez A, Bruhat. Laparoscopic treatment of endometriosis. Acta Obstet Gynecol Scand Suppl 1989;150:15–2.

10

Harmonic scalpel excision of endometriosis
Martin Robbins

Endometriosis can be treated medically or surgically. Medical treatment gives excellent short-term pain relief, but lesions persist and symptoms recur, therefore endometriosis must be approached surgically. Surgical treatment can be open or endoscopic. The improved illumination and magnification, and the ability to work close to the tissues, makes laparoscopy the preferred approach to this disease.

Endometriosis can be treated surgically by coagulation, vaporization and/or excision. There are several concerns with coagulation or fulguration regardless of whether the coagulation is performed with electrical, laser or ultrasonic energies. These methods cannot be used with lesions on the surface of the bowel or adjacent to the ureter or within peritoneal pockets. Importantly, there is no way of knowing if the energy penetrated to the full depth of the lesion for complete destruction.

Laser vaporization can completely remove superficial lesions with excellent results. It is essential to vaporize to normal tissue in order to avoid skip areas with residual disease.

Excision, regardless of the energy used, has several advantages. All involved areas are confirmed, by histology, as to whether there was or was not endometriosis present at those sites. Excising with wide margins, always staying in underlying normal areolar tissue, and removing all areas of associated fibrosis, gives the best possible chance of long-term pain relief and avoids subsequent surgeries. Complete removal of disease occurs if the dissection is carried into normal tissue. Postoperative medical suppression is unnecessary.

The harmonic scalpel and laparosonic coagulating shears are safe, easy to use and have a short learning curve. This chapter will review the use of ultrasonic energy in the surgical treatment of endometriosis.

Ultrasonic technology

The harmonic scalpel (Harmonic Scalpel; Ethicon Endo-Surgery, Cincinnati, OH) is a blade that vibrates 55,500 times per second over a distance of 50–100 μm. The harmonic scalpel enables the surgeon to make incisions with concomitant hemostasis and with minimal tissue injury. Laser, electrical and ultrasonic energy all achieve hemostasis through the process of coaptive coagulation. Coaptive coagulation is when tissue proteins are denatured producing a protein coagulum, which then seals coapted vessel walls. Laser and electrical energies denature proteins through the production of heat. The harmonic scalpel denatures tissue proteins mechanically. The harmonic scalpel blade couples with the tissue proteins and physically breaks the hydrogen bonds, thereby creating a protein coagulum. Protein coagulation occurs in the 50–100°C range. Tissue desiccation occurs at 150°C, and tissue charring occurs in the 150–400°C range. Therefore, as the temperature rises above 100°C there is no additional hemostasis, just increased tissue injury. The harmonic scalpel functions at approximately 80–100°C,[1] giving hemostasis while minimizing tissue injury. Cutting is achieved in two ways with ultrasonic energy. First, there is the cavitational effect of the ultrasonic energy, which physically disrupts the tissues. Second, there is the small sharp blade moving rapidly through the tissues.

The harmonic scalpel system includes a generator, handpiece, blade system, and foot pedal. The generator is a computer-controlled power supply, which is used to activate the handpiece. The electrical signal causes expansion and contraction of the piezoelectric ceramics in the handpiece, thereby transforming electrical energy into mechanical motion. The mechanical motion is then conveyed down the blade extender to the blade tip. The mechanical motion is amplified at the blade tip. The foot pedal has two power level options, variable and full. Full power is always level 5. Variable power is whatever power level the generator is set at.

There are several harmonic scalpel blade systems available:

Open surgery:
  Coagulating shears (CS) straight blade and CS curved blade.

Laparoscopic straight blades:
  5 mm ball coagulator, dissecting hook, sharp hook, and curved blade.
  10 mm ball coagulator, dissecting hook, and sharp hook.

Laparosonic coagulating shears (LCS):
  5 mm LCS, straight or curved blade.
  10 mm LCS.

The coagulating shears (CS), straight and curved blades, are for open surgery and could be used when endometriosis is excised at the time of laparotomy. The 10 mm straight blades and the ball coagulators are not used because the 5 mm blades work just as effectively.

Power level, blade geometry, tissue tension, and grip strength determine the balance between cutting and coagulation. Level 5, with blade excursion 100 µm, gives the most rapid cutting with the least coagulation effect. Level 3, with blade excursion 60–80 µm, gives slower cutting with more coagulation effect. Level 1, with blade excursion 50 µm, is generally not used and is mostly coagulation effect with extremely slow cutting. The generator is usually set at level 3 and the surgeon can then control the power level with the full and variable foot pedals. Full power is always level 5, and variable power is the power level the generator is set at.

Blade geometry is specific to the harmonic scalpel blade being used. The 5 mm hook blade (Fig. 10.1) has an inner concave sharp surface that gives efficient cutting; an outer convex blunt surface that gives more coagulation effect with slightly slower cutting; and the side surfaces are mostly coagulation effect. The 5 mm curved blade has a shear surface on both sides, which gives efficient cutting and an outer convex flat surface for coagulation effect with slower

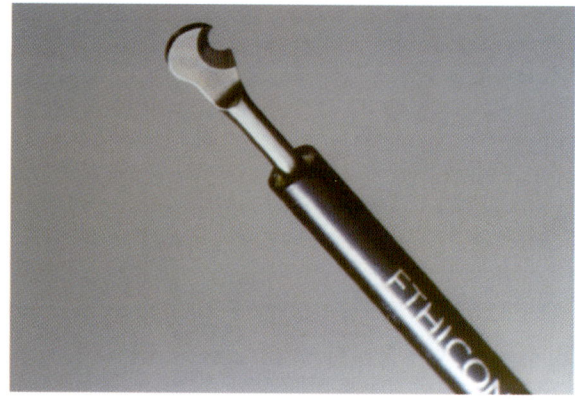

Figure 10.1

The 5 mm harmonic scalpel hook blade with sharp inner concave surface and blunt outer convex surface

cutting. The 5 mm blades are useful for endometriosis excision, cystectomy, adhesiolysis, ectopic pregnancy, ureterolysis, morcellation during a laparoscopic supracervical hysterectomy (LSH), and dissection of the retropubic space.

The 10 mm LCS (Laparosonic Coagulating Shears; Ethicon Endo-Surgery, Cincinnati, OH) has a shear surface for rapid cutting with minimal coagulation effect; a blunt surface for slightly slower cutting with more coagulation effect for 'hemostatic cutting'; and a flat surface for coagulation of large vessels and control of bleeding (Fig. 10.2). With the 10 mm LCS the blade is 15 mm in length and the blade can rotate so that the shear, blunt, or flat surfaces can be used against the inactive tissue pad. The 10 mm LCS is useful for all procedures where the harmonic scalpel can be used. Since there are now 5 mm alternatives, the 10 mm LCS is used less often.

The 5 mm LCS straight blade has a round blunt blade with an inactive tissue pad that rotates 360 degrees around the blade. Although it has a bevel on one side, the 5 mm LCS straight blade is slow at cutting, the coagulation effect spreads farther than it should, incisions are not as precise as they should be, and it should not be used for endometriosis excision. The 5 mm LCS straight blade is useful for lysis of vascular and omental adhesions, oophorectomy, and laparoscopic-assisted vaginal hysterectomy. The 5 mm LCS, straight or curved, will give excellent hemostatic cutting through thick tissue, such as the uteroovarian ligament.

The 5 mm LCS curved blade (Fig. 10.3) is excellent for excision of endometriosis. The curved blade has a shear edge on both sides that gives excellent cutting with effective hemostasis. The outer convex flat surface can be used for surface coagulation with slower cutting. The blunt tip of the blade can be used for more precise coagulation. The tissue pad and the blade rotate together. Therefore, depending on whether the curved blade is directed to the right or the left, the blade will be either above or below the tissue pad. The 5 mm curved LCS cuts more efficiently when the blade is below the tissue pad. It is also useful for hysterectomy (laparoscopic-assisted vaginal or supracervical), myomectomy, oophorectomy, cystectomy, dissection of the retropubic space, ureterolysis, and

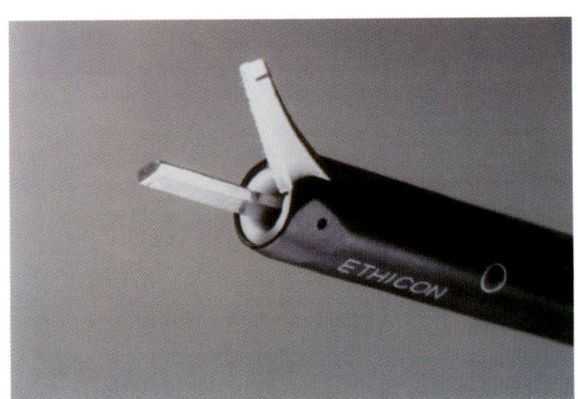

Figure 10.2
The 10 mm laparosonic coagulating shears with shear, blunt and flat blade surfaces and inactive tissue pad

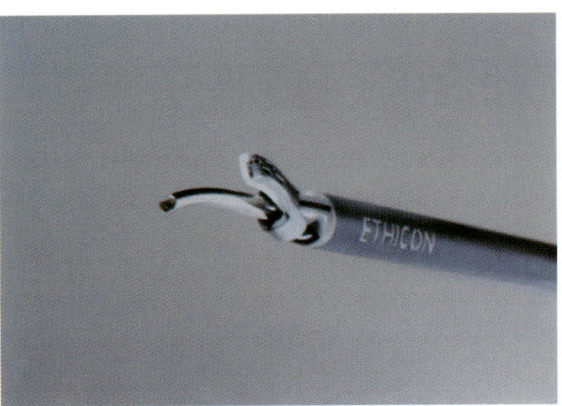

Figure 10.3
The 5 mm laparosonic coagulating shears curved blade with inactive tissue pad

dissection of the mesoappendix. There tends to be more bleeding when using the harmonic scalpel on the ovary, but this can be avoided by using slow energy to tissue to allow more time for more coagulation effect.

Cutting is more rapid with a tighter grip and when the tissue is held on tension. To coagulate and divide a vascular structure requires slower delivery of energy to the tissue. When using the LCS, 'slow energy' implies level 3, loose grip, tissue off tension, and a blunt blade surface if available. This allows time for the coagulation effect to extend lateral enough to give an adequate hemostatic pedicle on both sides of the cut. For avascular tissue you need rapid delivery of energy. When using the LCS, 'rapid energy' implies level 5, tight grip, tissue on tension, and a shear blade. This allows efficient cutting with as minimal coagulation effect as possible. Depending on the tissue being dissected you may choose to use any combination of these variables. For example, when cutting through tissue that looks more vascular, level 5 could be used with a slightly looser grip and holding the tissue off tension.

For excision of endometriosis you need the most rapid incisions with the least possible coagulation effect. The slower the cutting is, the more time the coagulation effect has to spread to adjacent tissues. Spread of coagulation effect can cause thermal injury if there is bowel immediately adjacent to the tissue being excised. Therefore, for endometriosis excision use a shear blade at full power, tight grip, with the tissue on tension. If intestines are densely adherent, it may be prudent to perform some of the dissection with sharp scissors with no energy.

The 5 mm harmonic scalpel hook or curved blades can safely coagulate vessels up to 1–3 mm in diameter.[2] Larger vessels should be coagulated first with the blunt or flat surface, and then transected. Lateral spread of coagulation effect with a 5 mm ultrasonic blade is up to 1 mm. The LCS is able to clamp, coagulate and divide larger vessels and unsupported vascular pedicles. The 10 mm LCS using the blunt blade can safely coagulate vessels up to 5 mm in diameter.[3] When transection of larger vessels is necessary, use power level 3 with a blunt surface and apply energy to coagulate and coapt the vessels in two or three adjacent areas. The pedicle can then be safely divided with an adequate pedicle of coagulated tissue on either side. After a single application of the 10 mm LCS the lateral zone of coagulation is less than 0.25–1.0 mm with the shear blade, and 0.75–1.5 mm with the blunt blade.[4] A study still needs to be done to document the tissue effects of the 5 mm curved LCS, but it appears to have a zone of lateral coagulation effect similar to the 10 mm LCS with the shear blade. Hambley et al compared the traditional scalpel, harmonic scalpel, electrosurgery, and carbon dioxide laser. Compared to the traditional scalpel, the harmonic scalpel caused less bleeding, and delayed tissue healing only minimally. Compared to the carbon dioxide laser and electrosurgery, the harmonic scalpel produced less secondary tissue injury and more rapid wound healing of skin incisions.[5]

Safety considerations

All energy forms and surgical modalities have the potential to cause harm. There are several characteristics of ultrasonic energy, which confer a good margin of safety.

Electrical energy from the generator is converted in the handpiece to mechanical motion. There is no electrical energy through the patient. Problems, such as capacitive coupling, direct coupling and insulation failures, are avoided.

There is no spray of ultrasonic energy. The harmonic scalpel only effects tissues it is in direct contact with. Therefore, ultrasonic energy can be safely maintained until all the coagulated tissues fall completely away from the blade. It is important to not pull the harmonic scalpel through the tissue, and to allow the energy time to work. This will avoid bleeding, prevent sticking of the tissues to the blade and keep the blade clean.

The oscillation of the ultrasonic blade is longitudinal. Energy is directed parallel to, and in the same direction as, the applied force. Therefore, if the harmonic scalpel is lifted away from the pelvic sidewall, no energy is directed downward. This allows the surgeon to safely dissect one tissue layer at a time and in close proximity to internal organs. The cavitational effect of the ultrasonic energy is called 'pneumodissection'. This facilitates the dissection of the tissue layers without distorting the anatomy.

Since the harmonic scalpel works in a lower temperature range, tissue desiccation and charring are minimized. There is minimal production of smoke. The small amount of vapor or steam settles out. Visualization is not impaired with the harmonic scalpel. Less surgical time is wasted on clearing smoke from the operative field. The harmonic scalpel does get warm but cools off quickly. Inadvertent brushing up against bowel wall is unlikely to cause harm. It is still important to avoid direct contact with bowel immediately after using the harmonic scalpel.

As with all surgical modalities there are several safety points that always apply. The patient's arms should be carefully tucked away. General endotracheal anesthesia with the patient adequately paralyzed is important. Preoperative bowel preparation helps to keep the bowel out of the way, and if bowel resection becomes necessary it is good to have prepped bowel. Instruments are moved only when they are in view. The active blade is positioned so that it is in clear view the entire time it is activated. When moving the blade it should be directed away from the pelvic sidewall or underlying vital structure. During the dissection, stop periodically to reorient yourself to the anatomy. During a deep pelvic sidewall dissection always identify and isolate the ureter. Hemostasis is always confirmed at the end of the surgery at low pressure and under fluid. Trocars are removed under direct vision.

Inspection and documentation

The entire abdomen and pelvis is first inspected carefully. All areas of disease are noted and documented with photographs taken before dissection begins. It is easier to identify subtle endometriotic lesions, such as vesicles, flame-type lesions, and brownish staining, before the appearance of the peritoneum becomes altered due to the tissue trauma.

It is essential to look at the undersurface of the ovary where it lies against the ovarian fossa. The superior surface of the ovary can appear normal while there is endometriosis and adhesive disease underneath the ovary. The abdominal wall is inspected for hernias. The upper abdomen, including the diaphragm and appendix, are examined for endometriosis. Incidental pathology of the appendix, such as carcinoid tumor, can be found with or without coexisting endometriosis.[6,7] In a patient with a history of multiple surgeries and chronic right lower quadrant pain it is appropriate to perform an appendectomy. In a patient with persistent central pelvic cramping a presacral neurectomy can be added to the procedure.

Studies on conscious sedation pain mapping have shown several interesting findings that are applicable to the surgical treatment of endometriosis.[8] Subtle lesions, such as clear vesicles, brownish staining, and flame-type lesions, can be more painful than the classic powder-burn lesions. Pain can be perceived up to 28 mm beyond the visible border of a lesion. Tissue touched on one side of the body may, at times, be perceived on the contralateral side. Therefore, identification of subtle lesions is essential, 2–3 cm margins are obtained on all specimens wherever possible, and both sides of the pelvis must be evaluated even if pain seems unilateral by history.

Coagulation

Coagulation is occasionally used, especially for superficial lesions of the ovary. When coagulating a lesion using ultrasonic energy, coagulation effect is maximized and cutting is minimized. There is an important difference between coagulating with ultrasonic energy and surface fulguration with electrical energy. With ultrasonic energy the blade will gradually burrow into the tissue leaving a defect that can be taken down to visible normal ovarian cortex. The ultrasonic blades that can be used for this purpose include the 10 mm laparosonic coagulating shears (LCS) using the blunt surface, the 5 mm LCS (straight or curved) using the tip or side, and the 5 mm hook using the side or the outer convex blunt surface. The blade is applied with light pressure on the tissue. A back and forth brushing technique, at either level 3 or level 5, is used until the desired depth of penetration has been achieved. This is a very easy, safe, and effective technique for superficial lesions involving the ovarian cortex. Deep invasive ovarian lesions need complete excision. Coagulation of small superficial lesions of the ovarian cortex is less traumatic to the ovary and avoids removal of any more ovarian cortex than necessary.

Excision

Excision of pelvic endometriosis starts with identifying and documenting all areas to be removed. It is necessary to delineate the lesion and note its location relative to the bladder, ureter, bowel and blood vessels. The uterus is elevated with a uterine manipulator. The ovary on the same side as the disease is lifted up with a forceps from the contralateral side. The LCS is used through the trocar site ipsilateral to the disease being excised. The LCS slides under and holds up the ovary. Normal peritoneum, approximately 2–3 cm beyond the border of the lesion to be excised, is then picked up by the grasping forceps and held away from the pelvic sidewall. The grasping forceps should only be holding peritoneum. The LCS incises the elevated fold of peritoneum to gain entry to the retroperitoneal space. A bubbling up, or cavitational effect, will often be seen as the harmonic scalpel gains entry into the retroperitoneal space. The initial peritoneal incision should be small so as to avoid bleeding when entering the retroperitoneal space. Once under direct vision it is safe to take larger, more efficient bites. Whenever the exact location of the ureter and nearby vessels is uncertain, it is better to stay with small cautious bites until the vital structures are identified. Time is often spent waiting to see ureteral peristalsis through the peritoneum. Time can be saved, and safety increased, by ureterolysis so that the ureter can be observed during the dissection. For superficial disease, ureterolysis is usually not necessary. For deep invasive disease with extensive fibrosis, ureterolysis is essential.

Pneumodissection by the ultrasonic energy further lifts the peritoneum, thereby facilitating the dissection into the retroperitoneal space. The LCS spreads the peritoneal opening and the grasping forceps is reapplied to the medial peritoneal edge. Excision is performed with the same traction/countertraction technique, regardless whether the energy source is laser, electrical or ultrasonic. The grasping forceps is positioned close to where the dissection is being performed. The LCS stays in normal tissue beyond the perimeter of the lesion being excised. The LCS stays in normal loose areolar tissue under the area being excised. Since the dissection is taken down to normal tissue, the resultant defect is the same regardless whether the disease was superficial or deep, and regardless whether the lesion was excised or vaporized.

When energy is applied, the LCS or harmonic scalpel is always lifted up away from the sidewall. Since the same instrument can both cut and coagulate, time is not wasted on changing instruments. Since ultrasonic energy has no spray, the LCS can only effect tissues it is in direct contact with. The LCS can be safely activated as it is applied to tissues and the energy maintained until the tissues are adequately coagulated and fall away from the blade. Wherever possible, full power is used with tissue on tension so that there will be minimal coagulation effect to adjacent tissues. Periodically during the dissection it is valuable to stop and reorient yourself to the anatomy. Ureteral peristalsis should be visualized and hemostasis confirmed when the procedure is completed.

Simple excision of mild endometriosis should be tried first (Figs 10.4, 10.5). As experience is gained and confidence increases, more difficult lesions can then be approached. Laparoscopic suturing is an important skill to acquire. A thorough understanding of pelvic anatomy is essential to the safe performance of these procedures. Anatomy is a topic that one never stops learning. Surgical procedures should be efficient but the focus should be on careful dissection of the anatomy and safe performance of the procedure. Nothing is gained by performing a quick procedure that does not remove all the endometriotic disease present. With time and practice, surgery becomes more efficient, and more difficult dissections are accomplished in less time. The harmonic scalpel and LCS are safe, easy to use instruments, and are an excellent modality with which to treat endometriosis.

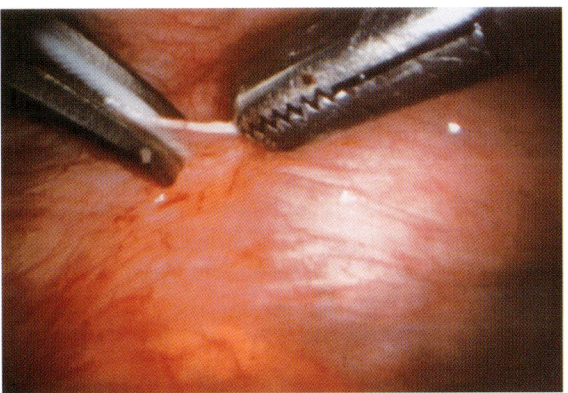

Figure 10.4
Left pelvic sidewall peritoneum is lifted up on tension to be incised with the 10 mm curved laparosonic coagulating shears. Reproduced with permission from Robbins ML, Excision of endometriosis with laparoscopic coagulating shears. J Am Assoc Gynecol Laprasc, 1999 May;6(2):199–203.

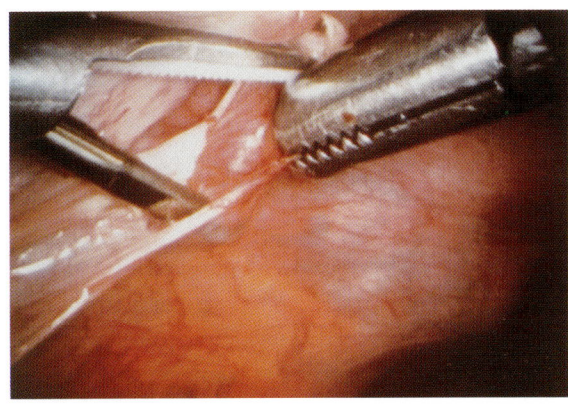

Figure 10.5
The left pelvic sidewall peritoneum has been opened and the retroperitoneal space is entered. The laparosonic coagulating shears spreads the opening while the grasping forceps is repositioned to hold the medial peritoneal edge. Reproduced with permission from Robbins ML, Excision of endometriosis with laparoscopic coagulating shears. J Am Assoc Gynecol Laprasc, 1999 May;6(2):199–203.

SURGICAL MANAGEMENT OF ENDOMETRIOSIS

Excision with ultrasonic energy in difficult situations

Ovary adherent to pelvic sidewall

In this situation, it is helpful to separate the ovary from the pelvic sidewall, and then approach these areas separately. At the time the first incision is made between the ovary and the adherent sidewall the location of the ureter is often not known. Entry into the retroperitoneal space is the essential first step. The ovary is lifted up on tension. An incision is made through peritoneum only, at the junction where the ovary meets the sidewall. When the retroperitoneal space is entered the ureter can be identified, then carefully isolated from the disease process, and kept in view during the dissection. Once in the right plane the ovary can be advanced with sharp and blunt dissection. The harmonic scalpel works well here since it only effects the tissues it is in direct contact with, at full power with a shear blade there is minimal lateral thermal spread, and there is no spray of energy.

Periureteral fibrosis

Endometriosis of the bladder flap and on the pelvic sidewall over the ureter is common, but invasive endometriosis of the ureter and/or bladder is seen in approximately only 1% of endometriosis cases.[9] The ureter and peritoneum comprise the first layer of the pelvic sidewall. But in a given patient, the ureter, on one or both sides, may lay close to the peritoneum or dive deeper in the pelvic sidewall. The ureter can, in most cases, be found fairly easily at the pelvic brim and then traced downwards. For deep invasive disease with extensive fibrosis, ureterolysis is essential (Fig. 10.6). I have found a curved dissector, such as the Everest bipolar dissector (BiCOAG Bipolar Dissecting Forceps, Everest Medical, Minneapolis,

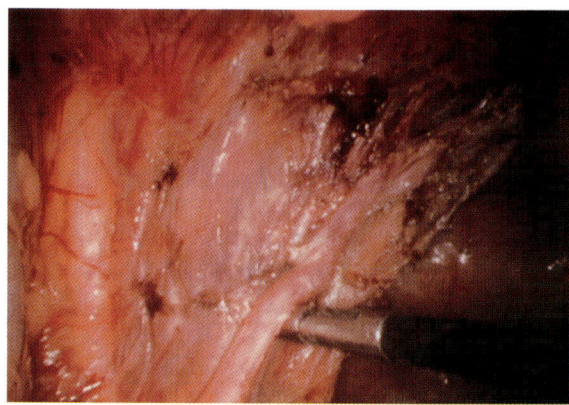

Figure 10.6
Left pelvic sidewall excision with left ureterolysis

MN), extremely helpful in dissecting the retroperitoneal space and isolating the ureter. If fibrosis is right up to the ureteral wall, a scissors without energy may be the safer approach. As long as the harmonic scalpel is not directly touching the ureter, using a shear blade with full power and lifting up away from the ureter, it is an excellent safe tool for this dissection.

Endometriosis over the external iliac vessels

Although working in this area is a cause for concern, excision here is actually relatively easy. The peritoneum is loose and visualization is good. The key point is to lift up, and incise, peritoneum only. As always, start in adjacent normal tissue. The cavitational effect of the ultrasonic energy will lift up the lesion with the peritoneum. Gently push down the underlying loose areolar tissue and work your way around the lesion.

Appendix

The mesoappendix can be taken with a stapler, bipolar cautery or the laparosonic coagulating shears (LCS). I use the 5 mm curved LCS at level

3 on the mesoappendix. I do not have to worry about bleeding from staple lines or lateral thermal damage. There can be bleeding if the vibrating ultrasonic blade bounces into the appendiceal vessels. Bleeding can be avoided by making sure the LCS is completely across the vessels before energy is applied. The base of the appendix is easily divided with endoloops or stapler. When endoloops are used, the LCS can be used to cut across the appendiceal base. The LCS will weld the specimen closed and coagulate the cut edge as it transects the appendiceal base, which has already been tied off. If the appendix looks abnormal, is difficult to get to, or if the patient has a history of Crohn's disease, then I would recommend asking a general surgeon to perform the appendectomy.

Intestinal involvement

Approximately 5–10% of patients with endometriosis have intestinal involvement, with over 70% involving the rectosigmoid colon.[10] Intestinal involvement is suspected preoperatively in less than half of the patients with intestinal endometriosis. The goal with intestinal endometriosis is complete excision of endometriosis and its reactive fibrotic component, and to restore normal anatomy. Treatment of colorectal endometriosis has been extensively reviewed by Jerby et al.[11]

For superficial implants without muscularis invasion, superficial excision is all that is needed and, when necessary, the area is oversewn. For lesions with deep infiltration into the muscularis and/or submucosal fibrosis, this can be treated with full-thickness disc excision and the defect is then closed. When there is a bowel nodule greater than 3 cm or multiple nodules, then laparoscopic segmental colectomy or proctectomy is done with end-to-end anastomosis (Figs 10.7–10.9).[11,12] Managing intestinal endometriosis is essential to getting the patient better and avoiding subsequent surgery. Gynecologists can manage superficial lesions of the bowel wall. For any significant bowel work a general and/or colorectal surgeon should always be involved. The LCS is very helpful with dissection of the pararectal space and mobilizing the mesentery of the bowel.

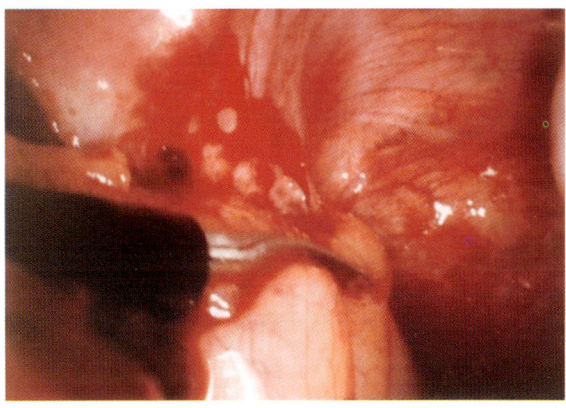

Figure 10.7

Deep invasive endometriosis of the rectosigmoid colon. The colon is densely adherent to the left uterosacral ligament and initially freed with scissors using no energy

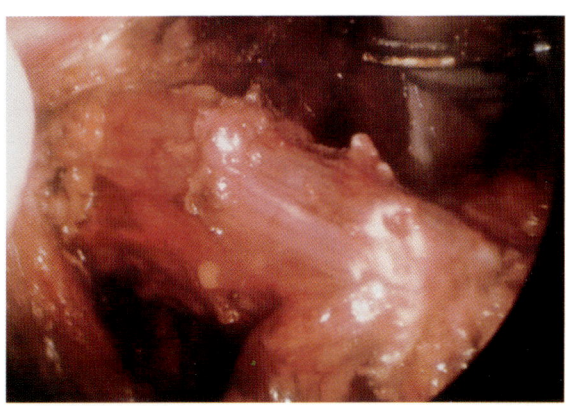

Figure 10.8

The longitudinal muscle fibers of the rectum are seen. The rectum has been completely mobilized distal to the areas of endometriosis

SURGICAL MANAGEMENT OF ENDOMETRIOSIS

Obliteration of the cul de sac

Two or more organs densely adherent are the hallmark of invasive endometriotic disease. Endometriosis is often found within the adhesions. Starting in normal tissue the disease needs to be removed en bloc, including the fibrosis between the organs. Often, a portion of the uterosacral ligaments needs to be excised with the specimen. Ureterolysis is generally necessary.

The LCS is safe and efficient at ureterolysis, dissecting out the uterosacral ligaments, and dissecting the disease off the rectal wall and the posterior aspect of the uterus. There is the risk of entering the bowel, but just separating the organs would leave disease on both sides. Traction/countertraction technique and always lifting up away from the bowel wall will help avoid problems. It may be necessary to oversew the bowel wall after the dissection is completed. A probe in the rectum, and a hand or probe in the vaginal canal will help delineate tissue planes. Inspection with fluid in the pelvis and air in the rectum can be done when the procedure is completed.

Bladder adherent to the uterus

Again, the endometriosis needs to be removed en bloc, including the fibrosis between the bladder and the uterus. The cavitational effect with the harmonic scalpel works nicely on the bladder flap peritoneum. Accessing the anterior uterine wall is more difficult because the serosa is more adherent. When there is extensive fibrosis between the bladder and uterus it may be helpful to periodically distend, retrograde via the Foley, the bladder to better delineate the bladder wall. Ultrasonic energy is a very safe energy

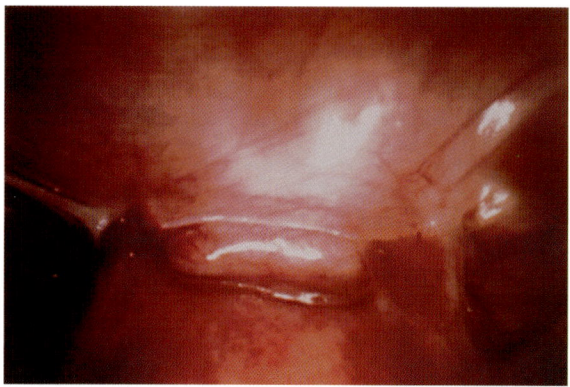

Figure 10.10
Invasive endometriosis of the bladder flap

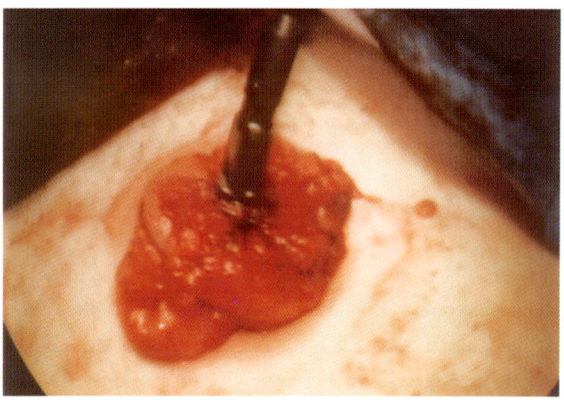

Figure 10.9
The colon has been exteriorized and the diseased bowel has been removed. The anvil of the circular stapler has been positioned in the proximal colon and is held in place with a purse-string suture

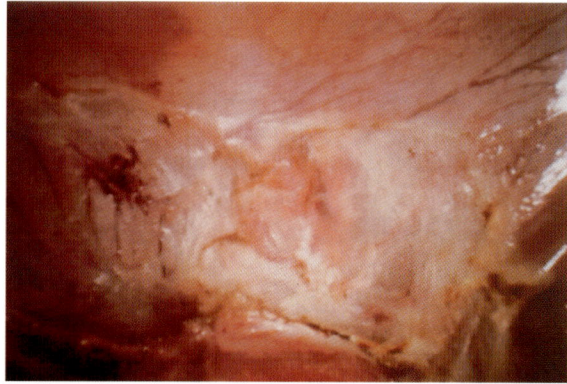

Figure 10.11
Completed excision of bladder flap endometriosis down to normal areolar tissue. The bladder wall is seen centrally

when working in this close proximity to the bladder (Figs 10.10, 10.11). It may be necessary to oversew the uterine wall after the dissection is completed.

Endometriosis on the diaphragm

For patients with cyclic chest pain and endometriosis on the diaphragm (Fig. 10.12) the disease must be excised if the patient is to get relief. A liver retractor is essential, but has to be handled gently so as to minimize subcapsular hematoma. Through-and-through holes in the diaphragm are well tolerated (Fig. 10.13) and at an abdominal pressure of 10 mmHg there was no drop in oxygen saturation. Holes were repaired with 2-0 Ethibond sutures tied intracorporeally (Fig. 10.14). One has to be very cautious when excising under the heart. This is another area where the harmonic scalpel is an excellent safe modality to use. When working close to the heart it was helpful to have a modality which was hemostatic, but with no electrical current through the patient. This dissection is always done in conjunction with general and/or thoracic surgeons. The gynecologist has a better understanding of endometriosis and can help guide the surgeons on how to best excise this disease.

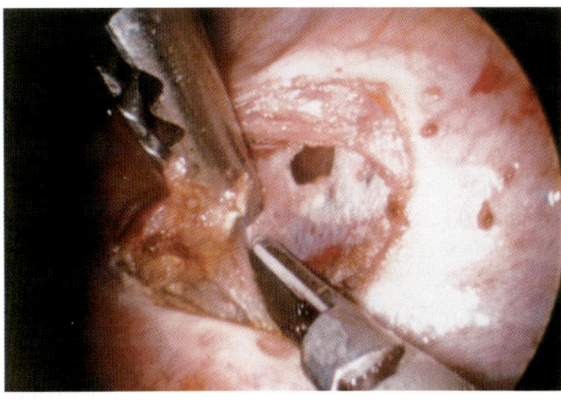

Figure 10.13
Endometriosis is excised from the right hemidiaphragm. A small opening into the right pleural space is seen

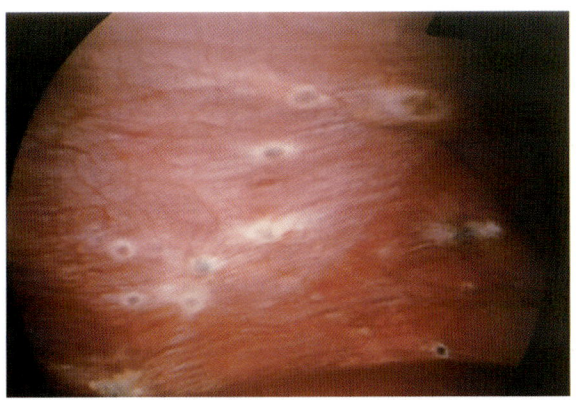

Figure 10.12
Clusters of endometriosis on the right hemidiaphragm

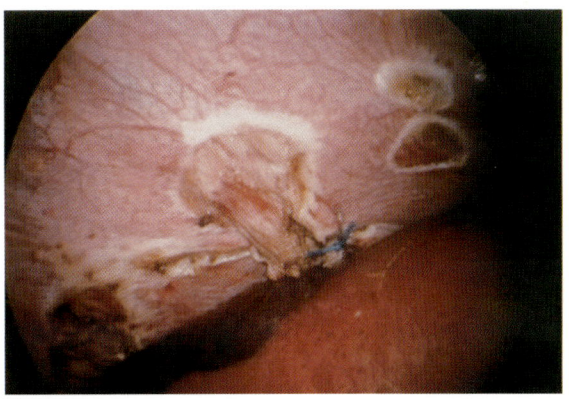

Figure 10.14
Completed excision of the right hemidiaphragm. Three openings into the right pleural space were repaired with 2-0 Ethibond

References

1. Fowler DL. Use of the harmonic in laparoscopic surgery. Abstract. XVIIIes Journées niçoises Pathologie et Chirugie Digestives Video-Laparoscopie, Nice, February 1995.
2. McCarus SD. Physiologic mechanism of the ultrasonically activated scalpel. J Am Assoc Gynecol Laparosc 1996;2(4):601–8.
3. Amaral JF. Cutting and coagulating with ultrasonic energy. Abstract. In: Third International Congress on New Technology and Advanced Techniques in Surgery, Luxembourg, June 1995.
4. Fowler DL. Use of the ultrasonically activated scalpel and shears in endoscopic surgery. Abstract. In: Third International Congress on New Technology and Advanced Techniques in Surgery, Luxembourg, June 1995.
5. Hambley R, Hebda PA, Abell E et al. Wound healing of skin incisions produced by ultrasonically vibrating knife, scalpel, electrosurgery, and carbon dioxide laser. J Dermatol Surg Oncol 1988;14:1213–17.
6. Heller DS, Reich H, Rosenberg J et al. J Am Assoc Gynecol Laparosc 1999;6(3):303–6.
7. Robbins ML, Sunshine TJ. Metastatic carcinoid diagnosed at laparoscopic excision of pelvic endometriosis. J Am Assoc Gynecol Laparosc 2000;7(2):251–3.
8. Demco L. Review of pain associated with minimal endometriosis. J Laparoendoscopic Surg 2000;4:5–9.
9. Nezhat C, Nezhat F, Nezhat CH et al. Urinary tract endometriosis treated by laparoscopy. Fertil Steril 1996;66:920–4.
10. Varol N, Maher P, Woods R. Laparoscopic management of intestinal endometriosis. J Am Assoc Gynecol Laparosc 2000;7(3):405–9.
11. Jerby BL, Kessler H, Falcone T et al. Laparoscopic management of colorectal endometriosis. Surg Endosc 1999;13:1125–8.
12. Redwine DB, Koning M, Sharpe DR. Laparoscopically assisted transvaginal segmental resection of the rectosigmoid colon for endometriosis. Fertil Steril 1996;65:193–7.

11

Ovarian endometriosis
David B Redwine

The ovaries are not the most common area of the pelvis to be involved by endometriosis, and almost all patients with ovarian disease will have disease in other pelvic or intestinal locations. Ovarian endometriosis is a marker for the presence of more severe pelvic and intestinal disease than exists in women without ovarian involvement.[1] Thus, one of the most important clinical features of ovarian endometriosis is that if a surgeon treats only ovarian disease, then incomplete treatment will almost certainly have occurred.

Sampson[2] postulated that endometrioma cysts might be due to invasion of a corpus luteum cyst by endometriosis from the ovarian cortex, while Russell[3] raised the possibility of embryonic Müllerian rests.

Symptoms

Ovarian endometrioma cysts may cause symptoms by several mechanisms in some cases but not others. Cysts of any size may cause ipsilateral pain or no pain at all due to stretching of the ovarian cortex. If the ovary is encased in adhesions that are stretched by growth of a cyst, then pain may occur. If an ovarian endometrioma cyst leaks, the chocolate-colored fluid is a potential irritant to the pelvis, in which case, patients may have an acute episode of severe pain that declines over several days, or even to the diaphragm, in which case, chest or shoulder pain may occur. Because women with ovarian endometriosis usually have other disease present, it is difficult to determine the precise contribution of the ovarian disease to the constellation of symptoms possible with endometriosis.

Superficial lesions of endometriosis on the cortex of the ovary appear to be asymptomatic.

Diagnosis

Superficial endometriosis of the ovarian cortex requires surgery for diagnosis. Ovarian cysts greater than 3 cm in diameter can potentially be felt on pelvic examination in patients of normal weight, while cysts of any size may be identified by imaging tests which may also suggest the nature of the fluid. Surgical diagnosis is somewhat inaccurate, as it has long been known that a corpus luteum cyst can masquerade as an endometrioma cyst.[2] Histology ultimately supplies the most accurate diagnosis.

Many endometrioma cysts are self-contained within the stroma and cortex of the ovary. Some 'endometrioma cysts' are actually collections of bloody fluid trapped between peritoneum and an adjacent adherent ovary, with a portion of the cyst wall being the normal ovarian cortex which is sometimes involuted around the fluid pocket. The relative frequency of each of these types of ovarian processes is not known. What is known, however, is that neither process alone is responsible for all lesions which may be termed 'endometrioma cysts'.

SURGICAL MANAGEMENT OF ENDOMETRIOSIS

Treatment

Endometrioma cysts do not respond well to medical therapy and surgery is the best treatment for resolution. Several surgical techniques are available. It is important that there are no obvious signs suggestive of ovarian malignancy before treating an endometrioma cyst. If doubt exists, a frozen section diagnosis during surgery may be helpful.

Superficial hemorrhagic adhesions may not be true endometriosis, and these are best treated by superficial desiccation by electrofulguration or similar mild ablative technique. These adhesions will be seen to shrink rapidly when treated.

Superficial lesions of endometriosis are typically less than 2 cm in dimension and can be treated by laser or electrovaporization or cortical excision. Some apparently superficial lesions may be located over a deeper small 'chocolate cyst' which may or may not be an endometrioma cyst.

Endometrioma cysts can be treated by either ovarian cystectomy or draining and ablation of the cyst wall. Ovarian cystectomy is associated with lower rates of recurrence or persistence of cysts,[4] since thermal ablation of the interior of large cysts to a consistent depth of complete destruction seems problematic.

A convenient site on the exposed ovarian cortex is chosen (Fig. 11.1). Since these cysts are frequently somewhat immobile because of underlying adhesions to the sidewall or uterosacral ligament, there usually is little choice in where the initial incision is made. Creating the incision alongside the mid portion of the adjacent fallopian tube will keep the dissection away from the fimbriae and protect them from inadvertent surgical damage. After the cortical incision is made, the cyst wall is exposed and it is punctured in turn, with the inevitable escape of chocolate-colored fluid (Fig. 11.2). The bloody fluid is suctioned and the pelvis and

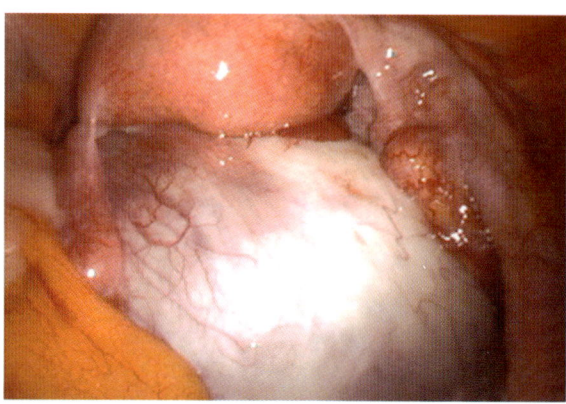

Figure 11.1

A large left ovarian endometrioma cyst is present. It is immobile because it is adherent to the underlying uterosacral ligament. This is not an ovarian pseudocyst after Runge/Hughesdon/Brosens. There is little choice of where to make an incision in the cortex. The incision obviously should not be made across the vessels of the mesovarium, and an incision too far around the side will be difficult to make and risks damage to the underlying bowel

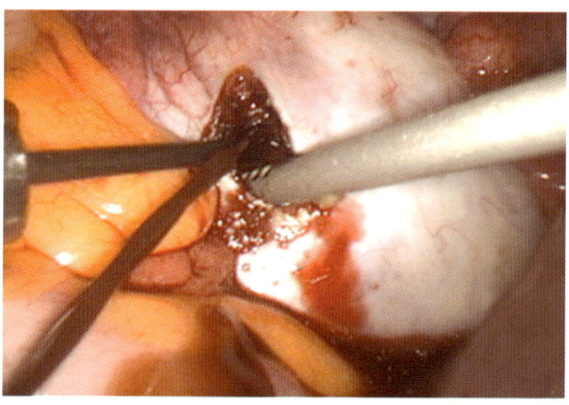

Figure 11.2

A cortical incision has been made in an area which is en face to the visual axis of surgery. The incision has been carried down into the underlying cyst and watery chocolate-colored fluid is spewing out under pressure

interior of the cyst are rinsed with irrigation fluid. The cyst wall can be visually inspected and much of it will be seen to be smooth, flat and colorless (Fig. 11.3), with endometriosis present

OVARIAN ENDOMETRIOSIS

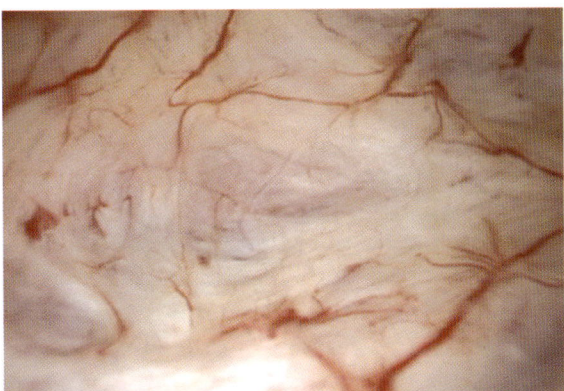

Figure 11.3

The interior of the cyst is composed largely of a fibrotic lining with no endometriosis

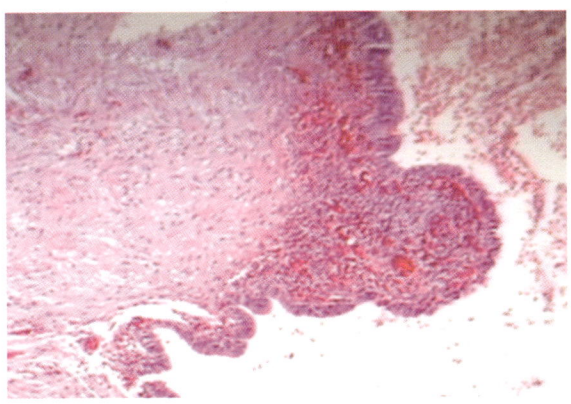

Figure 11.5

Microscopy of one of the reddish papules in Fig. 11.4 shows endometrium-like epithelium overlying a hemorrhagic stroma

only in discrete areas in a portion of the wall (Figs 11.4, 11.5). The cyst wall is then bluntly teased and dissected out of the ovarian stroma using two graspers. This is easy because frequently the cyst wall is fibrotic, which allows strong traction to be used during cystectomy. The healthy ovarian stroma is reddish in color compared to the greyish-white color of the cyst wall (Fig. 11.6). When the cyst is large (Figs 11.1, 11.7) the topography of its removal can be confusing. As the cyst is extracted, the ovarian cortex can become inverted and pulled out of the

incision site as well. It is important to maintain the cleavage plane which was initiated and to observe the medial side of the ovarian cortex to ensure that cortex is not being resected. Many endometrioma cysts are densely adherent to the adjacent uterosacral ligament (Fig. 11.8), and this correlates with the area of the cyst which is most difficult to remove as the cyst wall is fused to the cortex and both are fused to the uterosacral ligament. Continuing attempts at ovarian cystectomy through the initial cortical

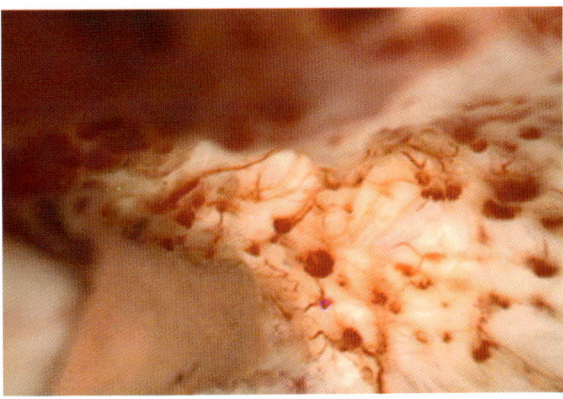

Figure 11.4

Endometriosis will be present as punctate reddish papules in certain areas of the cyst wall

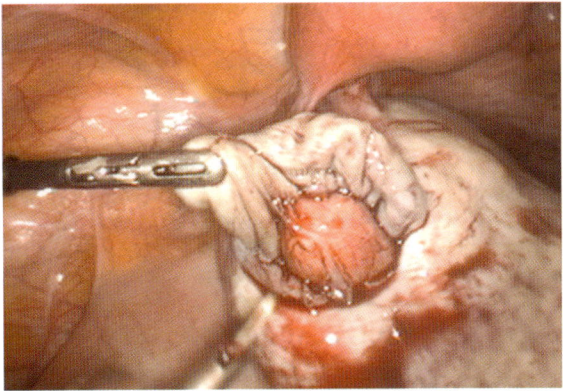

Figure 11.6

The greyish-white ovarian cyst wall is bluntly dissected away from healthy normal reddish ovarian tissue

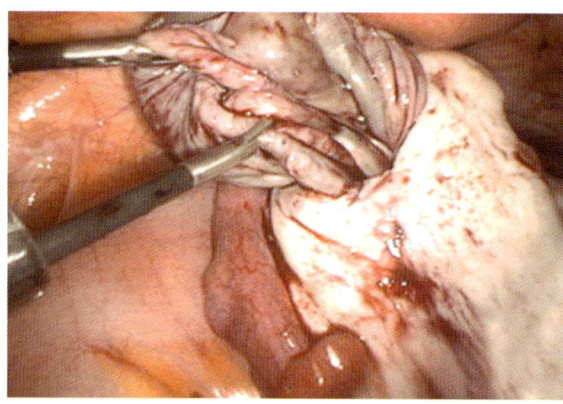

Figure 11.7

Large ovarian endometrioma cysts are easy to dissect out because the cyst wall is thick and fibrotic. At some point, however, progress will cease because the bottom of the cyst is fused to the uterosacral ligament

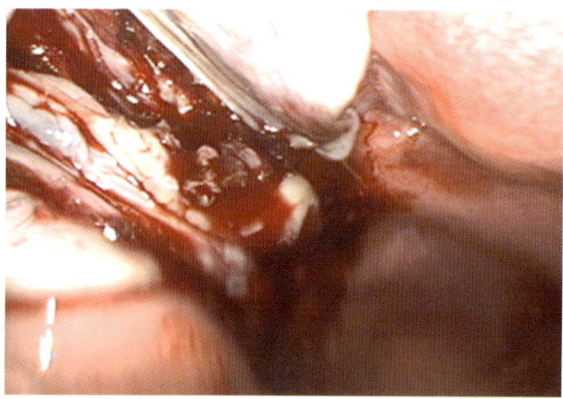

Figure 11.8

The left ovary is densely adherent to the left uterosacral ligament and the bottom of the cyst wall is fused at this point as well. This fusion of the cyst wall, ovarian cortex and uterosacral ligament is what will cause many easy cystectomies to become difficult

incision will be difficult or unsuccessful because of this area of mass tissue fusion. Once the surgeon realizes that ovarian cystectomy has reached a dead end because of this feature, it is frequently easier to attack the area of tissue fusion directly. The area of tissue fusion can be resected en bloc as one specimen which contains the uterosacral ligament, the area of the cortex adherent to the ligament, and the area of the cyst wall which is fused to each (Figs 11.9–11.11). This frees up the ovary considerably as well as the deepest part of the cyst wall which can now continue to be extracted easily.

If the ovary is not adherent, there frequently will be a stellate scarred area of previous cyst leakage. This corresponds to the site of attachment to the uterosacral ligament if a cyst were adherent as described above. It is at this point that endometriosis of the ovarian cortex may be present. This cicatrix of the cortex should be removed with adequate margins into normal cortical tissue, similar in effect to the en bloc resection described above for the point of mass tissue fusion. This will allow the chocolate-colored contents of the cyst to escape. After suctioning and irrigating the released fluid, the cyst

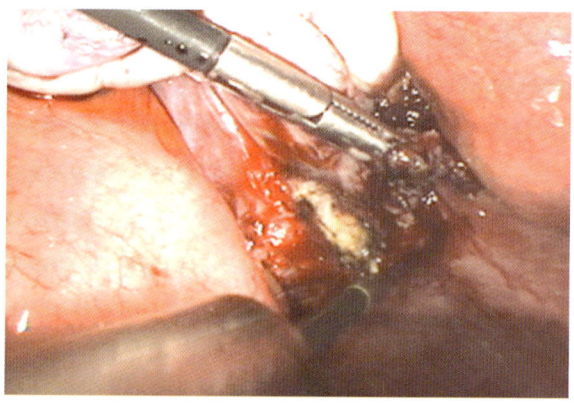

Figure 11.9

The fused, adherent part of the ovary is amputated from the remainder of the ovary. This allows the ovary to be freed up while the fused tissue is still attached to the uterosacral ligament for later removal with that ligament. This frame shows the beginning stage of this amputation process. The scissors have begun to make an electrosurgical incision across normal peritoneum just lateral to the left uterosacral ligament. The area of tissue fusion is held medially and anteriorly by the graspers in counter traction

OVARIAN ENDOMETRIOSIS

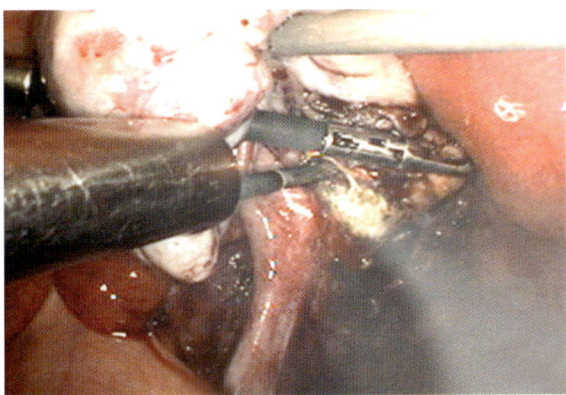

Figure 11.10
The incision across the left broad ligament continues until the scissors explore the normal retroperitonal space beneath the adherent ovary. The area of fusion is held by the graspers

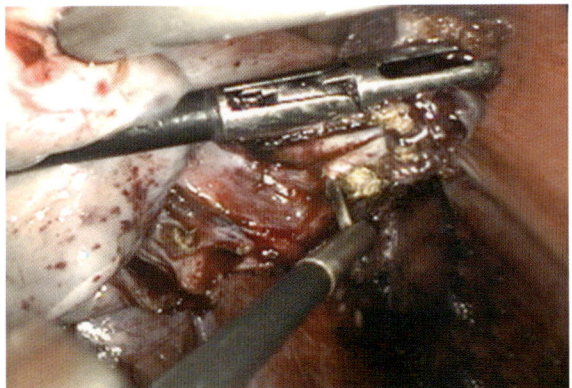

Figure 11.11
The remaining attachments of the ovarian cortex and cyst wall are amputated from the area of fusion still held in the graspers

If the ovary is adherent to the pelvic sidewall, the peritoneum hidden under the adhesions may harbor endometriosis. Retroperitoneal fibrosis immediately beneath the adherent ovary may invest the underlying ureter (Fig. 11.12), so difficult ureterolysis is sometimes necessary (Fig. 11.13). Surgery on the ovary combined with a sidewall dissection can produce dense postoperative adhesions which can cause the ovary to fuse to the underlying ureter, making reoperation more difficult. Suspending the ovary from the ipsilateral round ligament with a single suture of 3-0 Vicryl or similar small absorbable suture can keep the ovary from adhering to the sidewall (Fig. 11.14).

A variant of an ovarian endometrioma cyst consists of the Runge/Hughesdon/Brosens pseudocyst, in which bloody fluid is trapped between the adherent ovary and the pelvic sidewall. Continued production of bloody fluid by superficial endometriosis of the ovarian cortex

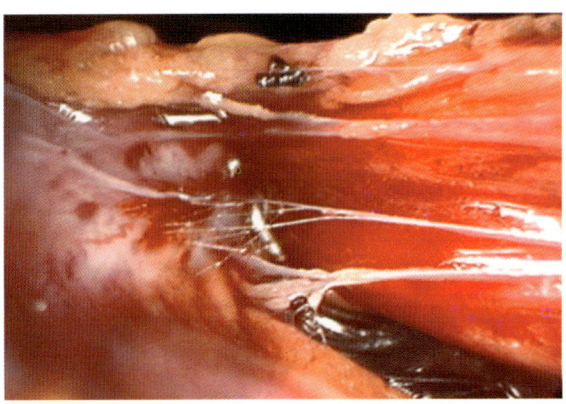

Figure 11.12
The right ureter is seen in close-up view in the right half of the frame. Tendrils of light fibrosis bind the ureter to the under surface of the peritoneum on the left half of the frame. The peritoneum is thickened, although that is not apparent from the image. Not visible out of the frame to the left is an ovarian endometrioma cyst which was itself adherent to the peritoneum. The tendrils of fibrosis in this case are mild and scanty, so ureterolysis will be easy

can be extracted through the opening that has been created. Sometimes the cyst wall will be difficult to grasp as it may remain somewhat fused to the cicatricial opening. In such cases, it is helpful to cut an incision into the normal cortex a few millimeters away from the opening. This provides a convenient traction 'handle' of normal cortex which allows easier entry into the plane between the cyst wall and the overlying cortex.

SURGICAL MANAGEMENT OF ENDOMETRIOSIS

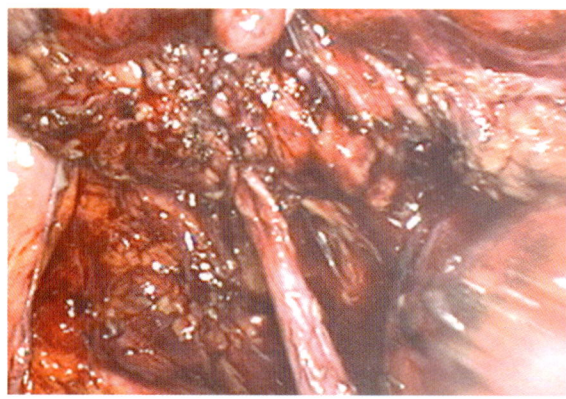

Figure 11.13
Sometimes, the retroperitoneal fibrosis involving the ureter can be massive. In this case, the left ureter seems to proceed directly into a retroperitoneal mass of fibrosis and adherent, invasive ovarian tissue

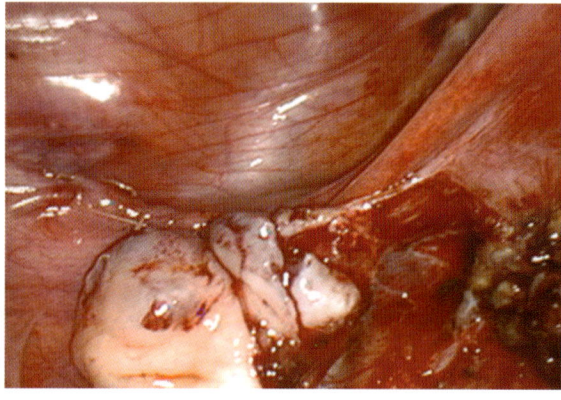

Figure 11.14
The left ovary has been suspended from the left round ligament using 3-0 Vicryl suture. A triangular hammock has been created so the ovary can be reconstituted and suspended with only one suture

causes accumulation of an increasing volume of fluid which is thought to progressively indent the ovarian cortex, resulting in a portion of the cyst wall being formed by ovarian cortex which is largely normal. The treatment of such a cyst consists simply of ovariolysis with freeing of the fluid and destruction of the areas of the cortex thought to represent endometriosis. The concept of formation of such a type of cyst is not new. Sampson[2] mentioned an earlier report by Runge from the German literature where this concept was proved by serial section study, which was later repeated by Hughesdon,[5] with the topic recently championed by Brosens.[6] It can sometimes be difficult to distinguish between these two morphologies of ovarian endometriosis, which can affect an intended conservative treatment.

A proposed benefit of the Brosens treatment of an ovarian endometrioma pseudocyst is that it preserves oocytes and ovarian function and thus protects fertility. This protective concept has been rendered a somewhat moot point since investigators have found that women undergoing ovarian cystectomy for treatment of endometriomas have a response to gonadotropins that is identical to women with only tubal factor infertility,[7] and others have found that the pregnancy rate is lower and the recurrence rate of cysts is higher if the ovarian cyst wall is not stripped out.[8]

Rarely, if a very large cyst or multiple endometrioma cysts are removed from an ovary, there will be but a paper-thin shell or shreds of cortex which may bleed and which is impossible to suture. In such a case, it may be best to perform a coup de grace and remove the remnant of ovarian tissue if the opposite ovary is salvageable.

Ovarian remnant syndrome

During difficult oophorectomy for removal of a densely adherent endometrioma, a portion of ovarian cortex may remain stuck behind to the sigmoid colon or pelvic sidewall (Figs 11.15, 11.16). This remnant of tissue can remain viable despite absence of a normal blood supply and undergo stimulation by pituitary hormones and regenerate sufficiently to be a continuing source

OVARIAN ENDOMETRIOSIS

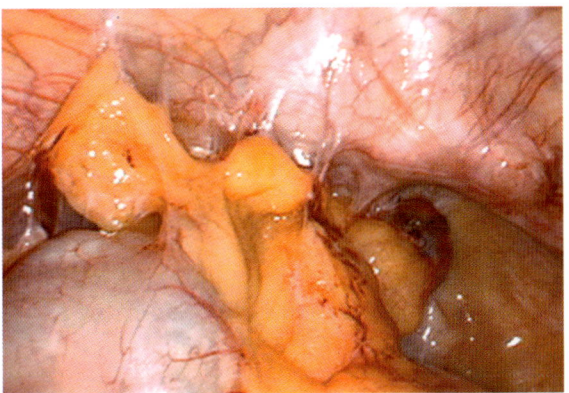

Figure 11.15

A cystic reddish ovarian remnant is seen adherent to the anterior sigmoid colon near the cul de sac

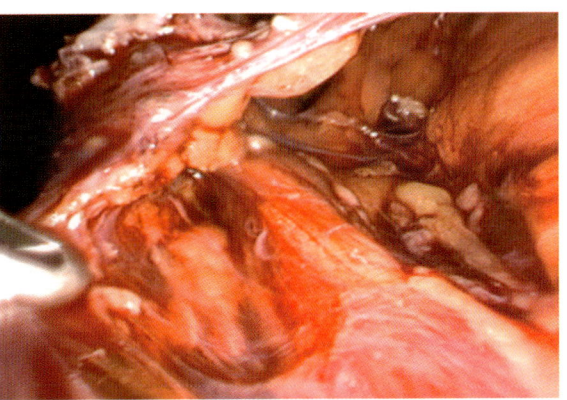

Figure 11.17

Retroperitoneal dissection beneath the ovarian remnant seen in Fig. 11.16. The right ureter is seen as it passes beneath the remnant, with retroperitoneal fibrosis binding it to the undersurface of the peritoneum immediately beneath the remnant. Ureterolysis will be necessary in such a case

of estrogen production or cyst formation. Ovarian remnants can also be a cause of pain, either by stretching of overlying adhesions by a cyst (Fig. 11.16), or by stimulation of residual endometriosis due to estrogen production. Prevention of the ovarian remnant syndrome is identical to its treatment: retroperitoneal dissection, frequently with ureterolysis, will allow removal of peritoneum of the pelvic sidewall with the adherent remnant or ovary still attached (Fig. 11.17).[9]

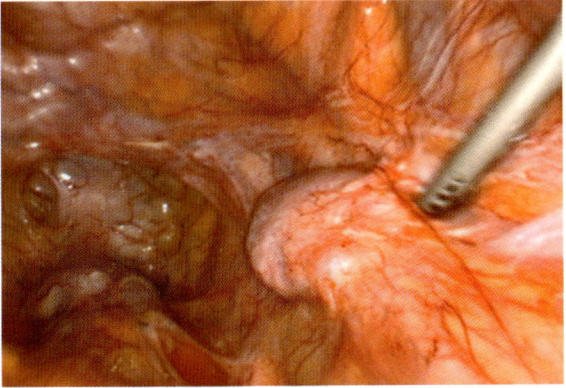

Figure 11.16

The suction irrigator points at an ovarian remnant of the right pelvic sidewall. Some ovarian remnants are endometriotic cysts

References

1. Redwine DB. Ovarian endometriosis: A marker for more severe pelvic and intestinal disease. Fertil Steril 1999;73:310–15.
2. Sampson JA. Perforating hemorrhagic (chocolate) cysts of the ovary. Arch Surg 1921;3:245–323.
3. Russell WW. Aberrant portions of the Muellerian duct found in an ovary. Johns Hopkins Hosp Bull 1899;10:8–10.
4. Fayez JA, Vogel MF. Comparison of different treatment methods of endometriomas by laparoscopy. Obstet Gynecol 1991;78:660–5.
5. Hughesdon PE. The structure of endometrial cysts of the ovary. J Obstet Gynaecol Br Emp 1957;44:481–7.
6. Brosens IA, Van Ballaer P, Puttemans P, Deprest J. Reconstruction of the ovary containing large endometriomas by an extraovarian endosurgical technique. Fertil Steril 1996;66:517–21.
7. Marconi G, Vilela M, Quintana R, Sueldo C. Laparoscopic ovarian cystectomy of endometriomas does not affect the ovarian response to gonadotropin stimulation. Fertil Steril 2002;78:876–8.
8. Beretta P, Franchi M, Ghezzi F, Busacca M, Zupi E, Bolis P. Randomized clinical trial of two laparoscopic treatments of endometriomas: cystectomy versus drainage and coagulation. Fertil Steril 1998;70:1175–80.
9. Rana N, Rotman C, Hasson HM, Redwine DB, Dmowski WP. Ovarian remnant syndrome after laparoscopic hysterectomy and bilateral salpingo-oophorectomy for severe pelvic endometriosis. J Am Assoc Gynecol Laparosc 1996;3:423–6.

12

Intestinal endometriosis
David B Redwine

History

The morphology of endometriosis ranges from the spectacular to the extremely subtle. Spectacular manifestations of any disease are most easily found, so the earliest descriptions of endometriosis naturally focus on cases with the maximal anatomic derangement and the most obvious physical and surgical findings. Endometriosis did not have a name at first because no one really knew much about it. Early cases of what might have been severe rectovaginal endometriosis were called 'posterior paravaginitis and parametritis with proliferation of epithelium.'[1] Surgeons finding extreme disease did not know by looking at it whether the nodular adhesive process they found was benign or malignant. The histological appearance, however, resembled a benign adenomyoma such as could be found diffusely or discretely in the uterine myometrium. Therefore, the earliest papers on endometriosis, including cases involving the intestinal tract, speak of the disease as an 'adenomyoma' to reflect the specific rubbery nodular morphology and microscopic appearance. 'Adenomyoma', 'deep endometriosis', 'severe endometriosis' and 'invasive endometriosis' are often used synonymously today which can seem confusing. The most impressive presentation of intestinal endometriosis is associated with obliteration of the cul de sac and associated rectal and vaginal involvement.

Early case reports

Stevens in 1910 presented to the Obstetrical and Gynaecological Section of the Royal Society of Medicine a case of adenomyoma of the posterior vaginal fornix.[2] On digital examination, the patient had two small hard nodules each about 6 mm in diameter. Excision was accomplished vaginally and was accompanied by 'some difficulty'. The histology was of interlacing bands of smooth muscle surrounding glandular structures resembling endometrium. There was no mention of accompanying severe rectal symptoms and the pelvic contents were not surveyed.

Cuthbert Lockyer in 1913 presented to the Royal Society two cases of adenomyomas invading the posterior vaginal fornix, one with 'teat-like' projections.[3] One patient was taken to surgery. Obliteration of the cul de sac with invasion of the anterior rectal wall by a benign adenomyomatous growth was found. The patient was treated by en bloc resection of the uterus still attached to the affected bowel segment, followed by diverting sigmoid colostomy. Illustrations of the gross and microscopic features of this case show unequivocally that this would be considered severe invasive endometriosis today. The rectal mucosa was intact. Lockyer guessed that this tumor must arise from rests of Wolffian duct origin, although he was to change his mind within two years. This must be one of the first reports in the English-speaking literature of endometriosis involving the intestinal tract.

DeJong, also in 1913, published a report of small bowel obstruction due to adenomyoma of the ileum.[4]

In 1914, Griffith presented a case of a pregnant woman with polyhydramnios and a tumor between the cervix and rectum, with invasion of the posterior vaginal fornix.[5] The tumor grew in size during pregnancy, and a vaginal biopsy showed glandular epithelium surrounded by decidual change which was surmised to arise from Müllerian duct rests. The tumor, as well as the uterine size, shrunk considerably after local implantation of radium for 20 hours.

Also in 1914, Leitch presented a case of an endometriotic nodule on the antimesenteric wall of the mid-sigmoid colon, 'the size of a Barcelona nut' which was found at surgery to be adherent to the posterior uterus, apparently without any rectal involvement.[6] After lysing the adhesions, the intestinal nodule was removed by segmental resection and anastomosis and microscopy clearly showed what today would be considered endometriosis invading the bowel wall to the submucosa. The area of the uterus to which the sigmoid had been adherent showed a fibrotic plaque which was removed and this also showed endometriosis. Leitch proposed that endometrium had migrated through the wall of the uterus and into the bowel wall, carrying with it the potential for formation of surrounding fibromuscular metaplasia. In the discussion that followed, Lockyer disavowed his former support of origin from Wolffian rests and introduced the concept of peritoneal epithelial metaplastic heteroplasia resulting from an inflammatory process, such as parametritis or 'pelvo-peritonitis'. Dr Leitch was unconvinced, having never seen any gross or microscopic evidence of inflammation. Leitch was also not swayed by Lockyer's previous argument for transformation from embryonic rests, stating that although fetal cells have some degree of totipotentiality: '(t)he cells composing (rests) manifestly age just the same as normal cells, and the embryonic potentialities for growth depart with their youth.' Leitch mentioned four cases of a similar condition which were reported by Sitzenfrey in 1909, but gave no reference.

Cullen published several papers between 1914 and 1920 which clearly illustrated and defined adenomyomas of the rectovaginal septum with obliteration of the cul de sac, rectal wall involvement and variable invasion of the cervix.[7–11] His usual treatment was by hysterectomy. This was performed by separation of the uterus from its lateral attachments followed by en bloc resection of the affected segment of rectum, with the uterus still adherent at the cervix to the anterior bowel wall, followed by colostomy. Occasionally, he would do staged procedures: a colostomy first, followed later by en bloc resection of the uterus and affected bowel segment. After performing this surgery on several patients, he concluded that: 'The removal of an extensive adenomyoma of the rectovaginal septum is infinitely more difficult than a (Wertheim) hysterectomy for carcinoma of the cervix.' This statement remains true today.

By 1922, Sampson had described adenomyoma of the appendix.[12] Sampson postulated, incorrectly, that intestinal adenomyomas occurred due to rupture of ovarian endometrioma cysts, with secondary seeding of the bowel, and that the cysts themselves were the result of reflux menstruation of endometrium first seeding the ovary resulting in a cyst. The existence of a leiomyomatous or adenomatous change in the bowel wall that could not be explained by implantation of endometrial epithelium apparently did not concern him, nor was he aware at that time of the multiple and often profound differences between endometrium and endometriosis which preclude consideration of endometriosis as an autotransplant.[13]

Endometriosis of the cecum is uncommon and the cecum is so large that obstructive symptoms are rare. This may explain why endometriosis of the cecum apparently did not enter the literature until much later.[14]

Sites of intestinal involvement

The sigmoid colon is most commonly involved, followed by the rectum, ileum, appendix and cecum (Table 12.1). There has been only one mention of endometriosis of the transverse colon, illustrated in schematic form.[15]

Some intestinal endometriosis is asymptomatic. Superficial disease of the bowel wall in any site does not typically produce symptoms, nor typically do small nodules less than 1 cm in diameter. Most disease of the appendix is asymptomatic, although cyclic catamenial right lower quadrant pain may rarely occur if the appendix is enlarged and hemorrhagic due to the effects of the disease. Intussusception of the appendix involved by endometriosis is a rare cause of abdominal pain, nausea and diarrhea.[16–20]

Table 12.1 Sites of intestinal involvement among 2473 patients treated at the Endometriosis Treatment Program, St. Charles Hospital, Bend, OR, USA

Intestinal site of involvement	No. of patients	% of 2473 total patients	% of 688 intestinal patients
Sigmoid	419	16.9	60.9
Rectum	322	13.0	46.8
Complete cul de sac obliteration	245	9.9	35.6
Partial cul de sac obliteration	35	1.4	5.1
No obliteration	42	1.7	6.1
Ileum	110	4.4	16.0
Appendix[a]	70	2.8	10.2
Cecum	38	1.5	5.5
Total patients with intestinal endometriosis	688[b]	27.8	100

[a] Some patients had previous appendectomy.
[b] The total of the column exceeds the total number of patients with intestinal disease because 200 patients had more than one intestinal site of involvement.

Symptoms

Symptoms due to lesions of intestinal endometriosis are related to their anatomic locations, depth of invasion of the endometrial-like glands and stroma with surrounding fibromuscular metaplasia ('adenomyoma'), and degree of distortion of the bowel wall and lumen. Since most patients with intestinal endometriosis frequently have endometriosis in multiple pelvic locations, it is sometimes difficult to know what symptoms are caused by the intestinal disease versus the pelvic disease.

Endometriosis involving the cecum only occasionally produces right lower quadrant pain[21] and will not cause symptoms of obstruction because the cecal diameter is so large. Endometriosis of the ileum can cause crampy right lower quadrant pain if the lumen is distorted, or symptoms of complete bowel obstruction and malnutrition in extreme cases. Bowel obstruction due to endometriosis is almost always due to ileal obstruction,[22] occasionally involving the ileocecal valve, although rare cases of rectosigmoid obstruction have been reported.[23]

Pain or intestinal cramping in the left lower quadrant before bowel movements can be caused by nodular endometriosis of the rectosigmoid colon, either because of partial mechanical obstruction or perhaps by impeding the transmission of peristaltic waves. Symptoms can worsen prior to and during menses and complete obstruction is rare.[24]

Rectal nodules of endometriosis occur most commonly in association with obliteration of the cul de sac (Table 12.1) and can cause rectal pain with each bowel movement throughout the month as well as rectal pain with flatus, intercourse, or sitting. In contrast, endometriosis of the cul de sac or uterosacral ligaments without rectal involvement may cause painful bowel movements primarily during menses. Some patients can be quite specific in their description of 'something between the vagina and rectum'. Occasionally, a woman may be so bothered by pain that they have examined themselves vaginally and felt tender nodularity. Some with obliteration of the cul de sac and rectal wall involvement may complain of low grade fever, particularly with menses. Alternating constipation and diarrhea may affect some,[25] with aggravation of either symptom possible during menses. Cyclic rectal bleeding during menses is highly suggestive of significant intestinal endometriosis, but is uncommon. With increasing severity of intestinal endometriosis, there is an increase of the clinical diagnosis of irritable bowel syndrome.

Intestinal perforation associated with endometriosis, sometimes fatal, has occurred in pregnant and non-pregnant patients.[26–29]

Diagnosis

Barium enemas, ultrasound exams, colonoscopy and magnetic resonance imaging (MRI) or computed tomography (CT) scans are only occasionally positive in cases of intestinal endometriosis. This is because the disease begins on the serosal surface and either remains there or invades the muscularis to some varying extent but rarely involves the mucosa. Positive preoperative scans or endoscopy depends on a sufficient degree of distortion of the affected intestinal site.[24, 30–33] Occasionally, endoscopy may reproduce the patient's pain when an intestinal nodule is reached.

Physical examination can suggest the possibility of intestinal involvement by the presence of cul de sac nodularity associated with exquisite tenderness that may reproduce the patient's pain. Not all nodularity that may be found during surgery will be palpable on pelvic examination.[34, 35] In some patients, the posterior vaginal fornix is invaded by endometriosis advancing from an underlying nodule of the rectum or uterosacral ligament. When present, vaginal endometriosis can manifest simply as epithelial piling (the 'teat-like' structures of Lockyer) without discoloration, epithelial piling with bluish papules, or full-thickness involvement with a reddish polypoid surface which sometimes is bleeding. These manifestations of vaginal endometriosis are frequently missed on vaginal speculum examination in the office because the speculum has been used solely to examine the cervix and obtain cytology. The speculum should be directed posteriorly to examine the posterior fornix in all patients.

The most accurate diagnosis of intestinal endometriosis occurs during surgery and each potential area of intestinal involvement can usually be seen easily with the laparoscope. After examining the upper abdomen and diaphragm, the cecum and appendix are viewed.

Endometriosis of the appendix most commonly manifests as a whitish scarred area, either in the midportion of the appendix or near its tip, which causes the appendix to curl toward the scarring. Hemorrhagic changes are uncommon. One of the first impressions the surgeon may get

INTESTINAL ENDOMETRIOSIS

is that the appendix cannot be straightened out even with traction (Fig. 12.1) as it appears to be curled upon itself.

Endometriosis of the cecum is the rarest site of intestinal involvement and is frequently manifest by an area of yellowish fibrosis of the anterior wall of the cecum, sometimes immediately adjacent to the base of the appendix. Cecal endometriosis is usually associated with some hemorrhagic changes associated with superficial sheets of adhesions which trap blood and cause the formation of hemorrhagic blebs (Fig. 12.2), and must be distinguished from the rare case of cecal hemangiomas (Fig. 12.3).

The small bowel should be examined from the cecum proximally for about 40 cm. This can frequently be done with one atraumatic grasper to run the bowel, although some cases may require two atraumatic graspers for efficient investigation. Like intestinal endometriosis in other sites, endometriosis of the ileum primarily occurs on the antimesenteric border (Fig. 12.4), sometimes in a linear pattern which is the result of embryologic patterning. In cases where certain areas are very biologically active, the ileum folds upon itself and can produce constriction of the lumen

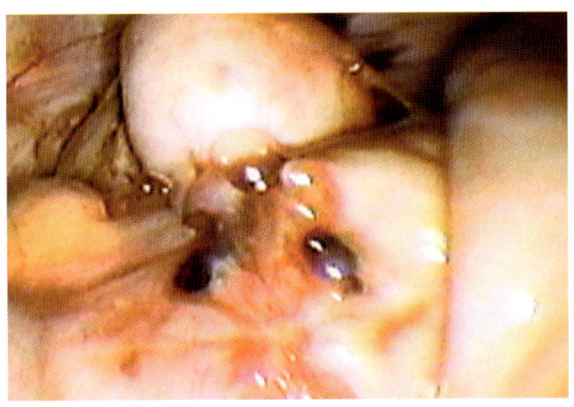

Figure 12.2
Endometriosis of the cecum and appendix. The swollen appendix is seen in the center top of the frame and hemorrhagic lesion of endometriosis of the cecum are located where the appendix joins the cecum. The wall of the cecum beneath the hemorrhagic changes is whitish and thickened

(Fig. 12.5). Occasionally, there are several discrete areas of such fibrotic folding, with normal bowel immediately adjacent to the nodules. There is usually no hypertrophy of the adjacent fatty mesentery. Frequently, there are associated smaller whitish plaques of superficial disease which can also be located on the antimesenteric

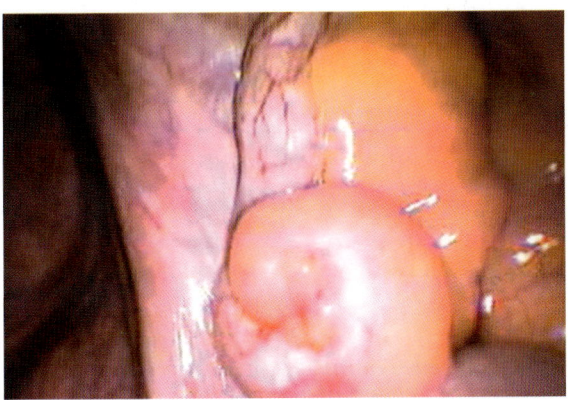

Figure 12.1
Endometriosis of the appendix. The tip of the appendix is thickened and curled upon itself. The visual appearance exhibits no significant hemorrhage

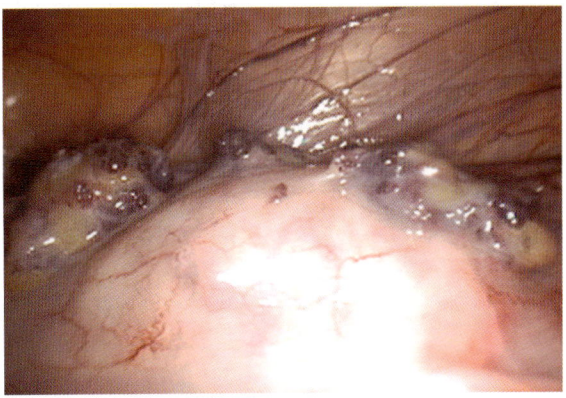

Figure 12.3
Superficial hemangiomas on the surface of the cecum are rare but could be confused with endometriosis since they are filled with dark red or purplish blood

SURGICAL MANAGEMENT OF ENDOMETRIOSIS

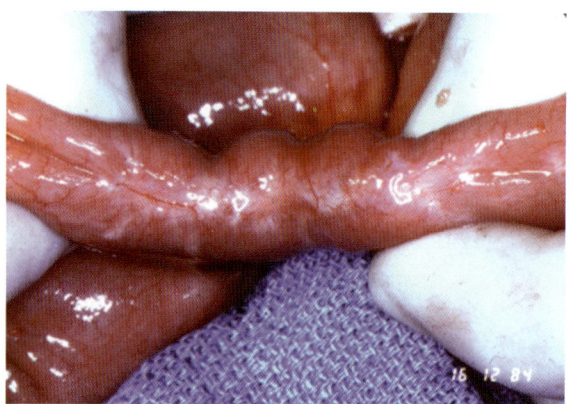

Figure 12.4
Endometriosis of the ileum is usually distributed along the exact antimesenteric border of the bowel. Note the small whitish nodules with subtle overlying neovascularity

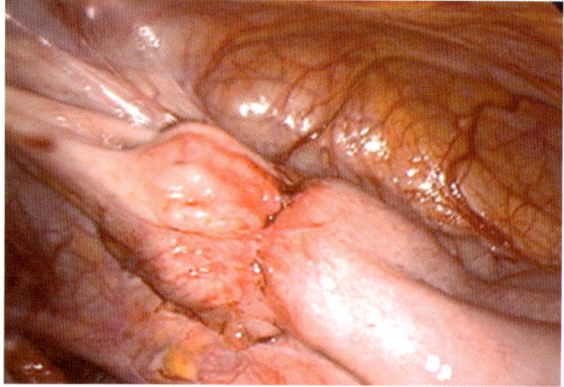

Figure 12.5
Obstructing lesion of endometriosis of the terminal ileum. This patient lost 25 pounds due to bowel obstruction over the course of 4 months. Intestinal barium studies were reported as negative and the patient was thought to have a psychogenic eating disorder. Nodules of endometriosis of the ileum tend to be discrete and are very firm

surface of the bowel, although some cases may display such small plaques on the sides of the ileal wall or on its mesentery. It is important to distinguish endometriosis of the ileum from Crohn's disease since both occur in the same region of bowel, although apparently never simultaneously. Crohn's disease manifests as an entire segment sometimes 15–20 cm in length of indurated, straight, hyperemic ileum with associated 'fat creeping' of the adjacent fatty mesentery completely along the length of the inflamed segment (Fig. 12.6). In either endometriosis or Crohn's disease of the ileum, mesenteric lymphadenopathy can be observed in the arc of mesentery draining the affected segment (Fig. 12.7).

Endometriosis of the sigmoid can be present as asymptomatic small superficial whitish or grayish macules with rare hemorrhagic change (Fig. 12.8). Like nodular ileal endometriosis, sigmoid nodules are located on the antimesenteric or anterior bowel wall and occur most commonly either immediately adjacent to the cul de sac reflection or in the mid-sigmoid several centimeters away. Rarely will two sigmoid nodules be present in the same patient. Sigmoid nodules are whitish due to the underlying fibromuscular hyperplasia and may have little or no hemorrhagic change. More commonly, the area of

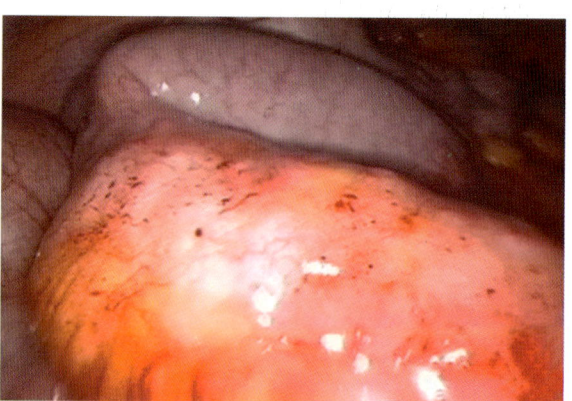

Figure 12.6
Crohn's disease of the terminal ileum involves several centimeters of bowel with a confluent erythematous change associated with a thickened bowel wall with reduced pliability. Notice the generalized hyperplasia of the appendix epiploica ('fat creeping') along the length of diseased bowel wall and the sudden change to normal bowel wall seen near the top of the frame

INTESTINAL ENDOMETRIOSIS

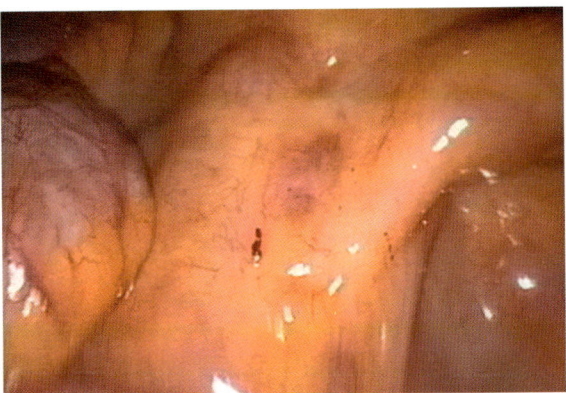

Figure 12.7
Either Crohn's disease or endometriosis of the ileum can be associated with mesenteric adenopathy, visible as discrete flesh-colored nodules within the mesenteric fat

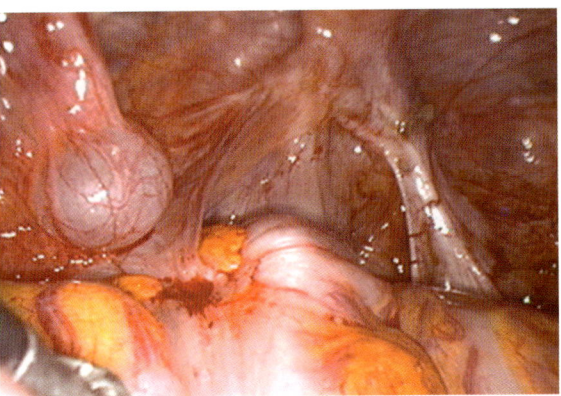

Figure 12.9
An endometriotic nodule of the mid-sigmoid colon is visible in the center of the frame. The bowel wall is nodular and whitish, particularly on the right side. In the midline of the anterior bowel wall, an area of hemorrhage is seen as well as localized hypertrophy of the appendix epiploica. This is the same patient with the ileal lesion seen in Fig. 12.4

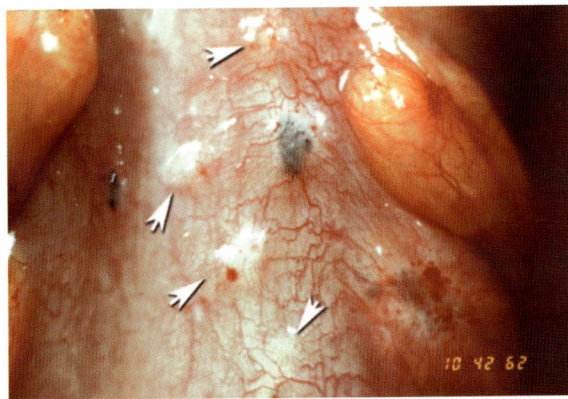

Figure 12.8
Superficial endometriosis of sigmoid colon. The four hemorrhagic lesions, two on the serosa and two on the appendix epiploica, catch the eye more easily than the four whitish nodules (arrows)

maximal fibrotic retraction of the anterior bowel wall in the center of the nodule will have hemorrhagic change and superficial sheets of hemorrhagic adhesions. There can be localized hypertrophy of the adjacent appendix epiploica on one or both sides of the bowel (Fig. 12.9).

Obliteration of the cul de sac occurs when the lower rectosigmoid colon is adherent to the posterior cervix and uterosacral ligaments. This condition is commonly associated with ovarian endometriomas which may hide the severe underlying pathology (Fig. 12.10). Although the morphology is one of adhesive change with slight overlying hemorrhagic changes along the line of adherence, obliteration of the cul de sac signifies the presence of invasive disease of the hidden surfaces, including the uterosacral ligaments, posterior cervix, and usually the anterior bowel wall. When the bowel is involved by nodular disease, the rectum will be rounded (Fig. 12.11). When the bowel wall is involved by little or no disease, the rectum will be flat as it joins the cervix (Fig. 12.12). Endometriosis of the vagina can occasionally be present with obliteration of the cul de sac. 'Endometriosis of the rectovaginal septum' may actually represent a slight misnomer which has been around for almost a century.[2,36] While extensive disease, such as can be found with obliteration of the cul de sac, can frequently be palpated between the fingertips during combined vaginal and rectal examination, the areolar tissue of the septum is

SURGICAL MANAGEMENT OF ENDOMETRIOSIS

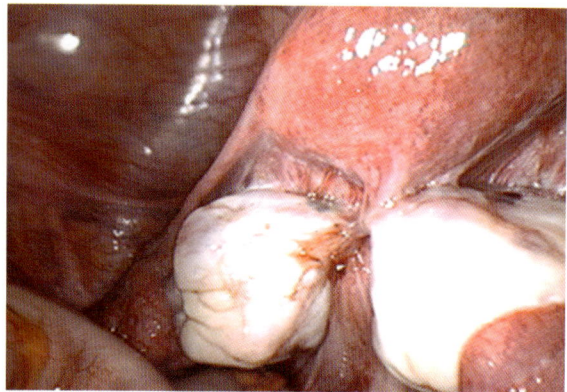

Figure 12.10
Bilateral ovarian endometrioma cysts are adherent in the midline to each other and to the posterior uterus. The rectum can be seen between the ovaries and seems to be pulled anteriorly out of its normal position. In fact, complete obliteration of the cul de sac is present, but largely obscured by the ovaries. Patients with ovarian endometriosis have an increased chance of intestinal involvement as well as an increased chance of more significant pelvic involvement

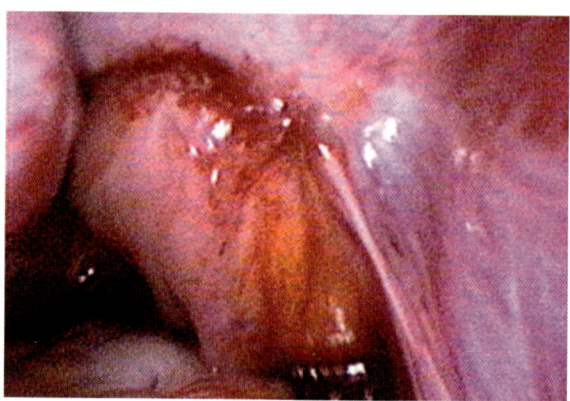

Figure 12.11
Complete obliteration of the cul de sac. There is only a little hemorrhagic change along the line of adherence of the rectum to the posterior cervix. The wall of the rectum is slightly rounded, indicating that it is involved by endometriosis, as are the uterosacral ligaments and posterior cervix

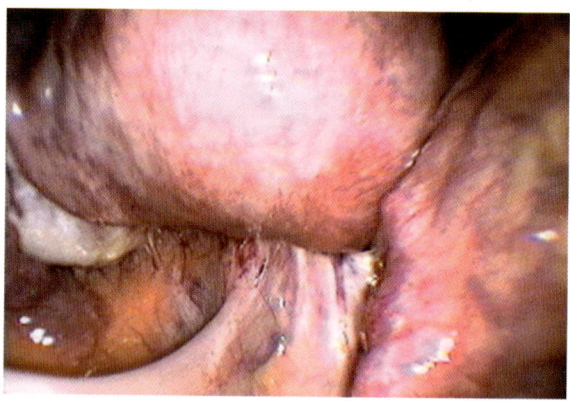

Figure 12.12
Complete obliteration of the cul de sac. The wall of the rectum is flat where it is adherent to the posterior cervix, indicating little or no involvement of the rectal wall by endometriosis

rarely extensively involved. Only at the end of the rectovaginal septum where the large nodule is physically intruding by its expansive growth will there be slight involvement by fibrosis associated with the advancing disease. Like endometriosis in many other pelvic areas, expanses of fatty tissue are largely spared from invasion by endometriosis.

Surgical treatment

Intestinal endometriosis may be treated by resections that are superficial, partial thickness, full-thickness or segmental. Most women with intestinal endometriosis will not require a segmental bowel resection. If bowel surgery is anticipated a preoperative bowel prep is given and prophylactic antibiotics are used. As the number of intestinal areas involved by endometriosis increases, the likelihood of a full-thickness or segmental bowel resection increase (Fig. 12.13). It is unnecessary to remove the pelvic organs to treat intestinal endometriosis successfully.

The wall of the intraperitoneal colon is composed of four layers: serosa, outer longitudinal muscularis, inner circular muscularis, and mucosa. Beneath the peritoneal reflection of the

INTESTINAL ENDOMETRIOSIS

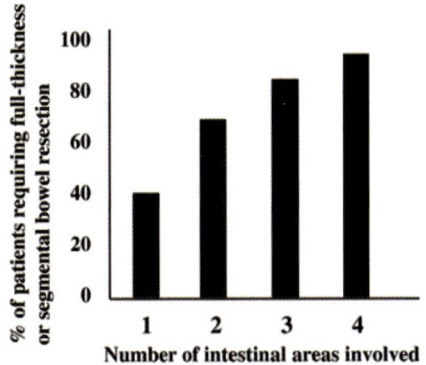

Figure 12.13

As the number of intestinal areas involved by endometriosis increases, the likelihood of a full-thickness or segmental bowel resection increases

cul de sac, the serosal layer is absent. The wall of the small bowel is similar but thinner. Thus, the muscularis of the small bowel behaves surgically as one layer. These layers of the bowel wall can be used to the surgeon's advantage during treatment of intestinal endometriosis since frequently a layer involved by endometriosis can be peeled away from underlying layers, resulting in a partial-thickness bowel resection which may denude the mucosa in some cases.

The techniques described below can be performed most effectively with a triple-puncture technique using 3 mm scissors passed down the operating channel of a 10 mm operating laparoscope, using either sharp dissection or high current density electroexcision using 90 watts of pure cutting current.[37] Surgery for intestinal endometriosis is dictated by the depth of invasion and the geographic distribution of disease, so various techniques are necessary, all guided in part by palpation of the bowel wall for nodularity.

Superficial lesions

Scissors cut perpendicularly into the normal bowel wall adjacent to the lesion, first entering only the outer layer of muscularis. The lesion is grasped and undermined, with the scissors working in a layer of muscularis. The dissection can quickly proceed beyond the lesion, so care must be taken to decide when to cut back out of the bowel wall. Suture reinforcement of the bowel wall with 2-0 silk is wise. Valuable practice can be gained by suturing even small defects in the bowel wall. To make internal suturing easy, two points must always be kept in mind: (1) The long end of the suture should be held in order to form an arch pointing toward the port through which the tying instrument is passed. (2) The short end of the suture should be placed immediately beneath where the knot will be tied (Fig. 12.14). This avoids reaching for the end of the suture, which can pull the suture through the tissue.

Mucosal skinning

Occasionally, a larger lesion will require dissection down to the mucosa for complete removal.

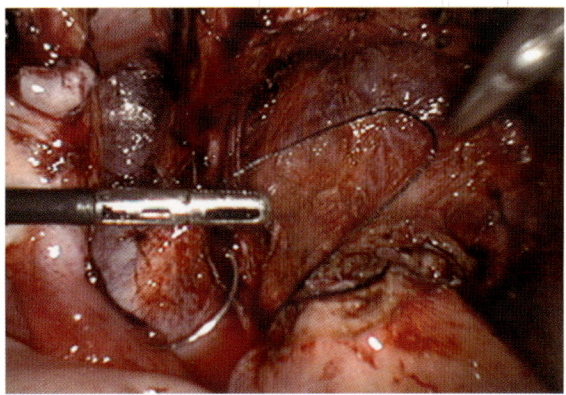

Figure 12.14

Intracorporeal knot tying is easy if simple steps are followed. The grasper on the left holds the suture so that the suture forms a loop whose axis of symmetry is directed toward the tying instrument, in this case the needle carrier coming through a right lower quadrant port. The short end of the suture is placed immediately below where the knot is to be tied for easy pick up

SURGICAL MANAGEMENT OF ENDOMETRIOSIS

If there is no submucosal fibrosis, both layers of muscularis can easily be peeled off the mucosa using sharp and blunt dissection (Fig. 12.15), a technique sometimes referred to as 'mucosal skinning'. Once the lesion has been completely undermined, the scissors are used to cut back out to the surface of the bowel. Be careful not to pass too far beyond the nodule before cutting back out. Interrupted 2-0 silk suture is used to close the serosa and muscularis in one layer. Antibiotic prophylaxis is optional.

Ileal resection

The ileum is most commonly involved in its terminal portion. A bulky mass effect of a nodule in the bowel wall may not be suggested by visible surface changes, but may be appreciated by palpation with graspers. Laparoscopic surgery on the ileum is possible, but is difficult due to the typical placement of accessory trocars for pelvic surgery. Scissors can be used to sharply excise the nodule within the muscularis by a mucosal skinning technique. With care, many nodules can be removed without penetrating the lumen. Most defects of the ileum should be closed with interrupted 3-0 silk since the bowel wall is thin to begin with.

Since the ileum is frequently involved by several lesions which may be superficial or deep, laparoscopic surgery can be tedious, even if additional appropriately placed trocars are inserted. In many cases, it is more efficient to mobilize laparoscopically the peritoneal attachments of the ileum and cecum so that the ileum can be delivered through a minilaparotomy incision where partial-thickness, full-thickness, or segmental bowel resections can be performed (Figs. 12.16–12.18). This minilaparotomy incision may be an enlargement of the right lower quadrant or umbilical trocar site. Occasionally, the ileum can be reached through a transvaginal approach if there is sufficient mobility (Fig. 12.19).

Full thickness disc resection of colon

If submucosal fibrosis is present, or if the nodule is large, entry into the lumen of the bowel

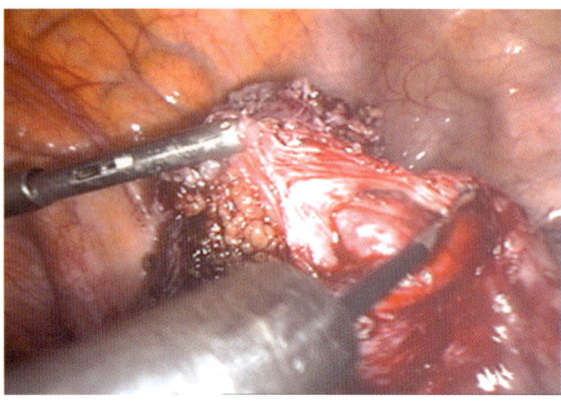

Figure 12.15
'Mucosal skinning' of the colon for treatment of intestinal endometriosis. The grasper on the left is holding a nodule of endometriosis which is being dissected away from the underlying mucosa. The 3 mm scissors are resting directly on the intact mucosa. Notice the linear striations of the circular inner muscularis layer

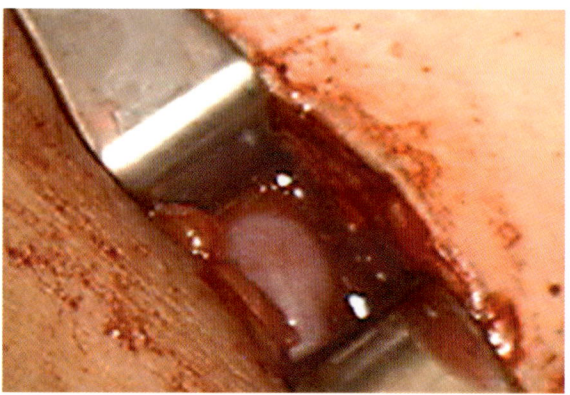

Figure 12.16
The right lower quadrant 5 mm trocar site has been enlarged slightly and the ileum is seen within the wound. This incision is 3 cm in length without retraction

INTESTINAL ENDOMETRIOSIS

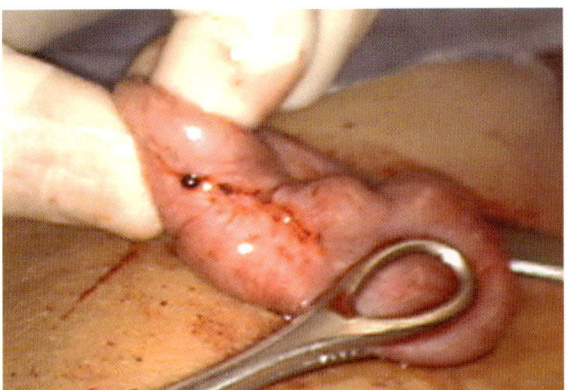

Figure 12.17
The ileum has been delivered onto the abdominal wall for resection of the linear deposit on the antimesenteric border

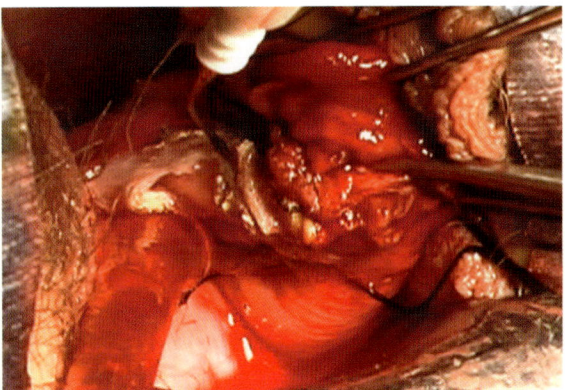

Figure 12.19
Transvaginal resection of ileal endometriosis by full-thickness resection. The affected loop of ileum has been delivered through the vagina in a patient undergoing laparoscopic hysterectomy. The electrosurgical needle has just made an incision into the bowel lumen which is seen near the end of the clear plastic suction tip. The nodule of the bowel wall is held by clamps seen on the right and silk traction sutures are in place on normal bowel wall around the nodule

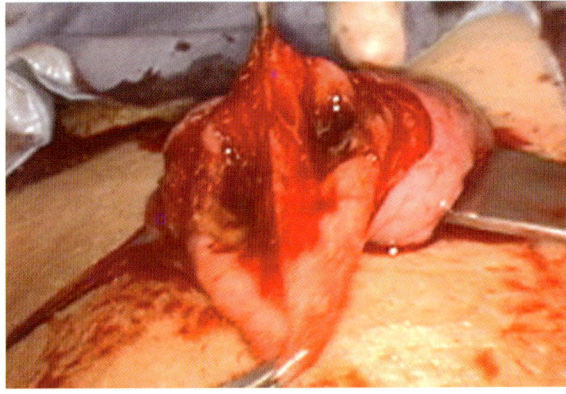

Figure 12.18
Ileal endometriosis has been removed by full-thickness resection. The proximal and distal bowel lumina are seen. Each angle of the intact mucosa on the mesenteric side of the bowel wall is held on traction by a clamp. The bowel is closed in two layers working from one angle to the other

may be inevitable. Entry into the bowel lumen allows palpation of the lesion through the mucosa as well, so the point at which the dissection begins to exit the bowel wall can be determined accurately. The mucosa can be closed with continuous 3-0 vicryl and the seromuscularis can be closed with interrupted 2-0 silk. The pelvis is filled with irrigation fluid and air can be injected into the sigmoid colon through a sigmoidoscope to check for air leaks. If leakage occurs, it must be stopped with more sutures.

Appendectomy

Monopolar appendectomy is simple and rapid. The appendiceal tip is grasped as the 3 mm monopolar scissors with 50 watts of coagulation current shave along the wall of the appendix where the vessels are quite small (Fig. 12.20). This cuts and coagulates the vessels simultaneously until the cecum is reached (Fig. 12.21). Three endoloops are applied around the base of the bare appendix and the scissors cut between the suture (Fig. 12.22). The scissors grasp the appendix and extract it out the 10 mm umbilical sheath. The appendiceal stump can be lightly electrocoagulated and buried beneath the surface of the cecum with a purse-string suture if desired.

SURGICAL MANAGEMENT OF ENDOMETRIOSIS

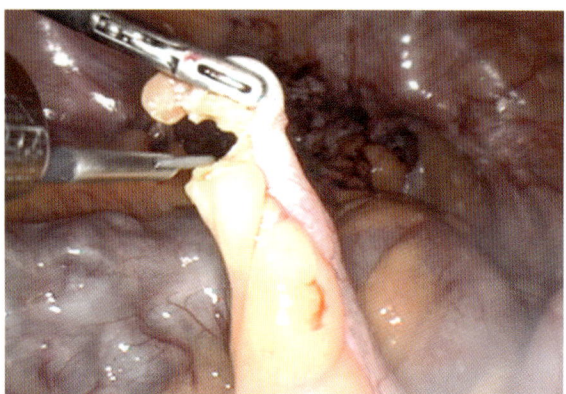

Figure 12.20
Monopolar laparoscopic appendectomy begins by shaving the mesentery of the appendix from the wall of the appendix. This is carried out immediately adjacent to the wall of the appendix where the vessels are smallest

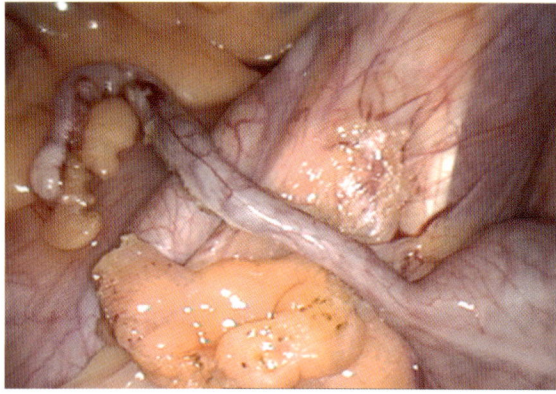

Figure 12.21
The appendix has been completely denuded of its mesentery which now rests alongside it

The following topics: obliteration of the cul de sac; rectovaginal endometriosis; and laparoscopic segmental bowel resection are covered in Chapter 9.

Conversion to laparotomy

While many cases of intestinal endometriosis can be managed successfully laparoscopically,

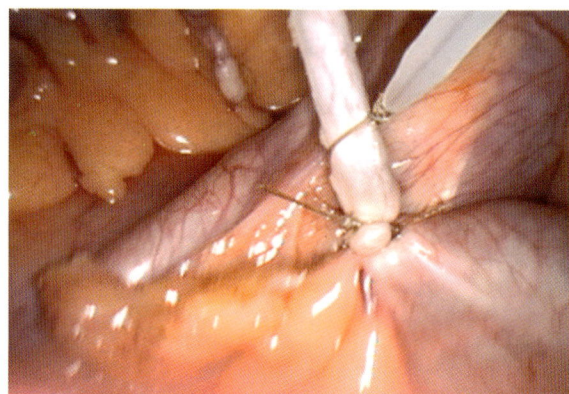

Figure 12.22
Two endoloop sutures have been placed adjacent to the cecum and the third is being placed just distal to these two. The appendix will be transected between these sutures. Since the appendix has been separated from its mesentery, it can be easily extracted through a 10 mm trocar sheath

laparotomy can still play an important role in treating intestinal endometriosis if the surgeon lacks the necessary laparoscopic skills.[38] Since patients with intestinal endometriosis frequently have extensive pelvic disease, bowel surgery for endometriosis may follow one to two hours of pelvic surgery for removal of invasive endometriosis and mobilization of the bowel. As the length of laparoscopic surgery increases, the energy level of the surgeon decreases, and surgery seems interminably long. Laparotomy may be selected if a lengthy surgery (i.e., over 4 hours) is anticipated. Also, laparotomy is far more efficient if two or more segmental resections are required in a single patient. In such patients, laparoscopic excision of all pelvic endometriosis and laparoscopic mobilization of the large bowel or ileum can allow the use of very small incisions for the remaining bowel surgery (Fig. 12.23).

In lengthy cases or cases involving extensive dissection or increased blood loss, a surgical drain left in the cul de sac can be helpful. Excess bloody irrigation fluid may otherwise drain

INTESTINAL ENDOMETRIOSIS

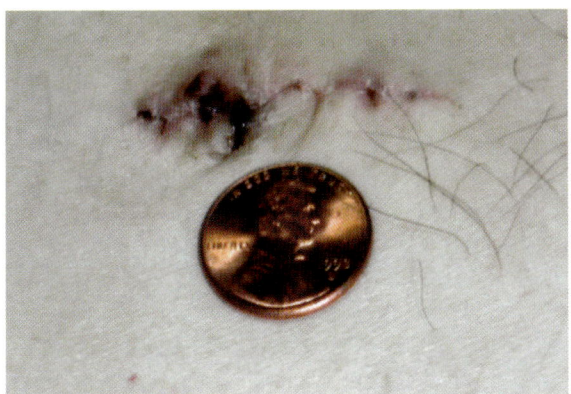

Figure 12.23
Laparoscopically assisted bowel resection can be done through small incisions. This patient underwent laparoscopic separation of the mesentery from the sigmoid nodule seen in Fig. 12.9. A segmental resection of the sigmoid with end-to-end hand-sewn anastomosis and a segmental resection of the ileocecal nodule seen in Fig. 12.4 with a stapled anastomosis were performed through this slightly enlarged umbilical incision

messily out of laparoscopy puncture sites for up to 18 hours following surgery, to the consternation and concern of the nursing staff. If such bloody irrigation fluid remains in the abdomen, it can be an occasional cause of mild postoperative temperature elevation which can confuse the postoperative clinical picture. A drain can also help detect postoperative bleeding or infection.

Postoperative care

No change in routine orders is necessary following partial-thickness bowel resection, and patients can be discharged the day of surgery if tolerating oral liquids and pain pills without vomiting, and if they are able to void and have stable vital signs. In patients with one or two full-thickness disc resections, clear liquids can be started the morning after surgery, and the patient can be discharged in the afternoon if stable. She should stay on a light diet until passing gas.

Following segmental bowel resection, the patient is given only ice chips by mouth until passing gas. Routine nasogastric suctioning is unnecessary. Flatus usually occurs on about the fourth postoperative day. Clear liquids are then begun. If this is tolerated, the patient can advance to full liquids and be discharged. At home, carbohydrates are added for a day or two, followed by white meat, then diet as tolerated. Such a diet provides low residue foods which are easily processed in the stomach and small intestine. The main dietary items to avoid in the early postoperative period are foods that are high in roughage, such as salads and vegetables, or foods that are high in protein, such as meat and beans. The volume of oral intake in the early postoperative period is also important, since even water in large volumes can challenge the intestines too much. Most patients will be on a regular diet by 10 days after surgery.

Complications

If significant postoperative gas pain or nausea occur, the patient should resume clear liquids until better and try to avoid narcotic pain pills. Narcotic pain pills can cause gastritis or stimulate the nausea center and may be the main problem in some patients. The patient should inform the doctor of unusual circumstances such as persistent vomiting, worsening pain or bloating, or fever so the possibility of complications can be considered. Dehydration due to decreased oral intake can sometimes confound the picture since the patient may have weakness or nausea on this basis. If the patient reports concerns by telephone, clinical information about presence of intestinal activity can sometimes be gained by having a family member listen for bowel sounds by pressing an ear against the patient's abdomen and by taking the patient's temperature. Information about dehydration can be gained by asking about urinary output over the last day or two.

If there is sufficient concern of a significant complication, the patients should be brought to the hospital for tests including blood tests, cultures if infection seems possible, as well as tests for integrity of the intestinal and urinary tracts. For rectal, sigmoid, cecal and some ileal resections, barium or water-soluble contrast enemas will give the fastest information about bowel leaks. Some radiologists may express concern that if a leak is present, the patient may be made sicker by the procedure, and may be hesitant to perform such a procedure. This concern is unfounded. Such a leak must be identified since it can be eventually fatal and if identified would lead to immediate surgery anyway to fix the problem and clean out the extravasated contrast material. Spiral CT scans with oral or intravenous contrast or intravenous pyelograms may be helpful in identifying urinary tract or small bowel problems. Simple upright x-rays of the abdomen can identify ileus with excess gas in the small bowel and excess air-fluid levels. Free air under the diaphragm could potentially be related to recent surgery but could indicate an intestinal leak.

Some patients might be so ill that extensive testing is pointless and urgent surgical evaluation is the best choice. If the patient is taken to surgery urgently with no imaging tests, indigo carmine should be injected intravenously during surgery since some patients might have simultaneous urinary tract damage. Underwater air pressure examination can help identify small leaks of the rectosigmoid colon. Larger leaks will be obvious by the presence of malodorous fecal-contaminated liquid. Occasionally, a suspected intestinal complication will not be found and the patient's clinical picture could actually be due to a urinary complication. If the surgeon focuses on the somewhat more worrisome possibility of an intestinal leak, the excess watery, cloudy fluid encountered during surgery could be misinterpreted as an early abscess.

During surgery, the actual repair to the bowel or urinary tract will frequently be in the hands of a general surgeon or urologist and such repairs are beyond the scope of this book. Small intestinal leaks operated quickly may require simple oversewing with sutures. Larger leaks may be treated by temporary diverting colostomy. Ureteral damage may respond to insertion of a stent, although small defects created by sharp injury may be stitched laparoscopically or at laparotomy. Larger ureteral defects may require reimplantation into the bladder, sometimes with a psoas hitch if a length of ureter must be resected. Bladder injuries can be oversewn at laparoscopy or laparotomy, or sometimes treated with a urinary catheter only. A surgical drain left in postoperatively can help identify what is happening in the abdomen after surgical repair of a complication. This can also be used to obtain intraperitoneal cultures later, or for postoperative irrigation. A drain allows simple bedside detection of ongoing urinary tract leaks by the injection of indigo carmine intravenously or through a catheter in the bladder.

The patient going through a surgical complication needs all the support she can get from family, friends and the treating staff. Although the surgeon responsible for a complication will naturally feel embarrassment and sometimes will want to avoid the patient and family, this is not helpful to anyone. The surgeon should not withdraw from the patient unless asked. Time at the patient's bedside will help provide an important part of the emotional support which will be helpful in the psychological healing which must accompany the physical healing. The patient will appreciate that her original surgeon is with her at every step of the process and has not abandoned her. Expressions of genuine concern and sorrow over what she is going through are entirely appropriate human responses. Concern over possible medicolegal action may cause some treating physcans to appear to withdraw, withhold information, and seem cold and uncaring. This escalates the possibility of legal action since it is easier to sue a boor than a friend. The facts of the case and what led to the complication can be fully and freely discussed with the patient without jeopardizing a legal defense later. The occurrence of a complication does not always signify medical negligence. Some complications are unavoidable and unrecognizable at surgery. Embarrassment and a desire for immediate self-punishment should not cause the surgeon to claim that the surgical care which preceded the complication was against the standard of care. The standard of care does not require perfection, since it is universally recognized by doctors, lawyers, judges and juries that perfection is impossible to obtain. The standard of care requires simply that the doctor has done what other reasonable physicians might do with the same disease process, or to have done what has repeatedly worked successfully in previous personal experience. It implies that certain guidelines or rules (not necessarily those that have been published) have been observed, that a rational game plan was developed and followed. The majority of medical and surgical practice is not supported by randomized controlled trials and never will be. Judgment, experience and flexibility are some of the hallmarks of the standard of care, and these are more important in surgical treatment than published journal articles or books. Publications represent opinions based on either the experience of an author or evidence usually from some type of observational study. As such, there will be many opinions possible about every step of a procedure, beginning with placement of incisions and trocars to postoperative feeding. Therefore, the standard of care does not exist in any book. The standard of care is not dictated by the practice of the majority, with the same thing done to every patient. This would ignore the fact that patients can be different. If the surgeon's judgment is to use one approach instead of another because of training, experience or the surgical problem at hand, then the standard of care is being fulfilled by consideration of the pertinent facts in choosing and performing a surgical step or an entire surgical procedure in accordance with basic surgical principles.

References

1. Meyer R. Quoted by Culbertson C, in Discussion of Cullen TS. Adenomyoma of the rectovaginal septum. JAMA 1916;67:401–6.
2. Stevens TG. Adenomyoma of the vaginal wall. Proc Roy Soc Med 1910;3:57–8.
3. Lockyer C. Adenomyoma in the recto-uterine and recto-vaginal septa. Proc Roy Soc Med 1913; 4:112–16 (plus Discussion).
4. DeJong RJ. Subserose Adenomyomatose des Dunndarms. Virchows Arch (Path Anat) 1913; 211:141–156.
5. Griffith WSA. Pregnancy with utero-rectal adenomyoma, with extensive decidual meaplasia. Proc Roy Soc Med 1914;6:389–92.
6. Leitch A. Migratory adenomyomata of the uterus. Proc Roy Soc Med 1914;6:393–8 (plus Discussion).
7. Cullen TS. Adenomyoma of the rectovaginal septum. JAMA 1914;62:835–9.
8. Cullen TS. Adenomyoma of the rectovaginal septum. JAMA 1916;67:401–6.
9. Cullen TS. Adenomyoma of the recto-vaginal septum. Johns Hopkins Hosp Bull 1917;28; 343–67.
10. Cullen TS. The distribution of adenomyomata containing uterine mucosa. Am J Obstet Gynecol 1919;80:130–8.
11. Cullen TS. The distribution of adenomyomas containing uterine mucosa. Arch Surg 1920;1: 215–83.
12. Sampson JA. Intestinal adenomas of endometrial type. Arch Surg 1922;5:217–80.
13. Redwine DB. Was Sampson wrong? Fertil Steril 2002;78:686–93.
14. Henriksen E. Endometriosis. Am J Surg 1955;90: 331–6.
15. Weed JC, Ray JE. Endometriosis of the bowel. Obstet Gynecol 1987;69:727–30.
16. Nissen ED, Goldstein AI. Intussusception of the appendix associated with endometriosis. Int J Gynaecol Obstet 1973;11:184–9.
17. Mann WJ, Fromowitz F, Saychek T, Madariaga JR, Chalas E. Endometriosis associated with appendiceal intussusception. A report of two cases. J Reprod Med 1984;29:625–9.
18. Sonnino RE, Ansari MR. Intussusception of the appendix and endometriosis. Henry Ford Hosp Med J 1986;34:61–4.
19. Panzer S, Pitt HA, Wallach EE, Thuluvath PJ. Intussusception of the appendix due to endometriosis. Am J Gastroenterol 1995;90: 1892–3.
20. Case 13–2000. Case records of the Massachusetts General Hospital. N Engl J Med 2000;342: 1272–8.
21. Aronchick CA, Brooks FP, Dyson WL, Baron R, Thompson JJ. Ileocecal endometriosis presenting with abdominal pain and gastrointestinal bleeding. Dig Dis Sci 1983;28:566–72.
22. Dmowski WP, Rana N, Jafari N. Postlaparoscopic small bowel obstruction secondary to unrecognized nodular endometriosis of the terminal ileum. J Am Assoc Gynecol Laparosc 2001; 8:161–6.
23. Cattell RB. Endometriosis of the colon and rectum with intestinal obstruction. N Engl J Med 1937;217:9–16 (plus Discussion).
24. Hepburn JJ. Endometriosis as a cause of acute intestinal obstruction. N Engl J Med 1937;217: 6–8.
25. Hauck AE. Endometriosis of the colon. Ann Surg 1960;151:896–902.
26. Yelon JA, Green JM, Hashmi HF. Endometriosis of the appendix resulting in perforation: A case report. J Clin Gastroenterol 1993;16:355–6.
27. Gini PC, Chukudebelu WO, Onuigbo WIB. Perforation of the appendix during pregnancy: A rare complication of endometriosis. Br J Obstet Gynaecol 1981;88:456–8.
28. Clement PB. Perforation of the sigmoid colon during pregnancy: A rare complication of endometriosis. Br J Obstet Gynaecol 1977;84: 548–50.
29. Bakri YN, Tayeb A, Amri A. Fatal perforation of endometriotic colon. Int J Gynecol Obstet 1992; 37:301 (Letter).

30. Colcock BP, Lamphier TA. Endometriosis of the large and small intestine. Surgery 1950;28: 997–1004.
31. Graham B, Mazier WP. Diagnosis and management of endometriosis of the colon and rectum. Dis Colon Rectum 1988;31:952–6
32. Harris RS, Foster WG, Surrey MW, Agarwal SK. Appendiceal diseae in women with endometriosis and right lower quadrant pain. J Am Assoc Gynecol Laparosc 2001;8:536–41.
33. Fedele L, Bianchi S, Zanconato G, Tozzi L, Raffaelli R. Gonadotropin-releasing hormone agonist treatment for endometriosis of the rectovaginal septum. Am J Obstet Gynecol 2000;183: 1462–7.
34. Chapron C, Dubuisson J-B, Pansini V, Vieira M, Fauconnier A, Barakat H, Dousset B. Routine clinical examination is not sufficient for diagnosing and locating deeply infiltrating endometriosis. J Am Assoc Gynecol Laparosc 2002;9: 115–9.
35. Redwine DB, Wright J. Laparoscopic treatment of obliteration of the cul de sac in endometriosis: Long term followup. Fertil Steril 2001;76: 358–65.
36. Martin DC, Batt RE. Retrocervical, rectovaginal pouch, and rectovaginal septum endometriosis. J Am Assoc Gynecol Laparosc 2001;8:12–17.
37. Redwine DB. Bowel resection for endometriosis. In: Tulandi T (ed) Atlas of laparoscopic technique for gynecologists. London: WB Saunders. 1994:121–9.
38. Coronado C, Franklin RR, Lotze EC, Bailey HR, Valdes CT. Surgical treatment of symptomatic colorectal endometriosis. Fertil Steril 1990;53: 411–16.

13

Rectovaginal endometriosis
Jeremy Wright

Rectovaginal endometriosis is perhaps the greatest gynecological surgical challenge, exceeding the complexity of gynecologic oncological surgery. If such disease represented cancer, it would be deemed inoperable, whereas endometriosis is benign and locally invasive and the only effective treatment is excision. The gold standard effective treatment is surgical removal of the disease from the body. Many have a long history of subfertility.[1] For the majority of women of childbearing age surgery can be accomplished with preservation of the uterus and adnexae. Pelvic endometriosis affects 5–7% of menstruating women.[1] The incidence of bowel involvement however varies greatly because of methods of case selection, with a reported incidence of between 3% and 34%.

Rectovaginal endometriosis is frequently associated with endometriosis elsewhere in the pelvis, particularly ovarian endometriomas and ovarian fossae endometriosis, which will require concurrent removal.[2–5] This chapter explores the presentation, clinical findings, pathology and treatment of this difficult manifestation of endometriotic disease.

Presentation

Women with rectovaginal endometriosis frequently present with severe backache, lower abdominal pain, dyschezia and constipation,[6] all of which can be aggravated before or during menses. They may also suffer with rectal pain with flatus, bowel movements and even sitting down. The frequent use of laxatives can give rise to diarrhoea, and some patients complain of diarrhoea during menstruation. Symptomatology is usually associated with severe dyspareunia and heavy and painful periods, during which time some patients may also report a slight temperature elevation. A detailed history will often find that the symptoms date from the patient's menarche and have been ignored or treated as primary dysmenorrhoea, often with oral contraceptives. One helpful distinguishing point is that with involvement of the rectum by endometriosis, patients frequently have pain with every bowel movement during the month, whereas patients with cul de sac or uterosacral ligament disease without rectal disease may complain of painful bowel movements only with menses.

When taking a history from these patients, it is useful to ask them to score their pain using a ranked ordinal scale or a visual analogue scale, or other quality of life measures. Preoperative symptom levels may easily be compared to postoperative levels to obtain an objective measure of symptom relief. Reports using such scales are rarely used in the literature to measure response of symptoms to treatment of rectovaginal endometriosis.[1,7]

Systemic upset is rare and general examination is usually normal apart from mild lower abdominal tenderness and tenderness over the sigmoid colon. Rectovaginal endometriosis is often associated with considerable psychological morbidity, a high dependence on family members, difficulties with relationships and underachievement associated with a poor sickness record in employment. Women with endometriosis are usually reluctant to undergo pelvic examination as they know this will be painful. However, examination of the pelvis is essential in aiding diagnosis.

Imaging techniques such as ultrasound, computed tomography (CT) and magnetic resonance imaging (MRI) may produce confirmatory evidence but are of themselves not diagnostic and interpretation of the findings can be difficult.[8–10] A normal scan result does not relieve the patient's pain nor eliminate the eventual need for surgical diagnosis and treatment. A positive scan result will usually show only ovarian cysts when they are present but will often fail to diagnose invasive disease of the pelvic floor and bowel wall. Thus, the scan may bias the surgeon to look for and treat only ovarian cysts and leave possibly highly symptomatic disease behind.

Pelvic examination

Speculum examination is sometimes useful and should concentrate on the area of the posterior vaginal fornix by tipping a bivalve speculum posterior to the cervix. The speculum is opened so as to expose the epithelium of the posterior fornix. In this area, rectovaginal disease may be seen invading the vaginal epithelium from an underlying nodule of the uterosacral ligament or rectal nodule. Vaginal endometriosis can be identified by disruption of the normal rugae in the overlying vagina and by epithelial piling, distortion, possibly small bluish cysts and occasionally larger polypoid reddish lesions (Fig. 13.1). It is always retained between the confines of the uterosacral ligaments and the space between them. This type of lesion is frequently missed on speculum examination in the office because only the cervix is visualized.

A thorough but gentle pelvic examination is necessary. Bimanual examination should assess size, position and mobility of the uterus, followed by an assessment of adnexal tenderness and the presence of any ovarian enlargement. The remainder of the examination should only be performed by monomanual vaginal digitation and careful observation of the facial expression and body language of the patient as she reacts to palpation of the cul de sac and uterosacral ligaments. Women with this condition will usually at least grimace, if not cry out and push up on the table away from the examining finger. The uterosacral ligaments should be gently palpated for any nodularity, which may be exquisitely tender. Palpation of the pouch of Douglas will often reveal a tender fixed nodule of endometriosis which may seem to involve the rectovaginal septum.[11] This can frequently be confirmed by rectal examination or by concomitant rectal and vaginal palpation, although this is uncomfortable and may cause the patient some distress. Not all nodularity which might be

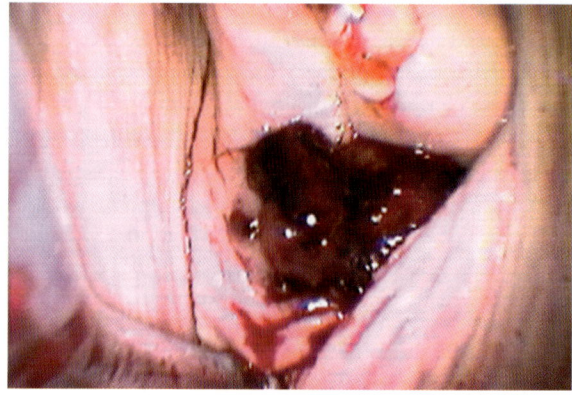

Figure 13.1

Endometriosis of the posterior vaginal fornix. By courtesy of David B Redwine

noted later at surgery will necessarily be found on pelvic examination.[2,12]

Indications for osmotic and mechanical bowel prep include symptoms or pelvic examination suggesting colon involvement by endometriosis, known bowel involvement or obliteration of the cul de sac or ovarian endometrioma cysts. Bowel preparation is recommended but can sometimes be problematic since the colon is frequently filled with watery fluid which can contaminate the pelvis if full thickness bowel resection is performed.

Etiology and pathogenesis

The etiology and pathogenesis of endometriosis remains controversial, but there is general agreement between the major theorists that rectovaginal endometriosis is different in morphology and histology from peritoneal disease, and most likely to arise from tracts of embryologically patterned rests of Müllerian tissue within the uterosacral ligaments, rectovaginal septum and anterior bowel wall.[6, 13, 14] There is a variation in oestrogen receptor and progesterone receptor content in this tissue compared to eutopic endometrium, suggesting different regulatory mechanisms for rectovaginal endometriosis as well as a different origin compared to peritoneal disease. The concept of embryologically patterned metaplasia is crucial to the surgical management of the condition since if all disease and all tracts which may form disease are removed, the disease can be cured surgically. If the disease were caused by retrograde menstruation, one would expect rapid regrowth following surgical excision.[15,16] As it is, a protracted clinical response can be expected to excision of endometriotic tissue when undertaken in specialist centres. The disease process seems to begin, often in a field effect, in parenchymal structures, such as the uterosacral ligaments, posterior cervix and anterior bowel wall. While many cases may invade the posterior vaginal fornix, the fatty and areolar tissue of the rectovaginal septum itself is not a site of origin, nor a site of frequent involvement. Thus, the term 'endometriosis of the rectovaginal septum' may be slightly in error.

Surgical diagnosis by laparoscopy

The majority of patients with the symptoms of endometriosis will be advised to undergo a diagnostic laparoscopy which needs to be adequate and thorough. The following points may help to identify what is required:

- The patient must be appropriately placed with her buttocks well over the edge of the operating table so that vaginal, uterine or rectal manipulation is not impeded.
- The patient must be put in sufficiently steep Trendelenburg to allow proper inspection of the pouch of Douglas. This should routinely include assessment of rectal tethering or mobility, which can be achieved by placing a ring forceps within the rectum and observing its mobility.
- Laparoscopic inspection should include the whole of the pelvic peritoneum including both ovarian fossae and the anterior and posterior cul de sacs. This requires manipulation of these structures and moving the bowel out of the posterior cul de sac. This cannot be carried out using a suprapubically placed Verres needle.
- Ideally, a laterally placed 5 mm port should be employed to allow access for a subsequent irrigation probe. Laterally placed ports, however, run the risk of epigastric injury. As these

vessels are very constant in position they can usually be avoided. The inferior epigastric vessels are always situated in the triangle between the obliterated umbilical vessels and the insertion of the round ligament and can usually be identified visually by examining them laparoscopically through the anterior parietal peritoneum.

- The laterally placed ports should be inserted when the abdomen is fully inflated and the point directed medially. This can either be under direct vision or by supporting the abdominal wall from the peritoneal side by holding the laparoscope just medial to the point of insertion of the 5 mm trocar and directing the trocar so it passes directly under the laparoscope into the pneumoperitoneum. Control of the tension on the abdominal wall ensures that there is no rapid or explosive insertion of the trocar leading to possible damage to underlying viscera or great vessels.
- Following inspection of the pelvic peritoneum, a suction irrigation probe or laparoscopic forceps should be used to palpate the pouch of Douglas and uterosacral ligaments for areas of nodularity,[17] while the uterus is upwardly displaced by a uterine manipulator. Nodular endometriosis is classically hard so the probe will appear to 'click' over it. Ideally, there should be concomitant excision biopsy of all these areas of endometriosis, but there are few centres where the equipment and expertise exist to undertake this procedure, and in these circumstances, a biopsy of at least one of the endometriotic lesions should be taken to confirm histologically the diagnosis, so that the patient can be advised to seek the appropriate specialist help.
- The cecum, appendix and terminal ileum should all be examined since if obliteration of the cul de sac is present, there is a possibility these other bowel areas could be involved.

Rectovaginal disease may not be associated with florid flame haemorrhages or active vascular change (Fig. 13.2). Occasionally, an apparently small vascular lesion of the uterosacral ligament may be the tip of a large rectovaginal nodule. The associated fibromuscular metaplasia and fibrosis give a yellowish or whitish appearance, occasionally with overlying haemorrhagic discolorations. Frank rectovaginal endometriosis will be diagnosed by the presence of dense adhesive fibrotic disease with obliteration of the pelvic cul de sac. Involvement of the rectum can be identified visually as the 'rounded rectum' indicating a round bulge in the rectal wall at the point of attachment to the posterior cervix (Fig. 13.3) as the uterus is held in extreme anteversion. Rectal involvement is absent or superficial if the rectum is flat at its point of adherence to the posterior cervix.[18]

Sometimes, the presence of bilateral ovarian cysts meeting in the middle of the pelvis and dense peritubal adhesions with tethering of the sigmoid colon to the fundus of the uterus and the left pelvic side wall will make a complete initial visual survey impossible.

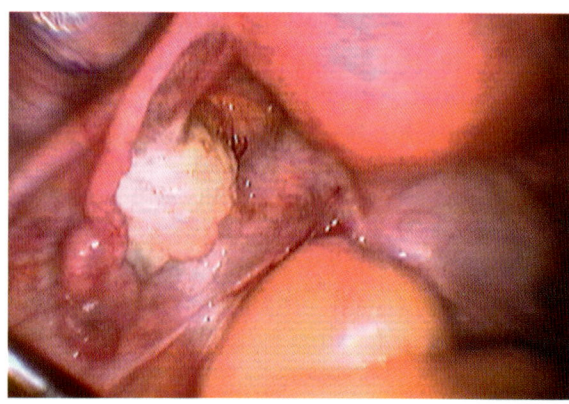

Figure 13.2

Laparoscopic appearance of the patient with the vaginal lesion in Fig. 13.1. Although the cul de sac is completely obliterated, the overall appearance seems quite innocuous at first glance. By courtesy of David B Redwine

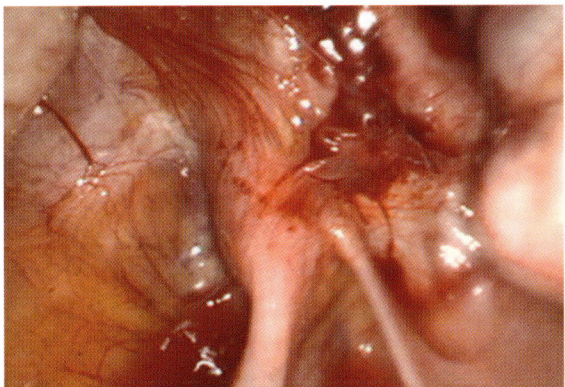

Figure 13.3
Another case of complete obliteration of the cul de sac with haemorrhage and neovascular change. The rectum is confluently and densely adherent to the posterior cervix with no obvious surgical plane. Note the round bulge in the rectal wall indicating involvement of the muscularis by endometriosis. The left ovary is normal in the upper left of the frame while the right ovary is cystic and adherent to the right uterosacral ligament. By courtesy of David B Redwine

Treatment

The pathology is that of dense fibrosis or fibromuscular metaplasia with relatively small areas of endometriosis (Fig. 13.4), which are poorly responsive to hormones. In bowel lesions, there may be striking hypertrophy of smooth muscle reminiscent of the changes seen in adenomyosis of the uterus.[19,20] Hormone manipulation does little to suppress the disease, despite the presence of oestrogen and progesterone receptors.[21,22] Even if there is some suppression during hormone therapy, symptoms resume once hormone suppression is stopped. Many clinicians view obliteration of the cul de sac as an adhesive process only: the colon is stuck to the back of the cervix and it must be unstuck. The important consideration for surgery is that the adhesive process is the result of inflammation from underlying invasive endometriosis. This invasive endometriosis involves the uterosacral ligaments, posterior cervix, cul de sac, and usually the anterior wall of the rectum. Accordingly, surgeons who treat only the adhesions will fail in any attempt at treating the disease. Some surgeons may observe obliteration of the cul de sac, describe 'dense adhesions' and attempt to dissect the rectum from the cervix to 'restore normal anatomy'. Such treatment completely misinterprets the pathology and leaves 100% of invasive disease behind as well as a broad, raw area extending from the posterior cervix and down across the cul de sac and on to the anterior rectal wall. The depth of invasion associated with obliteration of the cul de sac can extend several centimetres beneath the visible surface, and just because this is not visible to the surgeon's eye does not make it acceptable for the surgeon not to think about it. This depth of invasion makes thermal ablation techniques, such as laser vaporization or electrocoagulation, inappropriate choices for surgical treatment.

The most efficient technique for treatment of obliteration of the cul de sac is en bloc resection[23] using unipolar electro-diathermy delivered

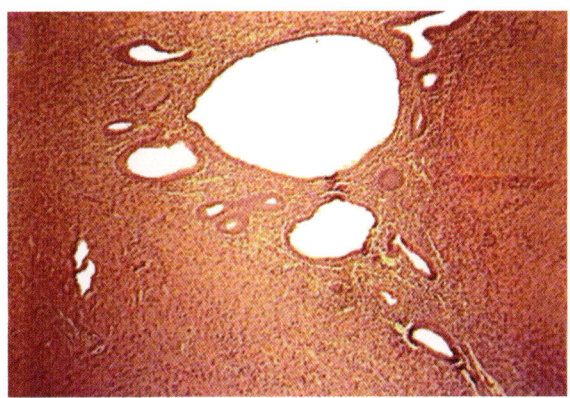

Figure 13.4
The histology of obliteration of the cul de sac shows relatively sparse glands and stroma of endometriosis surrounded by relatively avascular fibromuscular metaplasia. By courtesy of David B Redwine

SURGICAL MANAGEMENT OF ENDOMETRIOSIS

by 3 mm hook scissors which are utilized via an operating laparoscope. High power settings (90 watts cut, 50 watts coag) allow a high current density beneath the tip of the active electrode with rapid cutting of tissue by vaporization and little lateral thermal spread.

With involvement of the vaginal mucosa it is helpful to first delineate this (Fig. 13.5), using a vaginal approach prior to laparoscopy. Using a pencil electrode and coagulation current, the nodule is outlined by incision of the vaginal mucosa. The incision is then extended into the softer tissue of the rectovaginal septum followed by blunt finger dissection laterally and inferiorly.

The laparoscopic procedure should begin with the excision of other areas of endometriosis, such as endometriomas or other pelvic sidewall disease. This begins to isolate the obliterated cul de sac in the bottom of the pelvis. Following any ovarian surgery, the ovaries can be suspended from the round ligaments using an absorbable suture, such as 3-0 Vicryl, as this will both improve access to the posterior cul de sac and prevent the ovary becoming adherent to the denuded pelvis postoperatively. The stitch will dissolve when the pelvic peritoneum has regrown, thus preventing dense adherence of the ovary into the cul de sac.

Laparoscopic dissection of the cul de sac begins with incisions lateral and parallel to the uterosacral ligaments in relatively normal non-fibrotic peritoneum (Figs 13.6, 13.7), followed by blunt undermining of the uterosacral ligaments. A transverse incision (Fig. 13.8) is created across the cervix or uterine body above the line of adherence of the bowel. Intrafascial dissection with electrosurgery is then carried down the posterior cervix towards the rectovaginal septum, with the dissection proceeding more deeply if hidden pockets of chocolate-coloured fluid are found (Fig. 13.9), indicating more deeply invasive endometriosis. The uterosacral ligaments are transected at the cervical insertions in this process and the dissection is continued caudally down the rectovaginal septum until normal areolar tissue of the rectovaginal septum is clearly identified. No attempt has been made to dissect in the plane between the rectum and cervix.

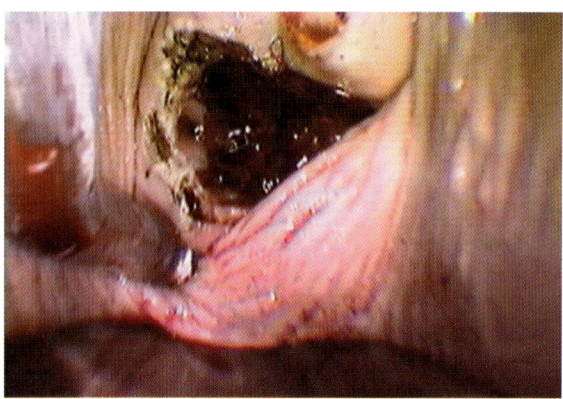

Figure 13.5
Treatment of rectovaginal endometriosis begins by incising the vaginal mucosa around the vaginal lesion. This incision goes just into the rectovaginal septum. The incision immediately adjacent to the cervix hugs the cervix tightly and does not usually enter the rectovaginal septum. By courtesy of David B Redwine

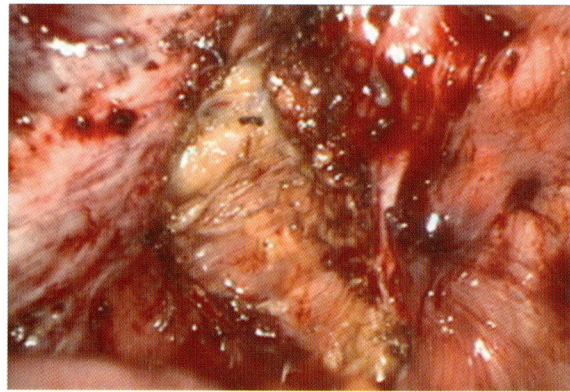

Figure 13.6
An incision has been started through relatively normal peritoneum lateral to the left uterosacral ligament. This incision goes only through the peritoneum, exposing retroperitoneal areolar tissue. By courtesy of David B Redwine

RECTOVAGINAL ENDOMETRIOSIS

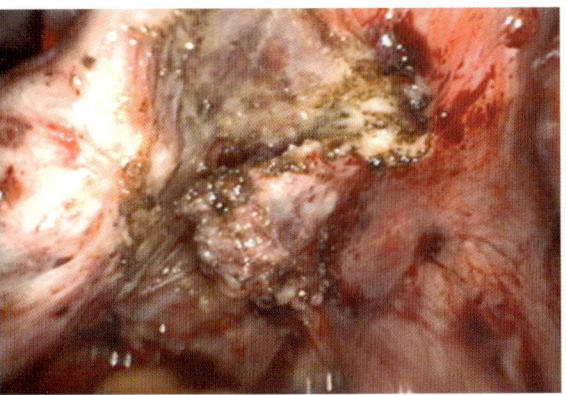

Figure 13.7
The peritoneal incision in the left broad ligament has been extended alongside the left ovary, which is on the left edge of the frame, and toward the left uteroovarian pedicle, which is out of view at the top centre of the frame. The incision then passes alongside the left edge of the uterus and begins to enter the lateral edge of the cervix where the yellowish white tissue of the cervical stroma is seen. This process has isolated endometriosis of the left broad ligament and left uterosacral ligament toward the centre of the pelvis. The cul de sac remains obliterated along the right side of the frame. By courtesy of David B Redwine

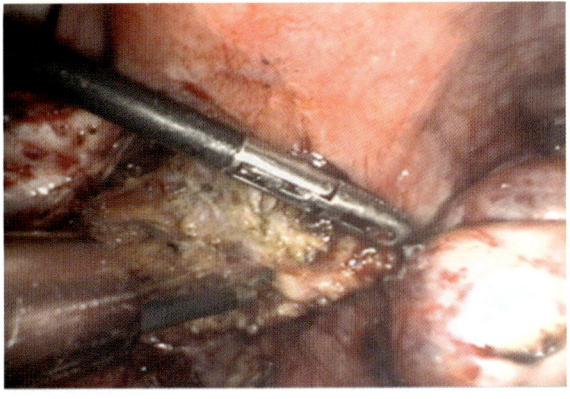

Figure 13.8
A transverse incision is begun across the posterior cervix above the point of attachment of the rectum. The grasper has a nodule of the left uterosacral ligament on medial traction. By courtesy of David B Redwine

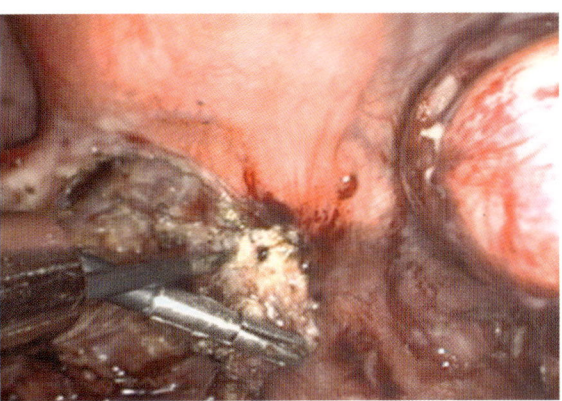

Figure 13.9
This is the same case shown in Fig. 13.8. The scissors have cut through a buried cystic area of endometriosis which is shown by the small brownish spot of chocolate-coloured fluid released from a microcyst. This indicates that the dissection must go even deeper in this area to ensure no endometriosis is left behind. By courtesy of David B Redwine

Instead, the cul de sac remains obliterated but comes to lie eventually on the anterior wall of the rectum as one mass containing the uterosacral ligaments, the posterior cervix and the obliterated cul de sac (Figs 13.10, 13.11). The lateral fatty attachments of the rectum to the pelvic sidewall are severed (Fig. 13.12) with the result that all the diseased area is now isolated centrally onto the rectum. The fatty tissue overlying the bowel wall adjacent to the nodule is shaved away further isolating the nodule and exposing normal bowel wall for later suturing (Fig. 13.13).

If the endometriotic disease involves the vaginal mucosa, the dissection is slightly altered. Since the central portion of the vagina is involved by the nodule which also involves the posterior cervix, the intrafascial dissection down the posterior cervix is postponed, because the plane of dissection will be more fibrotic and obscured due to the vaginal lesion. Instead, after transecting one or both uterosacral ligaments, the vagina is entered on the right or left side of

SURGICAL MANAGEMENT OF ENDOMETRIOSIS

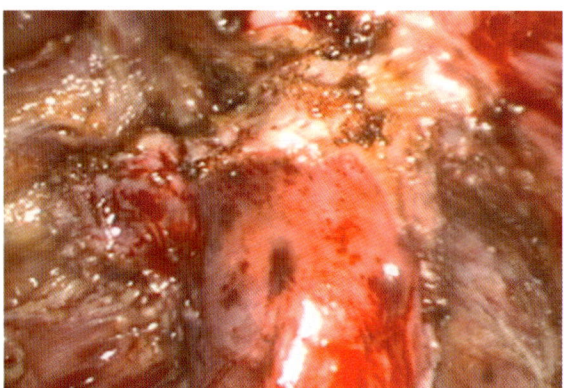

Figure 13.10
The obliterated cul de sac has been outlined by lines of incision laterally through the peritoneum of the broad ligaments as well as by a transverse incision across the posterior cervix anteriorly. The cul de sac itself remains obliterated and no effort is made to try to find a plane between the rectum and cervix. An intrafascial dissection down the posterior cervix toward the rectovaginal septum will shave the outer 1 mm or 2 mm off the posterior cervix. By courtesy of David B Redwine

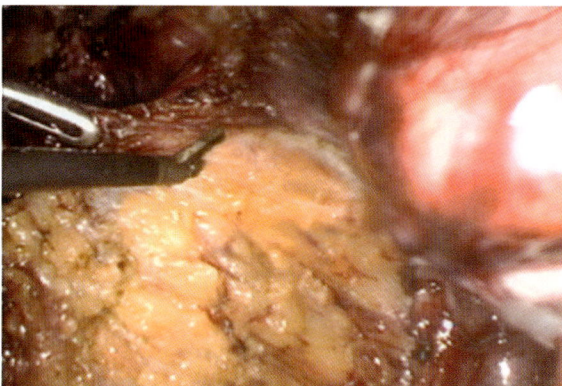

Figure 13.12
The lateral fatty attachments of the rectum to the right pelvic sidewall are severed along the length of affected bowel, working near the bowel wall. The same process will be repeated on the left side. By courtesy of David B Redwine

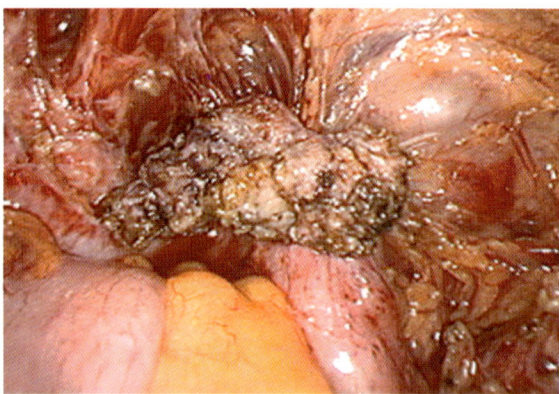

Figure 13.11
The cul de sac remains obliterated but now has been mobilized onto the anterior rectal wall by en bloc resection. The normal rectovaginal septum and vestiges of the deeper normal uterosacral ligaments and lateral attachments of the upper vagina are seen in the right upper corner of the frame. This patient did not have vaginal endometriosis, which would have required initial lateral entry into the upper corners of the rectovaginal septum, which is shown in Fig. 13.14. By courtesy of David B Redwine

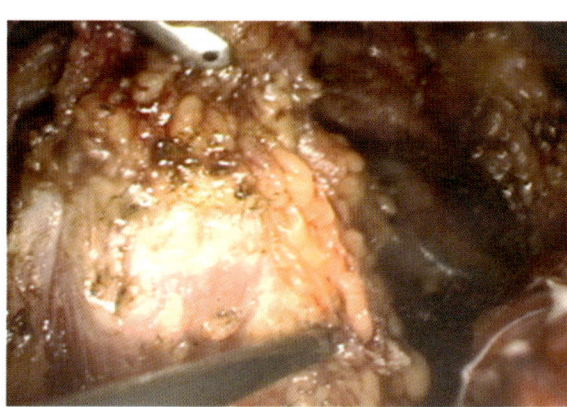

Figure 13.13
The grasper at the top of the frame is holding the edge of the rectal nodule. The scissors are used to dissect the fatty tissue away and expose normal bowel wall, which appears slightly pinkish in this frame. By courtesy of David B Redwine

the apex, alongside the vaginal nodule (Fig. 13.14). The vaginal epithelial incisions that were previously created help guide the vaginal entry. Once the vagina has been entered from the side, it is easier to ensure that the rectovaginal nodule can be removed completely under direct vision, working immediately adjacent to the posterior lip of the cervix at first, then following the epithelial incision line with the dissection to ensure that the vaginal lesion has been incorporated on to the mass which remains attached to the bowel wall. The normal rectal wall distal to the nodule is exposed by dissection of its areolar tissue. It is important that all fatty tissue be cleaned from the wall of the bowel in areas where sutures will eventually be placed.

If the vagina is not opened, dissection is continued laparoscopically. The colonic wall has four layers: the serosa, outer longitudinal muscularis, inner circular muscularis, and mucosa. The serosa is absent distal to the peritoneal cul de sac reflection. These layers can be used to the surgeon's advantage. The hypertrophied muscular layers of the bowel frequently allow the surgeon to lightly peel the affected layers off the underlying mucosa by a technique called 'mucosal skinning' (Fig. 13.15). In many cases rectal mucosa is not penetrated during resection, in which case the seromuscular layer is closed with interrupted 2-0 silk. If dense submucosal fibrosis causes the mucosa to be penetrated during dissection, the mass of diseased tissue can be removed transanally with a ring forceps and a rectal repair undertaken; otherwise, the diseased tissue can be removed after slight enlargement of the 10 mm umbilical port. The defect to be repaired can be suspended between sutures which exit the lower incisions alongside the trocar sheaths (Fig. 13.16). The bowel is closed in two layers, the first being a running layer of 3-0 Vicryl beginning at one lateral angle and working toward the other (Fig. 13.17). Each end of the mucosal suture line is buried beneath the bowel wall surface using a purse-string suture of 2-0 silk (Figs 13.18, 13.19). The seromuscular layer is closed from each angle to midline with interrupted 2-0 silk (Fig. 13.20). The repair can

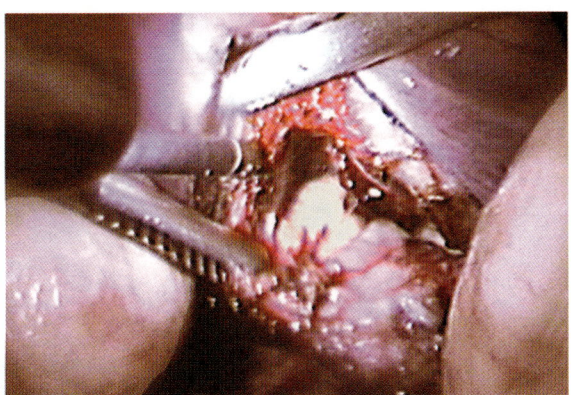

Figure 13.14

This patient had endometriosis of the vagina invading from a rectal nodule associated with obliteration of the cul de sac. The left vaginal apex has been entered laparoscopically to temporarily avoid the vaginal nodule in midline. The laparoscopic incision can then follow along the vaginal mucosal incision which was made from below (Fig. 13.5), resulting in positive complete separation of the vaginal disease from the posterior cervix and distal vagina. By courtesy of David B Redwine

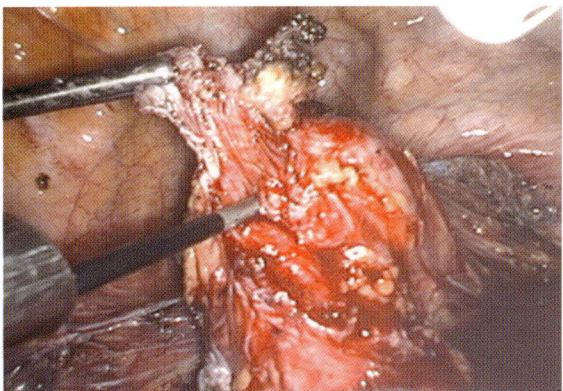

Figure 13.15

The 5 mm graspers at top are holding the right edge of an endometriotic nodule of the bowel wall. The 3 mm laparoscopic scissors working through the operating channel of an operating laparoscope is being used to bluntly separate the inner circular muscularis (seen as stripes of muscle tissue above the scissors) from the intact mucosa (seen as a reddish layer immediately below the silver hub of the scissors). By courtesy of David B Redwine

SURGICAL MANAGEMENT OF ENDOMETRIOSIS

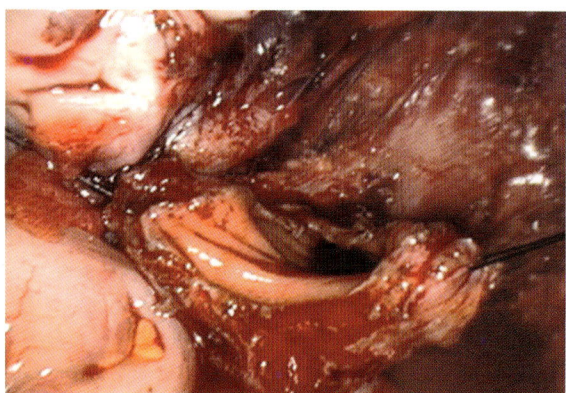

Figure 13.16
Angle sutures of 2-0 silk placed through normal seromuscularis are used to suspend the rectosigmoid colon following full thickness resection of a sizeable nodule. This may help prevent retained bowel prep liquid from running out of the bowel and contaminating the pelvis. By courtesy of David B Redwine

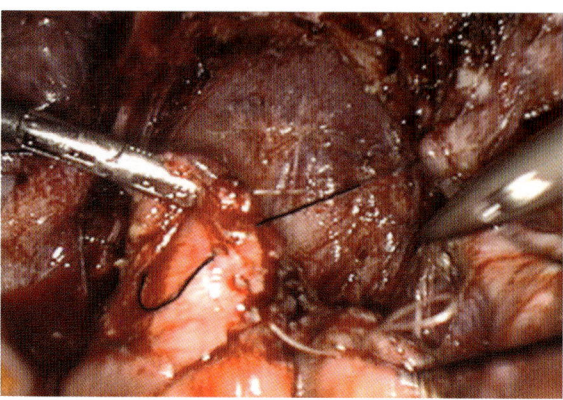

Figure 13.18
After the mucosa is closed, a purse-string suture of 2-0 silk is placed around each angle to bury the corners of the mucosal closure. By courtesy of David B Redwine

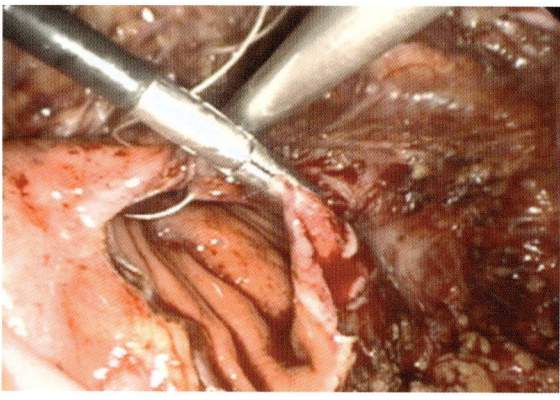

Figure 13.17
Full-thickness resections of the anterior bowel wall are repaired in two layers. Here, the mucosal closure is begun at the left angle, using running 3-0 Vicryl. As at laparotomy, it is easier to sew toward yourself. By courtesy of David B Redwine

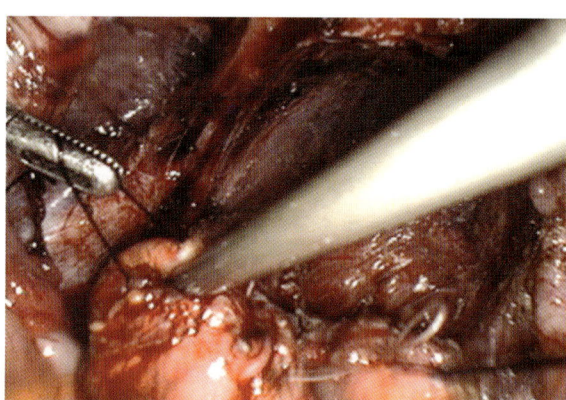

Figure 13.19
The mucosal angle is dunked beneath the seromuscular surface of the bowel and buried by the purse-string suture. This process is repeated on the opposite angle of the bowel before the intervening seromuscular layer is closed with interrupted 2-0 silk sutures. By courtesy of David B Redwine

be checked for leaks by underwater transanal air pressure examination. If surgery has been lengthy and copious irrigation used, a drain can be pulled through one of the 5 mm ports and placed into the cul de sac (Fig. 13.21) for postoperative drainage. This approach, associated with meticulous attention to haemostasis and peritoneal lavage, is associated with a very low morbidity.

Occasionally a patient with rectosigmoid endometriosis may have a lesion so large that segmental bowel resection is necessary. The steps of the procedure are identical to the point

RECTOVAGINAL ENDOMETRIOSIS

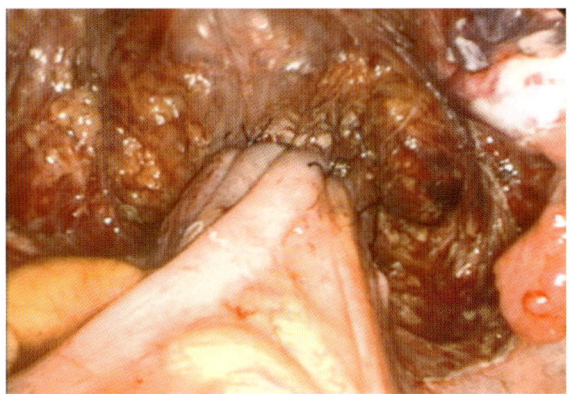

Figure 13.20
The appearance of the bowel after repair has been completed. Underwater air pressure examination or rectal injection of povidone-iodine can be used to ensure a safe repair. By courtesy of David B Redwine

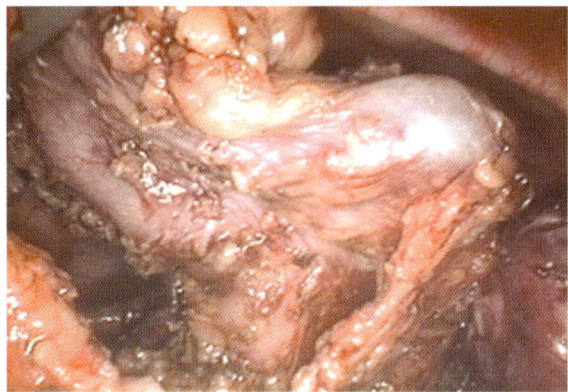

Figure 13.22
A segment of rectosigmoid colon whose anterior surface is involved by a large endometriotic nodule has been completely detached from its mesentery laparoscopically. A ring forceps passed transanally is seen distending the lumen on the right side of the frame. By courtesy of David B Redwine

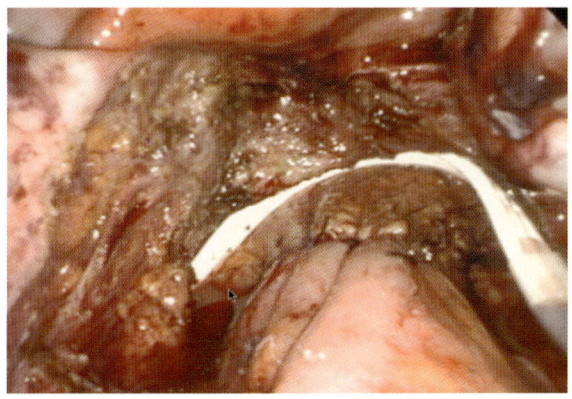

Figure 13.21
A 7 mm drain has been drawn through the right lower quadrant trocar site and placed in the cul de sac. With longer surgeries, more irrigation fluid will have been used and the drain will help it drain out more promptly. By courtesy of David B Redwine

of isolating the nodule to the anterior wall of the mobilized bowel. At this point, coagulation current is used to isolate the involved segment from its mesentery by coagulating and severing the mesentery immediately adjacent to the bowel wall (Fig. 13.22). The vessels of the mesentery are smallest and easy to coagulate as they enter the bowel wall, although occasionally a larger vessel will be encountered in the centre of the posterior bowel wall. These larger branches of the inferior mesenteric artery can still be controlled with a longer application of 50 watts of coagulation current. Since the segment which is being isolated will be removed, there is no concern over thermal damage to the bowel wall, although it is possible to avoid any thermal damage if the tissue is quickly coagulated before being bluntly stripped from the bowel wall. Once the mesentery has been completely separated from the segment to be removed, the normal distal bowel wall is stripped of its enveloping fatty tissue so clean muscularis is present 360 degrees around the bowel (Figs 13.23, 13.24). A linear endoscopic stapler is used to staple across this area of normal bowel wall just distal to the mass (Fig. 13.25). The umbilical incision is enlarged slightly and the proximal segment of rectosigmoid colon with the mass at its stapled end is delivered on to the abdomen (Fig. 13.26). The bowel wall is transected proximal to the mass,

SURGICAL MANAGEMENT OF ENDOMETRIOSIS

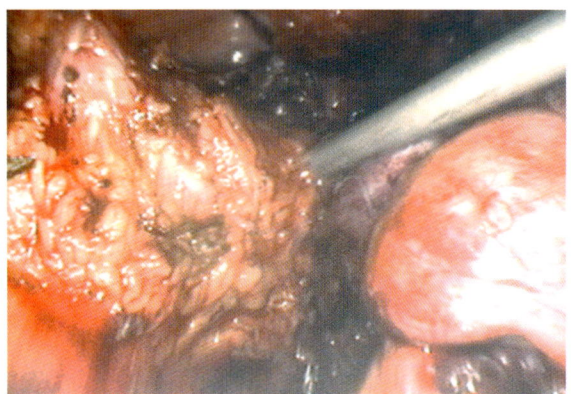

Figure 13.23
Fatty tissue is being cleansed from the wall of the distal normal bowel in preparation for segmental resection. A small area of normal bowel wall is just visible to the left of centre frame. By courtesy of David B Redwine

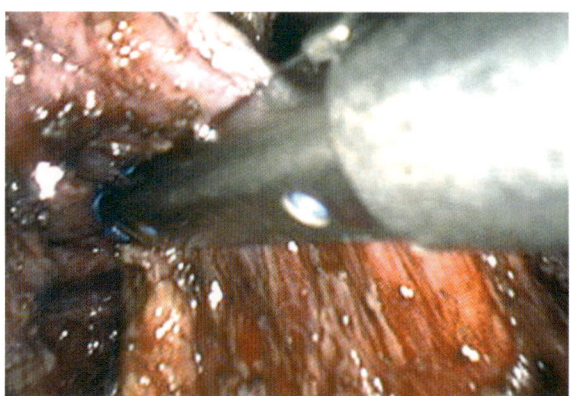

Figure 13.25
A linear stapler is used to transect the distal normal bowel just beyond the nodule. By courtesy of David B Redwine

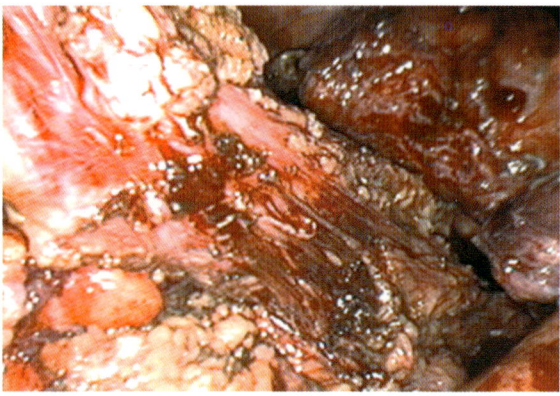

Figure 13.24
The normal distal bowel wall has been completely cleansed of investing fatty tissue. The edge of the large bowel nodule is seen in the upper left corner of the frame. By courtesy of David B Redwine

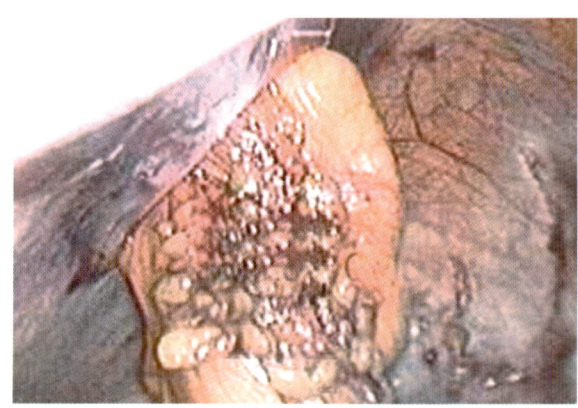

Figure 13.26
The proximal stump of the sigmoid colon has been delivered onto the abdominal wall through a slightly enlarged umbilical incision. By courtesy of Thomas L Lyons

then the anvil of a circular endoscopic stapler is placed into the normal bowel lumen and secured with a purse-string suture, then returned to the abdomen (Fig. 13.27). The mating spike of the stapler is now forced through the stapled rectal stump (Fig. 13.28), and the anvil fitted on to it using a laparoscopic grasper (Fig. 13.29). The stapler is then closed (Fig. 13.30), and fired and the anastomosis is complete. The tissue within the stapler should have two complete rings of tissue to ensure proper bowel repair. The integrity of the bowel can be checked with underwater air pressure examination.

Another technique which can sometimes be used with low lying rectal nodules is a transvaginal approach, particularly if hysterectomy is undertaken as well. This approach can be used

RECTOVAGINAL ENDOMETRIOSIS

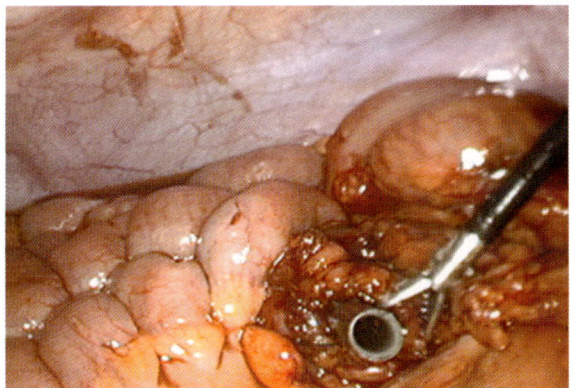

Figure 13.27
The proximal segment of sigmoid with the anvil head secured by a purse-string suture has been returned to the abdomen. This frame shows the shaft of the anvil head about to be grasped. By courtesy of David B Redwine

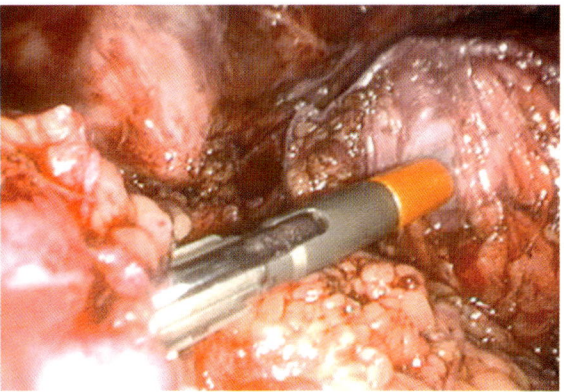

Figure 13.29
The anvil head is guided onto the shaft of the stapler until it locks in place. By courtesy of David B Redwine

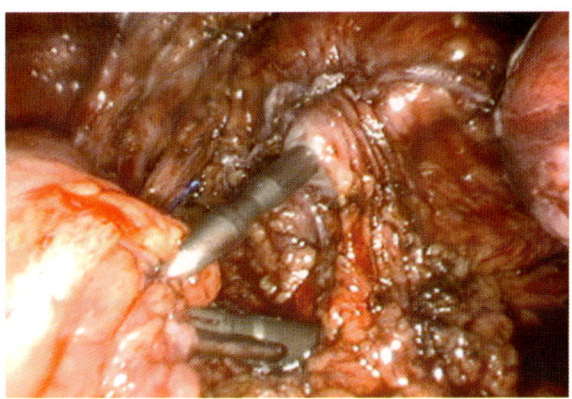

Figure 13.28
The pointed shaft of the stapler is advanced through the stapled rectal stump. By courtesy of David B Redwine

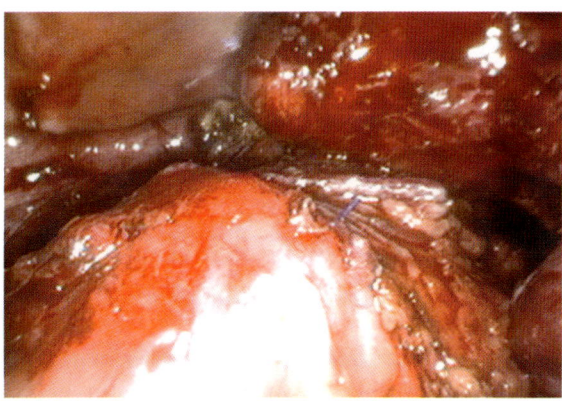

Figure 13.30
The stapler is screwed shut then fired to complete the anastomosis. By courtesy of David B Redwine

for anterior disc resection or repair, or even segmental bowel resections in some cases.[24,25]

Morbidity from bowel leakage is low when a deliberate decision is taken to perform full-thickness bowel resection for endometriosis. This is because the hole which is created is obvious and must be repaired. Where there is an attempt to dissect in the adhesive plane binding the rectum to the posterior cervix in an effort to avoid bowel entry, the likelihood of occult bowel injury is increased. Management of complications is discussed in Chapter 12.

Excision of rectovaginal disease with these techniques is associated with good symptom relief, low morbidity and a short one or two day hospital stay.[1,7]

Other forms of treatment for rectovaginal endometriosis have been described. A large series has been published by Nisolle and Donnez et al in Belgium.[26] Their surgical technique is based on the belief that endometriotic involvement of the rectum does not occur, despite decades of published evidence to the contrary. Plaque disease lying on the anterior wall of the rectum identified by double contrast barium enema is diagnosed as 'peri-visceritis'. Since no biopsy is typically taken from the bowel wall, this diagnosis is a presumption which many experts believe is incorrect. Using a carbon dioxide (CO_2) laser as a dissecting tool and staying within the boundaries of the utero-sacral ligaments, they dissect the rectum free from the posterior cervix. Once the rectum is freed, the vaginal adenomyoma is removed transvaginally and the defect sutured. Any residual endometriosis in the uterosacral ligaments is then ablated using the CO_2 laser to vaporize the tissue. No attempt is made to remove the plaque from the anterior bowel wall. Good symptomatic relief is claimed for this method, although objective measurement of symptom response was not mentioned. Leaving intestinal disease behind may be evidence that symptoms arise more commonly from the uterosacral ligaments and rectovaginal adenomyoma than from the rectal wall itself. The bowel lumen was entered on three occasions in their series with no significant morbidity resulting, since entry was identified and suture repaired.

Summary

There are few gynaecologists who have had sufficient training in complex laparoscopic techniques to feel confident to undertake rectal repair. There is an equally small number of coloproctologists who understand the pathology of endometriotic disease involving the bowel, particularly the disease of the seromuscular layer which rarely involves the mucosa and which can frequently be treated by limited disc resection. Women with a diagnosis of endometriosis of the bowel or rectovaginal septum, or those with a diagnosis of obliteration of the cul de sac, should be referred to specialist centres where this surgery can be carried out most successfully. Specialist surgical treatment centres for endometriosis should allow open access to surgeons wishing to learn these techniques, and where possible, have adequate supervised operative training, as well as training in the correct assessment of patients with this disease. Record-keeping in a standardized form allows valuable information on symptoms and signs to be collected and coded so that comparisons of treatment efficacy can be made.

References

1. Mathias SD, Kuppermann M, Liberman RF, Lipschutz RC, Steege JF. Chronic pelvic pain: prevalence, health-related quality of life, and economic correlates. Obstet Gynecol 1996; 87(3): 321–7.
2. Redwine DB, Wright JT. Laparoscopic treatment of complete obliteration of the cul-de-sac associated with endometriosis: long-term follow-up of en bloc resection. Fertil Steril 2001; 76(2):358–65.
3. Hemmings R, Bissonnette F, Bouzayen R. Results of laparoscopic treatments of ovarian endometriomas: laparoscopic ovarian fenestration and coagulation. Fertil Steril 1998; 70(3):527–9.
4. Jones KD, Sutton CJ. Laparoscopic management of ovarian endometriomas: a critical review of current practice. Curr Opin Obstet Gynecol 2000; 12(4):309–15.
5. Wright JT. The diagnosis and management of infiltrating nodular recto-vaginal endometriosis. Curr Opin Obstet Gynecol 2000; 12(4):283–7.
6. Garry R, Clayton R, Hawe J. The effect of endometriosis and its radical laparoscopic excision on quality of life indicators. BJOG 2000; 107(1):44–54.
7. Boog G, Penot P, Momber A. Ultrasound as a diagnostic aid in endometriosis. Contrib Gynecol Obstet 1987;16:119–24.
8. Dumontier I, Roseau G, Vincent B, Chapron C, Dousset B, Chaussade S et al. [Comparison of endoscopic ultrasound and magnetic resonance imaging in severe pelvic endometriosis]. Gastroenterol Clin Biol 2000; 24(12):1197–204.
9. Roseau G, Dumontier I, Palazzo L, Chapron C, Dousset B, Chaussade S et al. Rectosigmoid endometriosis: endoscopic ultrasound features and clinical implications. Endoscopy 2000;32(7): 525–30.
10. Momoeda M. [Recto-vaginal endometriosis]. Nippon Rinsho 2001;59(Suppl 1):192–5.
11. Stevens TG. Adenomyoma of the vaginal wall. Proc Roy Soc Med 1910;3:57–8.
12. Chapron C, Dubuisson J-B, Pansini V, Vieira M, Fauconnier A, Barakat H, Dousset B. Routine clinical examination is not sufficient for diagnosing and locating deeply infiltrating endometriosis. J Am Assoc Gynecol Laparosc 2002;9: 115–9.
13. Redwine DB. Mulleriosis: the single best fit model of origin of endometriosis. J Reprod Med 1988;33:915–20.
14. Halme J, Hammond MG, Hulka JF, Raj SG, Talbert LM. Retrograde menstruation in healthy women and in patients with endometriosis. Obstet Gynecol 1984;64(2):151–4.
15. Koninckx PR, Barlow D, Kennedy S. Implantation versus infiltration: the Sampson versus the endometriotic disease theory. Gynecol Obstet Invest 1999;47(Suppl 1):3–9 (Review, 87 refs).
16. Brosens I, Puttemans P, Deprest J. Appearances of endometriosis. Baillière's Clin Obstet Gynaecol 1993;7(4):741–57.
17. Martin DC, Hubert GD, Vander ZR, el Zeky FA. Laparoscopic appearances of peritoneal endometriosis. Fertil Steril 1989;51(1):63–7.
18. Redwine DB. Bowel resection related to endometriosis. In: Tulandi T (ed) Atlas of laparoscopic technique for gynecologists (2nd edn). London: WB Saunders, 1998:85–92.
19. Brosens I, Puttemans P, Deprest J. Appearances of endometriosis. Baillière's Clin Obstet Gynaecol 1993;7(4):741–57.
20. Bardos A. [Pathogenesis of endometriosis and notes on its histological diagnosis]. [Slovak]. Cesk Gynekol 1973;38(1):25–7.
21. Howell RJ, Dowsett M, Edmonds DK. Oestrogen and progesterone receptors in endometriosis: heterogeneity of different sites. Hum Reprod 1994;9(9):1752–8.
22. Jones RK, Bulmer JN, Searle RF. Immunohistochemical characterization of proliferation, oestrogen receptor and progesterone receptor expression in endometriosis: comparison of eutopic and ectopic endometrium with normal cycling endometrium. Hum Reprod 1995;10(12): 3272–9.
23. Redwine DB. Laparoscopic en bloc resection for treatment of the obliterated cul de sac in endometriosis. J Reprod Med 1992;37:695–8.

24. Redwine DB, Koning M, Sharpe DR. Laparoscopically assisted transvaginal segmental bowel resection for endometriosis. Fertil Steril 1996;65:193–7.
25. Varol N, Maher P, Woods R. Laparoscopic management of intestinal endometriosis. J Am Assoc Gynecol Laparosc 2000;7:405–9.
26. Donnez J, Nisolle M, Casanas-Roux F, Bassil S, Anaf V. Rectovaginal septum, endometriosis or adenomyosis: laparoscopic management in a series of 231 patients. Hum Reprod 1995;10(3):630–5.

14

Endometriosis of the urinary tract
David B Redwine

Bladder endometriosis

Many authors have reported many cases of endometriosis of the bladder,[1–9] with a particularly complete review of the literature after 1945 by Abeshouse.[10] Early reports frequently described the lesion as an adenomyoma of the bladder to reflect the histopathology seen under the microscope, with endometrial-like glands and stroma imbedded in fibromuscular metaplasia. Essentially, all reported cases represent spontaneous occurrence, and invasive bladder disease frequently coexists with significant invasive disease of the posterior pelvis. A case of full-thickness bladder endometriosis after Cesarean section has been reported,[11] although there was no intraoperative bladder injury.

Symptoms

Bladder endometriosis may be superficial or deep. Superficial endometriosis of the peritoneum overlying the bladder is common and is usually asymptomatic. It is important to remember that just as with any other area of involvement in the body, invasive endometriosis can masquerade as a 'superficial' lesion unless discrimination is made by palpation or surgical resection.

Endometriosis invading the muscularis of the bladder is uncommon, and disease involving the mucosa is extremely rare. Invasive lesions are composed of combinations of endometrial-like glands and stroma surrounded by fibromuscular metaplasia. For this reason, such lesions have been termed 'adenomyomas' of the bladder.[12] With invasion of the muscularis, endometriosis of the bladder may result in urgency, frequency, nocturia,[13] painful bladder spasm during voiding or either gross or microscopic hematuria.[14] These symptoms may be cyclic and increase during menses, although some patients may have a chronic lower level of symptoms throughout the month. Interstitial cystitis should be considered in the differential diagnosis.

Workup

Cystoscopy will infrequently be helpful in the diagnosis of bladder endometriosis because full-thickness penetration of the bladder wall is rare. Occasionally, cystoscopy may reveal a bluish tinge beneath the mucosa, but a negative cystoscopy does not rule out significant invasion of the muscularis. A case of bladder endometriosis associated with a 14 week sized fibroid uterus was associated with decreased bladder capacity and increased detrusor irritability. These abnormalities resolved after hysterectomy and removal of a small 4 mm endometriotic nodule of the bladder.[13] The relative contribution of the enlarged uterus to this clinical picture confounds the issue of which problem caused the symptoms.

As with most cases of endometriosis, surgery provides the most accurate diagnosis. While magnetic resonance imaging (MRI) scans are recommended by some, scans do not relieve symptoms nor eliminate the eventual need for surgical exploration if symptoms do not resolve with conservative therapy. Additionally, the depth of resection required will be obvious at surgery since the surgical dissection will occur in normal soft tissue adjacent to a firmer nodule of bladder disease. Thus, preoperative scans will not assist the surgeon in planning or executing surgery. Just because a type of scan is available does not make it always necessary, particularly with a disease like endometriosis, which depends so heavily on surgery for diagnosis and treatment.

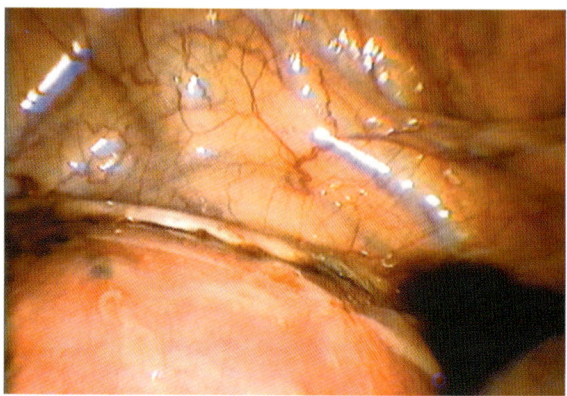

Figure 14.1

The peritoneum of the bladder exhibits rolling along its junction with the uterus, indicating significant endometriosis along this area, although bladder invasion is unlikely

Diagnosis

The principles of surgical diagnosis are identical whether performed at laparotomy or laparoscopy. Occasionally, peritoneal rolling will be seen across the uterovesical peritoneal fold (Fig. 14.1), and this frequently predicts only slight muscularis involvement. Invasive bladder disease that may result in full-thickness bladder resection can manifest as significant scarring and retraction of the bladder peritoneum with underlying nodularity and massive overlying hemorrhagic and exophytic changes (Fig. 14.2). Occasionally, a nodule of invasive bladder endometriosis may appear to be only a superficial hemorrhagic change (Fig. 14.3), with the nodule visible if the surface of the bladder is retracted (Fig. 14.4), or palpated, or if the bladder is filled with fluid instilled through a catheter.

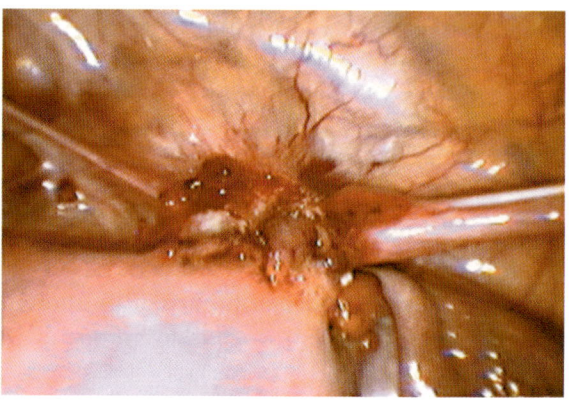

Figure 14.2

Florid invasive and exophytic endometriosis with massive distortion of the position of the round ligaments. Bladder invasion will always be present with disease having this appearance

easy and represents a good starting point for surgeons seeking to advance their skills. The bladder is easy to visualize and reach with laparoscopic instruments and is filled with a sterile fluid which keeps the risk of infection low. The surgeon must be able to perform intracorporeal suturing in some fashion to repair the bladder. The main risk in the surgical treatment of bladder endometriosis is possible damage to

Surgical treatment

The surgical treatment of bladder endometriosis by laparotomy or laparoscopy is essentially identical. Laparoscopic surgery on the bladder is

ENDOMETRIOSIS OF THE URINARY TRACT

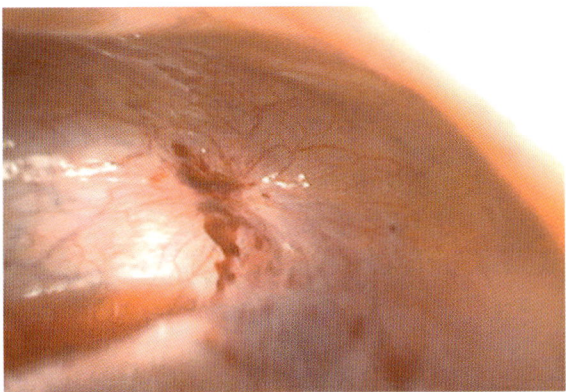

Figure 14.3

An innocuous-appearing lesion of the right bladder. This appears to be a superficial hemorrhagic lesion. Actually, it is a large invasive bladder nodule which will require full-thickness resection of the bladder

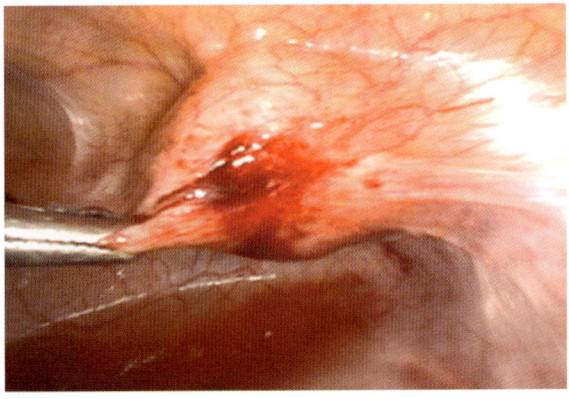

Figure 14.4

Traction on the innocuous lesion seen in Fig. 14.3 reveals an underlying large nodule over 2 cm in diameter

the portion of the ureter traveling within the bladder muscularis. Most cases of invasive endometriosis of the bladder do not encroach directly on the course of the ureter through the bladder muscularis or on the ureteral orifice.

Superficial endometriosis of the bladder peritoneum is easily treated by peritoneal resection without damage to the muscularis. Invasive bladder endometriosis will require partial-thickness resection of the muscularis or occasionally full-thickness resection resulting in partial cystectomy of the urinary bladder. This can usually be accomplished laparoscopically. Partial-thickness resections of bladder muscularis are reinforced with imbricating dissolving sutures which can be placed in running or interrupted fashion. If the sutures are placed with care within the outer layer of muscularis which has been damaged, there is little risk to the unseen ureters. Ureteral catheters are rarely helpful and are not mandatory.

Nodules of the bladder wall are approached first by dissecting into normal, soft bladder muscularis adjacent to the nodule (Fig. 14.5). The nodule is circumscribed and undermined by incising normal muscularis (Fig. 14.6), until it is removed entirely either by partial-thickness or full-thickness resection.

Even a large diameter full-thickness penetration of the bladder during surgery may not always be apparent to the surgeon (Figs 14.7, 14.8). Sometimes, the first notice of bladder penetration will be when the retention catheter bag is noted to fill with air, although neither this nor hematuria is always present during surgery.[15] Resection of large nodules will result in obvious

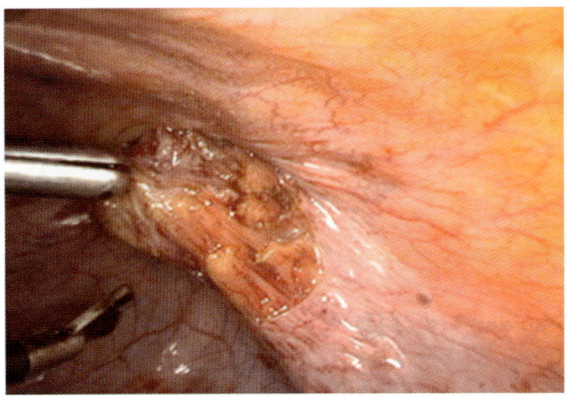

Figure 14.5

Electrosurgical incisions are created around the nodule in normal bladder muscularis

SURGICAL MANAGEMENT OF ENDOMETRIOSIS

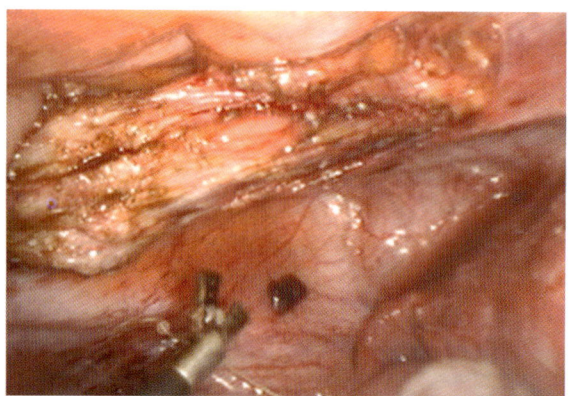

Figure 14.6

Full-thickness penetration of the bladder has just occurred

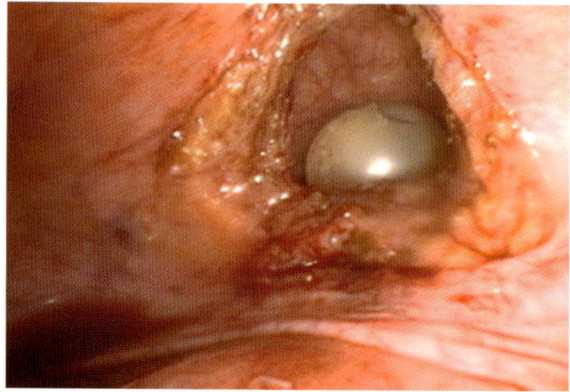

Figure 14.7

After resection of the nodule, a large bladder defect is obvious if the anterior edge of the defect is retracted anteriorly

entry into the bladder (Fig. 14.7). The ureteral orifices may sometimes be slightly hidden behind the rim of the posterior bladder wall, which needs to be retracted in order to view the jets of urine exiting the ureters (Fig. 14.9). Intravenous injection of indigo carmine may help identify the orifices more easily. It is mandatory to identify the ureteral orifices upon initial bladder entry to judge if the ensuing dissection may encroach upon them. The surgeon needs to be aware of the course of the unseen portion of the ureter within the bladder muscularis traveling posterolaterally away from the visible orifice. Since bladder endometriosis rarely involves the inferior wall of the bladder adjacent to the ureters and trigone, in most cases it is easy to repair the bladder in two layers without high risk of damage to the ureters. The mucosa can be repaired with absorbable suture, such as running 3-0 Vicryl (Fig. 14.10), while the muscularis is repaired with running 1-0 or 2-0 Vicryl. Interrupted sutures can also be used to repair the bladder, although this may take slightly longer. Once the bladder has been repaired, its integrity can be checked with instillation of irrigation fluid, with or without colored dye, injected through the catheter, although a retention catheter left in place postoperatively can allow

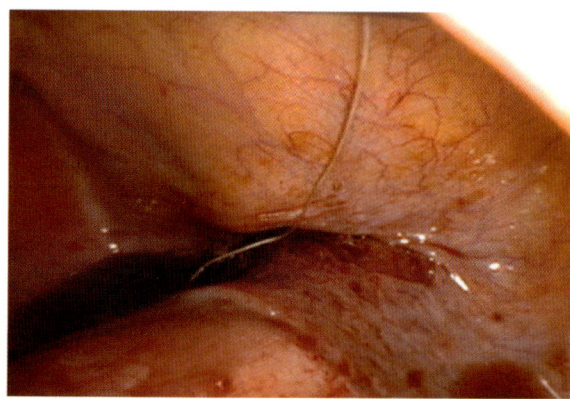

Figure 14.8

The large defect seen in Fig. 14.7 is virtually inapparent without traction on the bladder

even a poorly repaired bladder to heal. If the repair is perfectly watertight, the retention catheter can be removed when the patient is mobile, otherwise it should be left in for at least a week. If a surgeon may think it risky to remove the catheter soon after surgery, it should be kept in mind that suture repair of full-thickness bowel resections heal without any catheter bowel drainage or diversion. If the surgeon is concerned about possible constriction of the ureter by a stitch, cystoscopy can be done to

ENDOMETRIOSIS OF THE URINARY TRACT

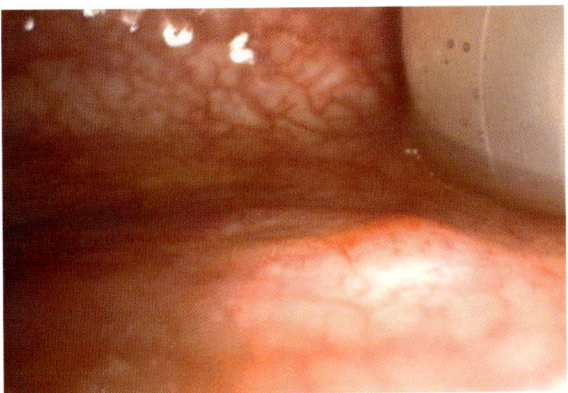

Figure 14.9
The left ureteral orifice is seen in the center of the frame, appearing like an oval crater on top of a hillock

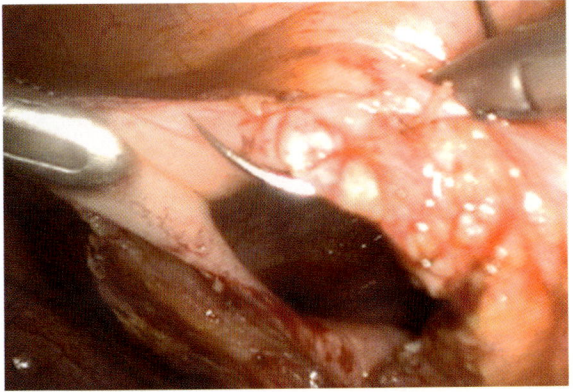

Figure 14.10
The bladder is repaired in two layers. Here, the mucosal closure with running 3-0 Vicryl is begun. The seromuscular layer is closed over this in running fashion with 3-0 Vicryl or similar suture

observe bilateral ureteral patency as shown by passage of indigo carmine. In rare instances, it may be preferable to pass ureteral catheters or to perform an intraoperative retrograde pyelogram to document ureteral patency.

One case of endometriosis involving the entire trigone has been encountered. This patient had multiple painful nodules palpable through the anterior vaginal wall, as well as associated severe pelvic disease with obliteration of the cul de sac. At laparotomy, it was necessary to remove the entire trigone from the level of the ureteral orifices down to the internal urethral meatus. The ureteral orifices were immediately adjacent to but not involved by the disease process and closure of the bladder left one ureter immediately anterior to the other, in an 'over and under' configuration. The patient had normal bladder function after removal of the catheter one week after surgery.

Laparoscopic resection of full-thickness bladder nodules has become fairly routine in many endometriosis treatment centers,[16] and is associated with a low morbidity rate.

Ureteral endometriosis

Ureteral endometriosis is less common than invasive endometriosis of the bladder and has been reported by many authors.[17–21]

Endometriosis invading the ureter is very rare and always results from extension of locally invasive disease from an adjacent uterosacral ligament nodule. More frequently, the ureter itself is not invaded by endometriosis, but is encircled by constrictive fibrosis related to invasive disease of the adjacent uterosacral ligament. When the diameter of the ureter is compromised either by extrinsic compressive fibrosis or actual invasion of the muscular wall of the ureter by endometriosis, hydroureter and hydronephrosis can occur with resultant flank pain which may occur or worsen during menses. In some cases, the stricture tightens so slowly that complete loss of kidney function occurs silently, sometimes with associated hypertension.[21]

Preoperative intravenous pyelogram, spiral computed tomography (CT) scan, renal scan, or intraoperative retrograde pyelogram may all be helpful in defining the extent of damage to the ureter and to renal function. For example, if the

SURGICAL MANAGEMENT OF ENDOMETRIOSIS

diameter of the ureter is seen to be small or non-existent, then resection of the involved portion of the ureter may be anticipated. In such a case, a urologist can assist by passing ureteral stents at the proper time during surgery. If renal function is already compromised or lost, this is helpful to know for medical and legal purposes so that unjust blame will not be assigned to surgical injury. If complete loss of kidney function seems apparent, laparoscopic nephrectomy may be a consideration.

Surgical treatment of endometriosis by removal of something else is rarely good practice, although this is favored by inexperienced surgeons. Thus, attempting to 'treat' ureteral obstruction by removal of the pelvic organs will frequently result in postoperative incredulity by the patient that her disease was left untouched and may invite further surgery since the obstructing nodule was left in place. Even in the absence of ovaries, invasive endometriosis may remain symptomatic because of the conversion of adrenal precursors into estrogen by the action of aromatase enzyme produced by the nodule itself.

Patients with ureteral obstruction due to endometriosis who have been treated by removal of the pelvic organs and retention of endometriosis may have involvement of the vaginal apex by disease invading from the underlying involved uterosacral ligament (Fig. 14.11). Surgery commences vaginally by circumscribing the lesion with electrosurgery until the soft areolar tissue of the rectovaginal septum is encountered (Fig. 14.12). This will make the last part of the upcoming laparoscopic surgery easier. The initial laparoscopic view (Fig. 14.13) will frequently seem normal, since all the invasive disease is retroperitoneal and bowel and omentum may be adherent to the pelvic surfaces, especially in the area overlying the active retroperitoneal nodule (Fig. 14.14).

Retroperitoneal fibrosis accompanying endometriosis may surround the ureter, requiring

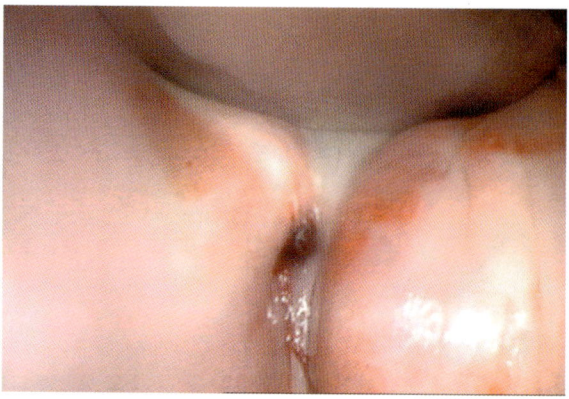

Figure 14.11

This patient had previous hysterectomy and castration. The apex of the vagina is involved by endometriosis invading from the region of the right uterosacral ligament, which in turn involved the ureter in retroperitoneal fibrosis

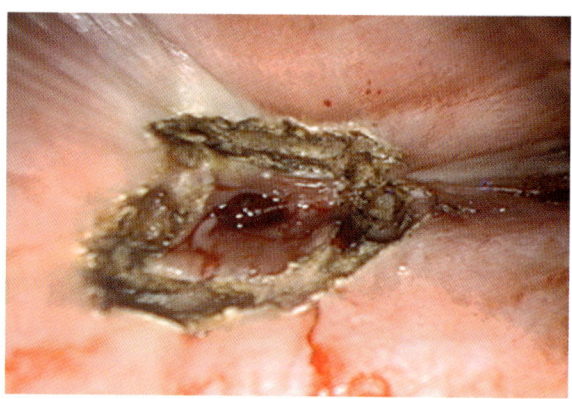

Figure 14.12

The vaginal lesion seen in Fig. 14.11 is circumscribed, the incision entering only into the rectovaginal septum

tedious ureterolysis. Frequently, this fibrosis will contain glands and stroma of endometriosis (Fig. 14.15), although sometimes the fibrosis seems to be only an intense reaction to adjacent disease. Ureterolysis is begun high on the pelvic sidewall in normal peritoneum anterior or posterior to the ureter. If an ovarian endometrioma cyst is adherent to the sidewall over a ureter, the retroperitoneal fibrosis can be surprisingly

ENDOMETRIOSIS OF THE URINARY TRACT

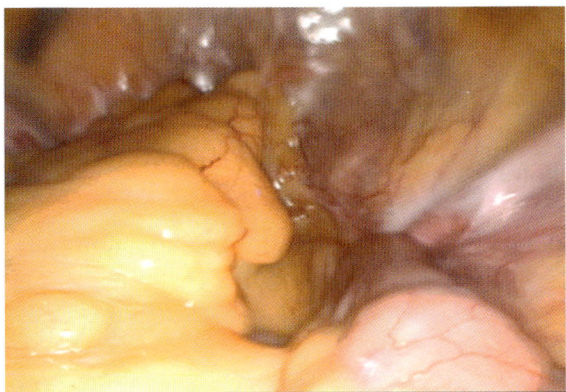

Figure 14.13
The laparoscopic view of the case seen in Figs 14.11 and 14.12 seems to be normal

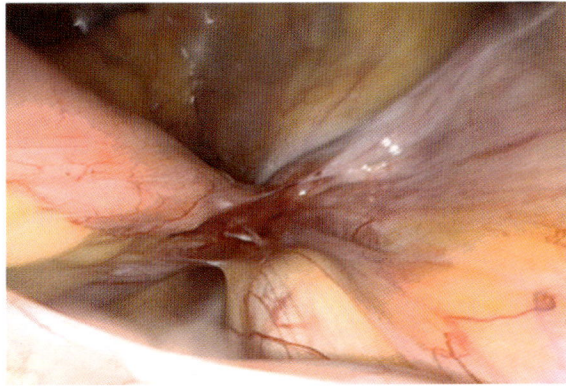

Figure 14.14
The ileum is adherent to the right uterosacral ligament. Note the right hydroureter in the bottom center of the frame, adjacent to the hemorrhagic area

pull the ureter strongly in one direction or another in order to obtain a line of attack against the fibrosis. Sometimes, the fibrosis will be isolated to an area immediately lateral to the uterosacral ligament, and probing the ureteral tunnel under the uterine artery will show that the ureter is freely mobile within this tunnel, in which case further ureterolysis toward the bladder is unnecessary. It will sometimes be necessary to sacrifice branches of the internal iliac artery, most commonly the uterine artery (Figs 14.18, 14.19), in order to completely free the ureter, and these can be controlled either with monopolar or bipolar coagulation or with sutures. Ureterolysis will be necessary immediately against the muscular wall of the ureter and occasionally small bleeding vessels on the surface of the ureter may require control by careful electrocoagulation applied in a very brief burst using a small active electrode. Bipolar electrocoagulation around the ureter may be problematic since many coagulator paddles are too large to apply a small energy footprint, so the risk to the ureter may be increased. Periureteral fibrosis may involve up to 4 cm of the length of the

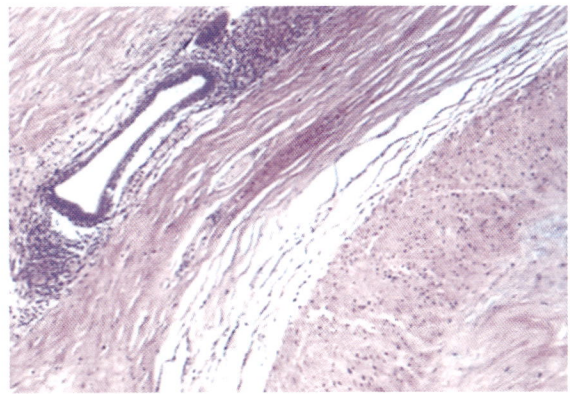

Figure 14.15
Periureteral fibrosis often harbors endometriosis. The adventitia of the ureter on the left upper side of the frame contains endometriosis. The muscular wall of the ureter is in the right lower side of the frame

intense (Fig. 14.16) and the ovary will need to be freed and suspended from the adjacent round ligament with 4-0 Vicryl so it will not impede visualization during an already difficult dissection. Sharp and blunt dissection combined with occasional cutting with short bursts of electrosurgery or laser will allow the ureter to be progressively freed up. A vessel loop may be helpful for ureteral traction (Fig. 14.17), although more commonly an atraumatic grasper can be used to

SURGICAL MANAGEMENT OF ENDOMETRIOSIS

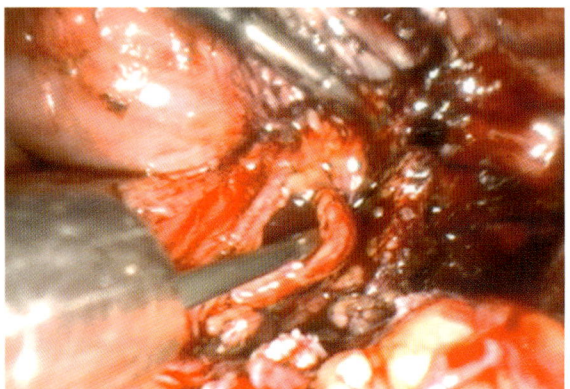

Figure 14.16
The left ovary is seen in the upper left corner of the frame, just beneath the shaft of the graspers. It is densely adherent to the left broad ligament. Dense retroperitoneal fibrosis has entrapped the ureter which is being placed on stretch by the 3 mm scissors

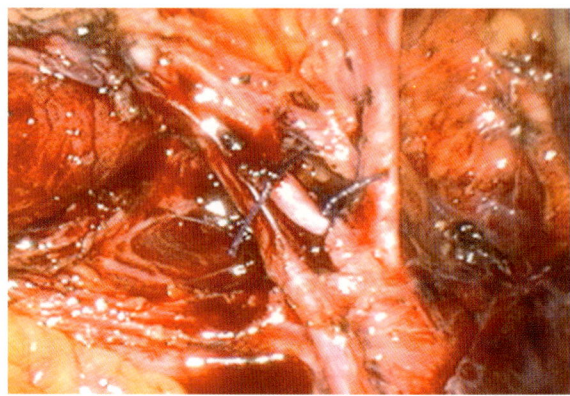

Figure 14.18
The right uterine artery is densely adherent to the right ureter lateral to the right uterosacral ligament. The artery has been ligated prior to transection

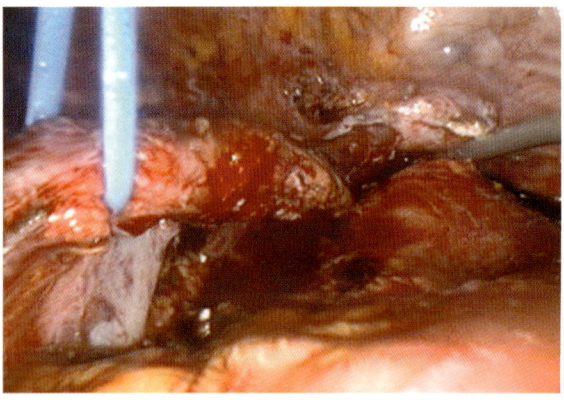

Figure 14.17
A vessel loop can sometimes be helpful in gentle traction on the ureter

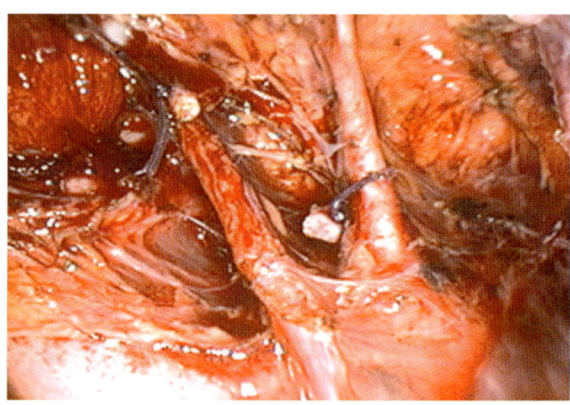

Figure 14.19
After transection, the right ureter is more visible and the distal uterine artery can now be dissected away from the ureter, thus completing the ureterolysis

ureter and may extend down to the edge of the base of the bladder. When the uterus is in place, the uterosacral ligament nodules will need to be amputated from the uterus while still encircling the ureters (Fig. 14.20).

In rare cases, the muscularis of the ureter will be invaded by endometriosis which may penetrate to the lumen with resultant partial or complete occlusion (Fig. 14.21). In such a case, resection of a portion of the wall of the ureter is necessary. The dissection to free up the ureter is much more difficult than the resection of the ureter and its repair. The dissection should seek to find fatty tissue deep to the ureter on its anterior, lateral and posterior sides (Fig. 14.22). When the nodule is put on traction, retroperi-

ENDOMETRIOSIS OF THE URINARY TRACT

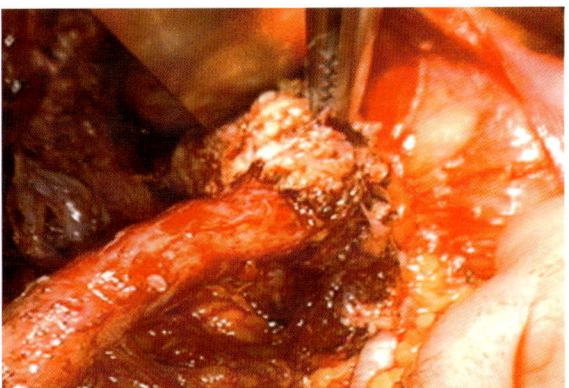

Figure 14.20
The right ureter is involved by dense fibrosis associated with endometriosis. The mass being grasped consists of endometriosis as well as the lateral side of the cervix and right uterosacral ligament

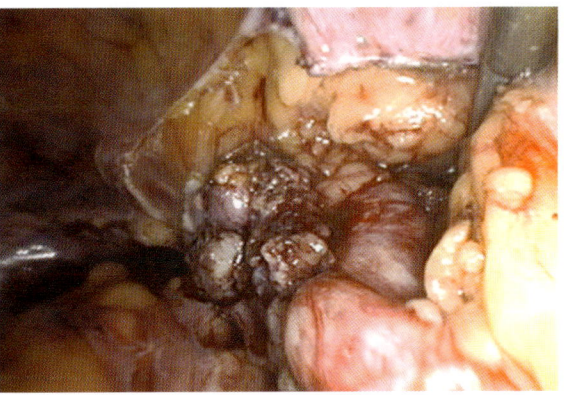

Figure 14.22
In this patient with previous hysterectomy and removal of the ovaries, the right ureter is in the bottom center of the frame and is massively dilated. Retroperitoneal dissection has begun to isolate a mass involving the stump of the right uterosacral ligament

toneal areolar tissue will exhibit straight lines of tissue pleats which will converge on the nodule (Fig. 14.23). These straight tissue pleats can be severed without undue risk to the ureter. However, as the nodule is approached, the fibrosis will encircle the ureter tightly and it will be necessary to operate directly on the ureter

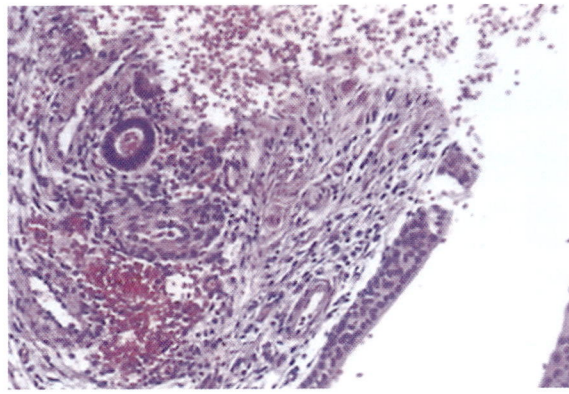

Figure 14.21
This is the case seen in Fig. 14.20. The endometriosis to the left side of the frame has invaded the wall of the ureter. The epithelial lining of the ureter is seen in the lower right of the frame. The left ureter was involved by an identical process

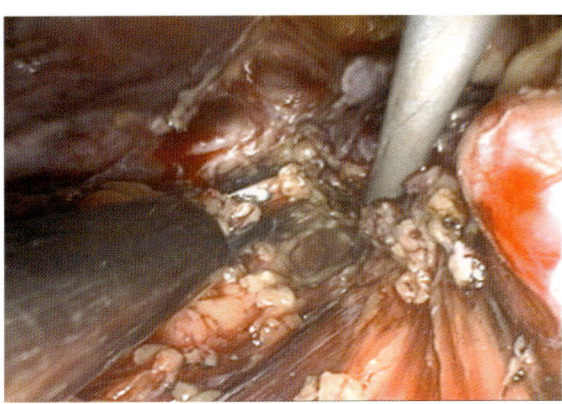

Figure 14.23
The right uterosacral ligament mass is separated from the right side of the rectum

(Fig. 14.24). The nodule must be completely separated from the ureter (Fig. 14.25).

Ureterolysis should extend at least 1 cm in each direction beyond the segment to be removed so that normal distal ureter is visible and available for suture. The segment to be resected will be apparent as a strictured area (Fig. 14.26) which may have a gristly texture

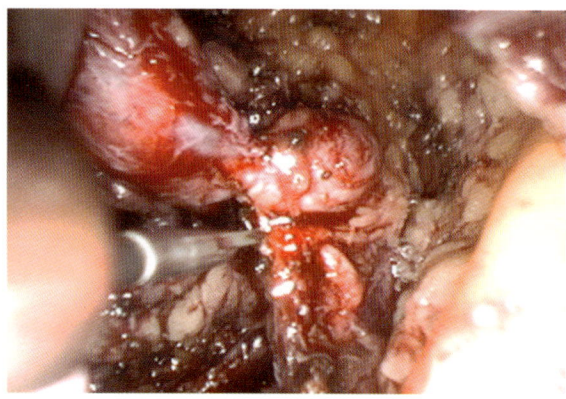

Figure 14.24

The ureter has been almost completely freed from the right uterosacral ligament mass posteriorly and laterally. The tight fibrosis associated with the mass had produced an area of severe ureteral constriction

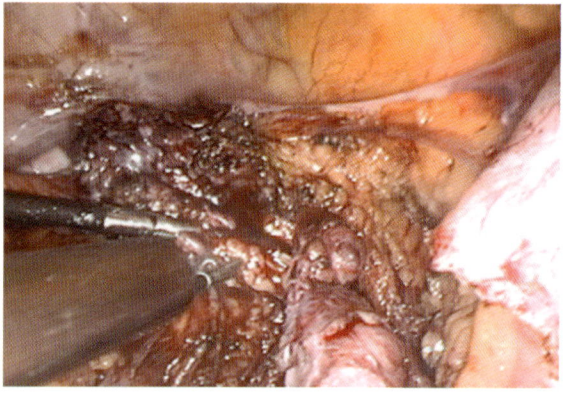

Figure 14.25

The last medial attachment of the mass to the ureter is severed

when brushed with an atraumatic grasper. The ureter proximal to the stricture may be obviously dilated while the distal ureter will appear normal in diameter (Fig. 14.27). Intravenous indigo carmine should be given before the segmental resection of the ureter is begun. The urologist should be present and performing cystoscopy with a double-J ureteral stent ready for passage in a timely manner. The ureter is cut proximal to the stricture with electrosurgical cutting current, cold scissors, or laser. The immediate exit of indigo carmine dye will give reassurance that no obstructive lesion has been left behind in the proximal segment. The cut edge of the proximal ureter can be inspected and should have a consistent thickness circumferentially since invasion of the wall of the ureter by endometriosis would be manifest by a thicker area. The diameter of the cut to the proximal ureter will be larger than normal and the wall may appear to be slightly thinned. The strictured area is now grasped and put on traction superiorly and the ureter is transected distal to the stricture. Sometimes, it will be necessary to trim the distal ureter further to ensure removal of all endometriosis. Since the resected segment typically measures less than 1.5 cm in length, primary anastomosis is usually possible. The urologist now passes a guidewire through the distal stump of the ureter and the gynecological surgeon grasps the wire and feeds it into the proximal stump (Fig. 14.28). The stent is advanced over the guidewire (Fig. 14.29) and intraoperative fluoroscopy is done to prove proper placement. The urologist is now free to leave the operating room after as little as 10 or 15 minutes of work. The ureter is reunited with four or five sutures of 4-0 Vicryl applied in each quadrant (Fig. 14.30). The first stitch usually accomplishes a rough approximation which can be reinforced properly with other stitches. The ends of sutures which have already been applied should be kept somewhat long so they can be grasped to help rotate the ureter in order to apply subsequent stitches. The stitch can pass through just the muscularis or can pass through the mucosa as the surgeon wishes. It has not been necessary to spatulate the distal stump to accommodate the larger diameter of the proximal stump. The stent is removed in the urologist's office after six weeks.

Bypass of the ureteral obstruction by redirection of the ureter via a psoas hitch may not be

ENDOMETRIOSIS OF THE URINARY TRACT

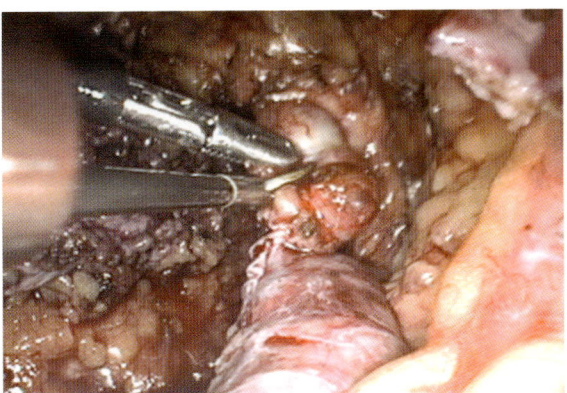

Figure 14.26
The strictured segment of the ureter is being excised. The scissors are cutting across normal distal ureter

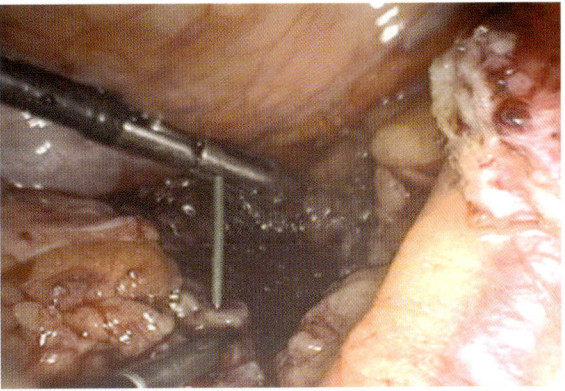

Figure 14.28
After removal of the stricture segment, a guidewire is passed by cystoscopy through the right ureter and is being delivered into the proximal segment of ureter by the graspers

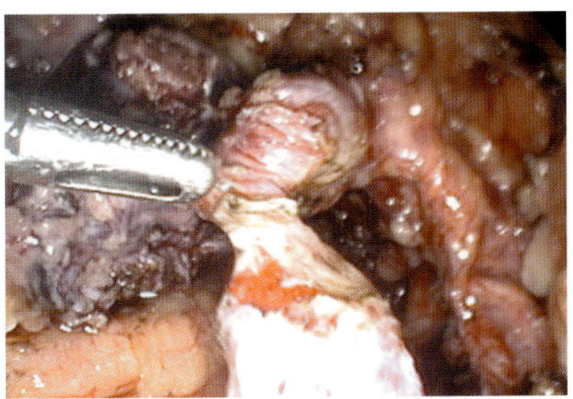

Figure 14.27
The graspers are holding the proximal edge of the strictured segment. An incision has begun across the proximal normal ureter

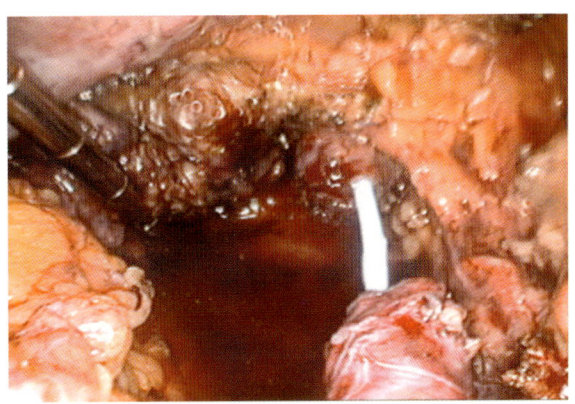

Figure 14.29
The double-J stent is passed over the guidewire before suturing the ureter

good practice. While this will relieve ureteral obstruction, the uterosacral ligament nodule responsible for the ureteral obstruction remains highly symptomatic for non-urologic reasons and will require reoperation. In one woman with previous left nephrectomy because of left ureteral obstruction by endometriosis, the right ureter was bypassed around the obstructing right uterosacral ligament nodule. The bypassing right ureter was reinvaded and was almost completely obstructed anew by the nodule that had not been removed.

Renal endometriosis

Endometriosis of the kidney is very rare and may cause back pain or hematuria which does not always occur with menses. Some cases can

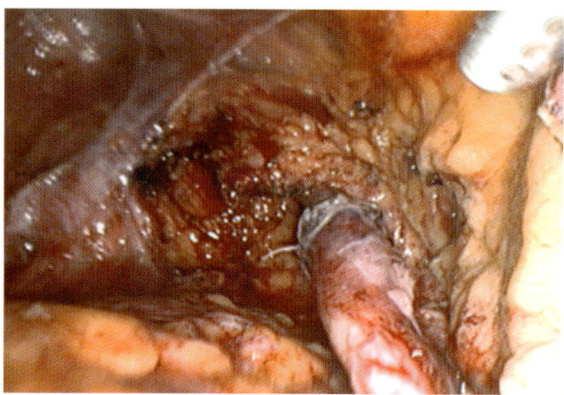

Figure 14.30

Four quadrant sutures of 4-0 Vicryl have been placed to complete the ureteral anastomosis

be asymptomatic and discovered incidentally at autopsy. Some symptomatic cases have been diagnosed by nephrectomy.[22,23]

A 40-year-old woman had a 10 month history of left flank pain and swelling and a painless mass in the left upper quadrant. There was no change of the pain or the mass with menses. The urinalysis showed minimal proteinuria but no red blood cells. Intravenous pyelogram showed a marked abnormality of the left kidney. At nephrectomy, the middle of the left kidney was replaced by a 9 cm cystic mass which was partially filled with chocolate-colored fluid. Smaller cysts were present within this mass which were filled with clear fluid. The mass was found to contain glands and stroma typical for endometriosis.[23]

One patient with daily hematuria and back pain was found by a combination of angiography and ultrasonography to have a 4 cm cystic lesion of the left kidney.[24] Needle biopsy of the lesion showed glandular fragments and cuboidal epithelium which could not have been of renal origin. At laparoscopy, a 1.5 cm endometrioma cyst was removed from the left ovary but no other endometriosis was seen. Symptomatic treatment with progestins for 6 months was only partially successful and repeat laparoscopy showed three sites of pelvic endometriosis, each only 1 mm in dimension. Nafarelin given by daily nasal inhalation for 11 months caused cessation of back pain and hematuria within one month and reduction of the left renal cystic lesion to 2 cm with only red and white blood cells found on repeat needle biopsy. Five months after cessation of nafarelin therapy, symptoms recurred and cystoscopy showed blood coming from the right ureteral orifice. Nafarelin was resumed for 8 months and the patient remained symptom-free for at least 41 months following treatment.

References

1. Judd ES. Adenomyomata presenting as tumor of the bladder. Surg Clin North Am 1921;1:1271–8.
2. Schwartzwald D, Mooppan UMM, Ohm HK, Kim H. Urology 1992;38:219–22.
3. Hyler DS, Baluch JD, Taylor RR. Intramural vesical endometriosis. J Reprod Med 1994;39:832–4.
4. Donnez J, Spada F, Nisolle M. Bladder endometriosis or adenomyosis? Diagnosis and management. In: Donnez J, Nisolle M (eds) An atlas of operative laparoscopy and hysteroscopy. Carnforth, UK: Parthenon, 2001:103–12.
5. Donnez J, Spada F, Squifflet J, Nisolle M. Bladder endometriosis must be considered as bladder adenomyosis. Fertil Steril 2000;74:1175–81.
6. Fedele L, Piazzola E, Raffaelli R, Bianchi S. Bladder endometriosis: Deep infiltrating endometriosis or adenomyosis? Fertil Steril 1998;69:972–5.
7. Nezhat C, Nezhat F. Laparoscopic segmental bladder resection for endometriosis: a report of two cases. Obstet Gynecol 1993;81:882–4.
8. Dubuisson JB, Chapron C, Aubriot FX, Osman M, Zerbib M. Pregnancy after laparoscopic partial cystectomy for bladder endometriosis. Hum Reprod 1994;9:730–2.
9. Chapron C, Boucher E, Fauconnier A, Vicira M, Dubuisson JB, Vacher-Lavenu MC. Anatomopathological lesions of bladder endometriosis are heterogenous. Fertil Steril 2002;78:740–2.
10. Abeshouse BS, Abeshouse G. Endometriosis of the urinary tract: A review of the literature and a report of four cases of vesical endometriosis. J Int Coll Surg 1960;34:43–63.
11. Buka NJ. Vesical endometriosis after cesarean section. Obstet Gynecol 1988;158:1117–18.
12. Donnez J, Spada F, Squifflet J, Nisolle M. Bladder endometriosis must be considered as bladder adenomyosis. Fertil Steril 2000;74:1175–81.
13. Goldstein MS, Brodman ML. Cystometric evaluation of vesical endometriosis before and after hormonal or surgical treatment. Mt Sinai J Med 1990;57:109–11.
14. Masson JC. Surgical significance of endometriosis. Ann Surg 1935;102:819–33.
15. Lamaro VP, Broome JD, Vancaillie TG. Unrecognized bladder perforation during operative laparoscopy. J Am Assoc Gynecol Laparosc 2000;7:417–19.
16. Nezhat CH, Malik S, Osias J, Nezhat F, Nezhat C. Laparoscopic management of 15 patients with infiltrating endometriosis of the bladder and a case of primary intravesical endometrioid adenosarcoma. Fertil Steril 2002;78:872–5.
17. Lucero SP, Wise HA, Kirsh G, Devoe K, Hess ML, Kandawalla N, Drago JR. Ureteric obstruction secondary to endometriosis. Br J Urol 1988;61:201–4.
18. Gantt PA, Hunt JB, McDonough PG. Progestin reversal of ureteral endometriosis. Obstet Gynecol 1981;57:665–7.
19. Abdel-Shahid RB, Beresford JM, Curry RH. Endometriosis of the ureter with vascular involvement. Obstet Gynecol 1974;43:113–17.
20. Case 49 – 1987. Case records of the Massachusetts General Hospital. N Engl J Med 1987;317:1456–64.
21. Davis OK, Schiff I. Endometriosis with unilateral ureteral obstruction and hypertension. A case report. J Reprod Med 1988;33:470–2.
22. Rosdy E, Sagi T, Torok P. Endometriose der niere. Urologe A 1979;18:22–5 (English summary).
23. Marshall VG. The occurrence of endometrial tissue in the kidney. J Urol 1943;50:652–6.
24. Hellberg D, Fors B, Bergqvist C. Renal endometriosis treated with a gonadotrophin releasing hormone agonist. Case report. Br J Obstet Gynaecol 1991;98:406–7.

15

Diaphragmatic endometriosis
David B Redwine

First reported in 1954 by Brews,[1] symptomatic endometriosis of the diaphragm is rare, with less than 30 cases reported in the world's literature. Most of these cases are contained in two series.[2,3] The right diaphragm is involved 27 times more frequently than the left. Bilateral disease is rare, occurring in only two of 28 cases. The age range of women with symptomatic diaphragmatic disease is 19–43, with an average age of about 34 years. There can be a delay of several years in diagnosis after symptoms appear.

Symptoms can be classic and consist of ipsilateral chest and shoulder pain which first appear during menses. Symptoms may extend earlier before menses as time passes, with some patients experiencing chronic mild symptoms with severe aggravation before and during menses. The pain can radiate up the neck or into the arm on the affected side and may feel like a muscular type of ache. When the pain is most severe, it can cause pain with breathing or lying down. Rarely, a patient may have to sleep in a sitting position and most will have to limit daily activities when the pain is at its worst. Heat, massage, and analgesics are used in an effort to relieve the pain.

The diagnosis of diaphragmatic endometriosis is initially suggested by symptoms, since imaging tests will usually be negative. Pleural effusions and pneumothorax are rarely diagnosed in these patients.[4] Surgery is necessary to confirm the suspicion of diaphragmatic disease, and this can be done laparoscopically. It is necessary to view the entire surface of each hemidiaphragm. A laparoscope placed through an umbilical port can view only the anterior portion of the right diaphragm because the large volume of the liver hides the posterior diaphragm from view (Fig. 15.1). While small, flat 'sentinel' lesions may be visible, the most highly symptomatic lesions will be located on the posterior half of the diaphragm.[2] The left diaphragm can be seen virtually in its entirety. The operating table can be placed into reverse Trendelenburg position to allow the liver to drop away from the diaphragm, but still the entire posterior diaphragm will not be seen in all

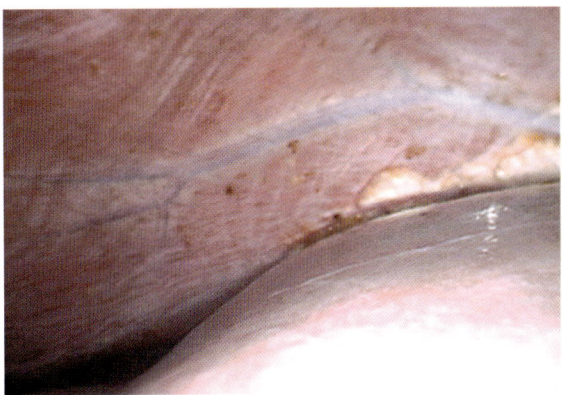

Figure 15.1

The right hemidiaphragm and liver seen with a 10 mm laparoscope maximally inserted through an umbilical sheath. The anterior and mid-diaphragm can be seen, but the posterior diaphragm is not visible

SURGICAL MANAGEMENT OF ENDOMETRIOSIS

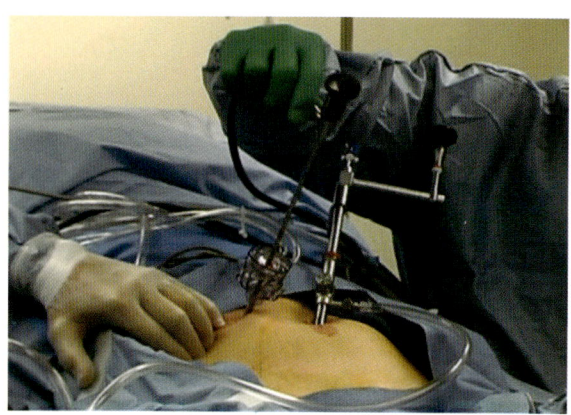

Figure 15.2
Exterior view of a 5 mm laparoscope inserted just inferior to the right costal margin in order to visualize the posterior diaphragm

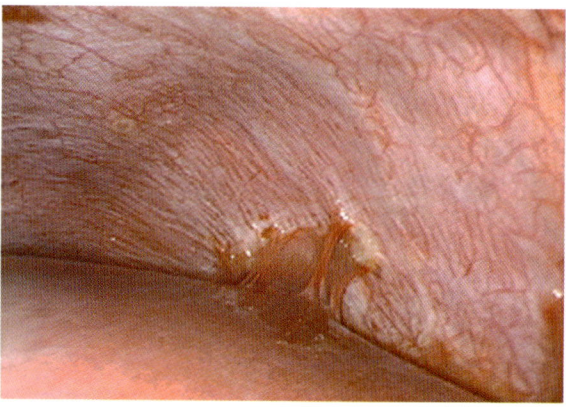

Figure 15.4
Endometriosis of the right leaf of the diaphragm with adhesions to the liver surface

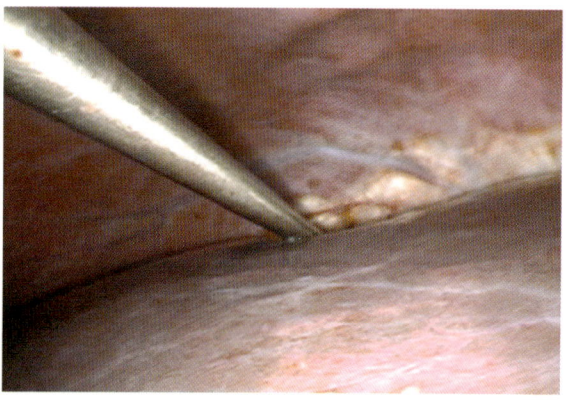

Figure 15.3
Laparoscopic view showing how much farther over the liver the 5 mm laparoscope can advance using the subcostal incision. The entire diaphragm can be seen

patients. The best way to view the right posterior diaphragm in its entirety is to insert a 5 mm port subcostally in the mid-clavicular line (Fig. 15.2). This allows a 5 mm laparoscope to be advanced much further over the dome of the liver than a laparoscope in an umbilical port site so that the entire diaphragm can be viewed (Fig. 15.3). Symptomatic endometriosis of the diaphragm exists as single or clusters of nodular lesions ranging up to 1.5 cm individually, spread across up to 10 cm of the surface of the diaphragm, usually in a swathe somewhat parallel to the posterior chest wall. Some lesions will exhibit adhesions to the adjacent liver surface (Fig. 15.4).

Treatment requires laparotomy and diaphragmatic resection for the best results.[2] Medical therapy has been ineffective in most cases where it has been used, and castration may not relieve symptoms in all patients.

The surgical procedure is straightforward. If unilateral disease is present, a subcostal laparotomy incision is used on the involved side. If bilateral disease is present, a midline epigastric incision is used. A self-retaining retractor is applied to the wound, and the liver is manually retracted inferiorly (Fig. 15.5), and the falciform ligament is lysed. Superficial lesions can be removed by partial thickness resection using electrosurgery or scissors (Fig. 15.6). Since the diaphragm is only a few millimeters thick, and since symptomatic nodules exceed the thickness of the diaphragm,[2] full-thickness diaphragmatic resection will be necessary. Long Allis clamps

DIAPHRAGMATIC ENDOMETRIOSIS

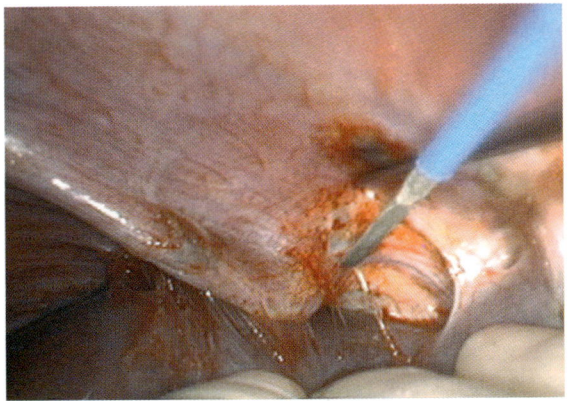

Figure 15.5
With the surgeon's fingers retracting the liver inferiorly, the adhesions are put on stretch and can be lysed with electrosurgery

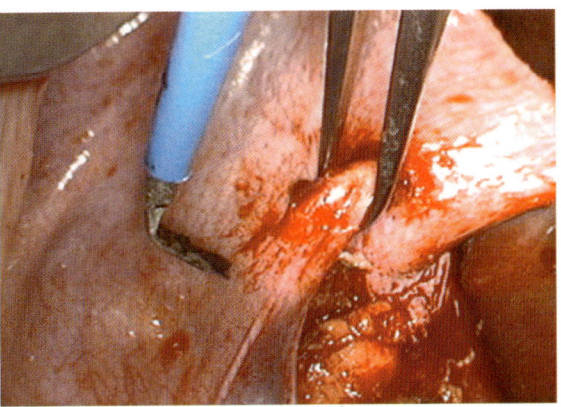

Figure 15.7
Full-thickness resection of the diaphragm is necessary to treat symptomatic disease. A nodule of endometriosis is grasped with an Allis clamp and pulled toward the abdominal incision while the electrosurgical pencil is ready to begin the resection

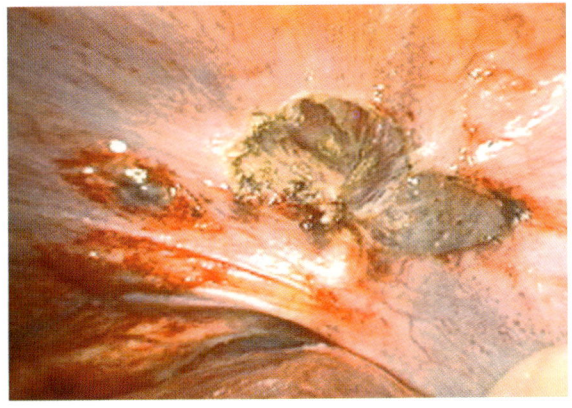

Figure 15.6
Some superficial lesions of the diaphragm can be removed by partial-thickness resection

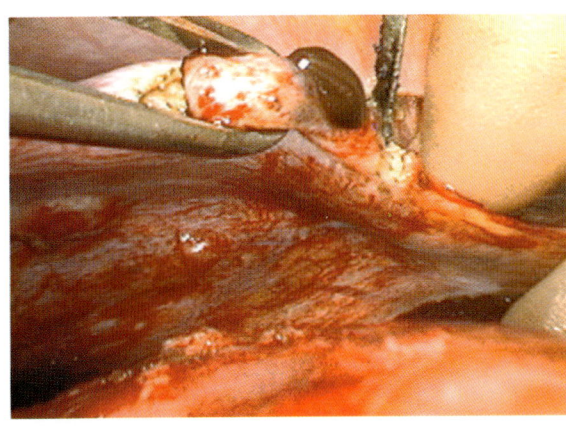

Figure 15.8
Electrosurgery is used to begin the resection adjacent to the nodule. Note that some thick chocolate-colored fluid has been forced out of the cystic lesion grasped by the Allis clamp

are used to grasp the affected diaphragm and pull it away from the underlying lung (Fig. 15.7). The pleat of tissue created between the jaws of the Allis clamp is incised next to the nodular disease (Fig. 15.8), using electrosurgery or scissors. The normal diaphragm alongside the lesions is then incised on both sides of the lesions (Fig. 15.9) until the full thickness of the diaphragm is penetrated (Fig. 15.10), and the segment of involved diaphragm is resected (Fig. 15.11). Occasionally the full-thickness diaphragmatic lesions (Fig. 15.12) may be adherent to the underlying lung (Fig. 15.13). Separate areas of resection are sometimes required for non-contiguous lesions (Fig. 15.14).

SURGICAL MANAGEMENT OF ENDOMETRIOSIS

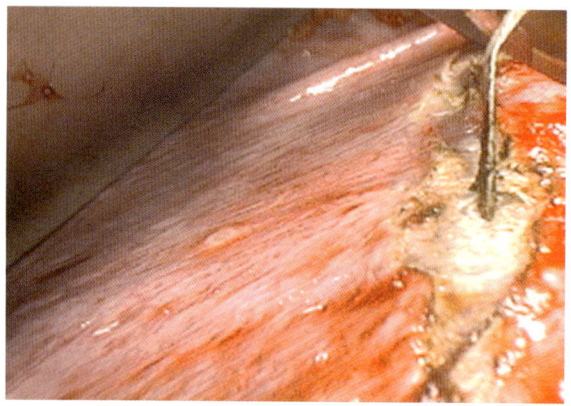

Figure 15.9
With the diaphragm pulled strongly anteriorly, the lesions on the right of the frame can be isolated with an electrosurgical incision alongside

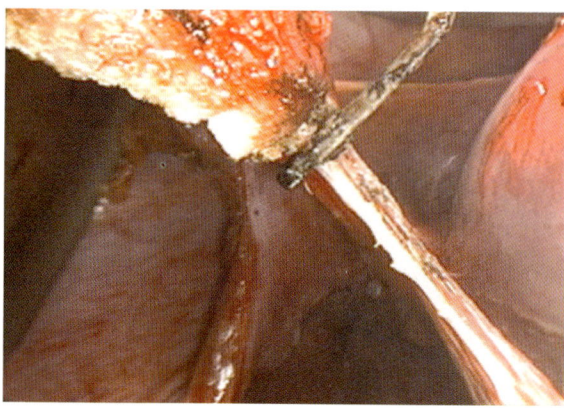

Figure 15.11
The piece of diaphragm carrying one area of endometriotic lesions is almost completely excised

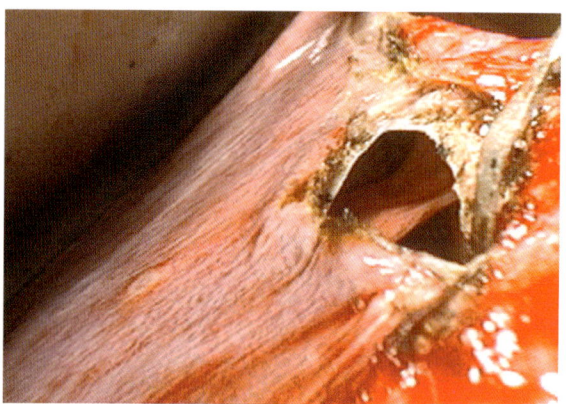

Figure 15.10
The incision quickly becomes full thickness since the diaphragm is so thin. The base of the right lung is seen through the defect

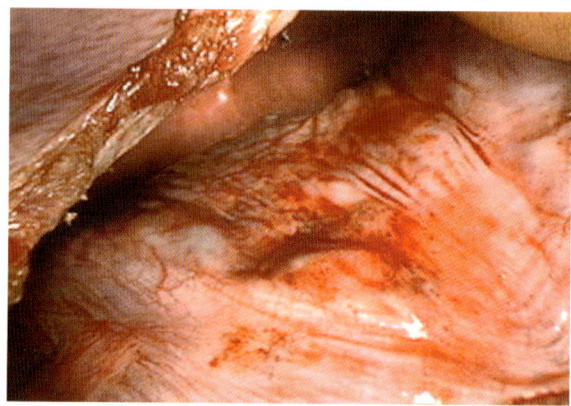

Figure 15.12
The pleural surface of the diaphragm can be examined after full-thickness penetration has occurred. Hemorrhagic neovascularity and nodules of endometriosis are seen penetrating the full-thickness of the diaphragm

The laparoscope can be advanced into the chest cavity (Fig. 15.15) to examine for thoracic endometriosis, which would rarely coexist with diaphragmatic endometriosis. The diaphragmatic defects are closed using a running permanent suture. Before the last suture is tied, a soft catheter is placed into the chest cavity and the anesthesiologist maximally inflates the lungs while the catheter is removed and the suture tied.

This eliminates the bulk of any pneumothorax. Postoperative chest x-rays are unnecessary in asymptomatic patients and would likely show a small pneumothorax. Postoperative fluoroscopy of diaphragmatic function was normal in two patients,[2] and there seems to be no morbidity from diaphragmatic resection, especially given the severe symptoms present before surgery.

DIAPHRAGMATIC ENDOMETRIOSIS

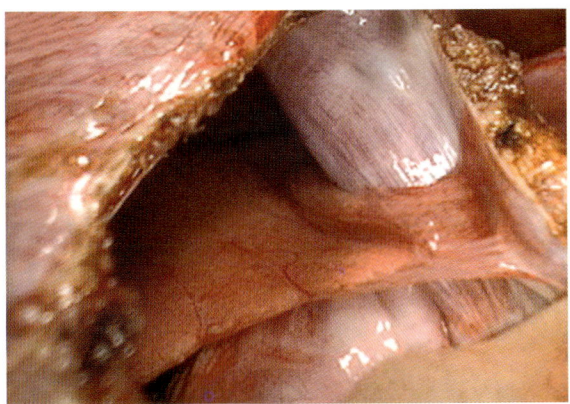

Figure 15.13
The base of the right lung is adherent to the pleural surface of the right diaphragm due to the inflammation of full-thickness endometriosis

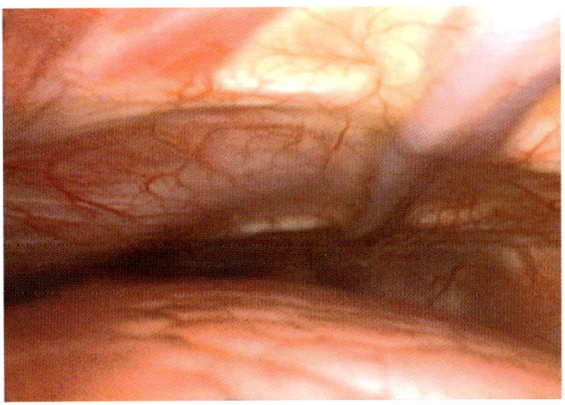

Figure 15.15
The laparoscope can be advanced into the thorax for transdiaphragmatic thoracoscopy. The anterior surface of the right lung is seen in the bottom third of the frame. The parietal surface of the right thorax is seen in the top half of the frame. The vessel is the right internal thoracic artery, which is also known as the internal mammary artery. This artery is a continuation of the inferior epigastric artery which is well known to pelvic surgeons

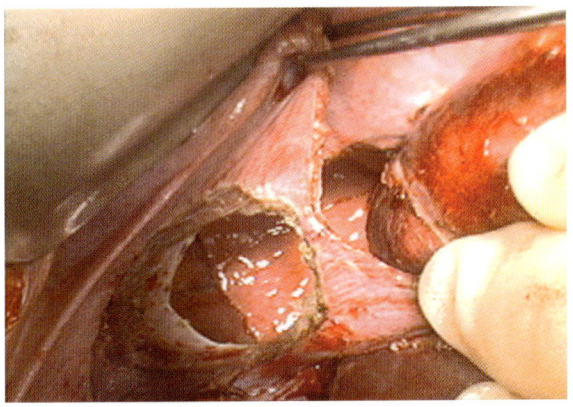

Figure 15.14
After complete removal of all diaphragmatic endometriosis by full-thickness resection, one or more defects will have been created

Symptomatic relief following diaphragmatic resection approaches 100%,[2] and is much more effective than laparoscopic laser vaporization of endometriosis through an umbilical port.[3] The lower symptom response seen with laser vaporization may be due to incomplete visualization of the diaphragmatic lesions and incomplete destruction. Indeed, since 100% of the cases of symptomatic diaphragmatic endometriosis in one series[2] were associated with full-thickness disease, thermal ablation techniques seem contraindicated.

References

1. Brews A. Endometriosis of diaphragm and Meig's syndrome. Proc Roy Soc Med 1954;47:461–8.
2. Redwine DB. Diaphragmatic endometriosis: diagnosis, surgical management, and long-term results of treatment. Fertil Steril 2002;77:288–96.
3. Nezhat CH, Seidman DS, Nezhat F, Nezhat CR. Laparoscopic surgical management of diaphragmatic endometriosis. Fertil Steril 1998;69:1048–55.
4. Bhaumik J, Hefni MA. Endometriosis of the liver and diaphragm: is the diagnosis often missed? Gynaecol Endosc 2002;11:155–8.

16

Conservative excision of endometriosis at laparotomy

David B Redwine

Before the availability of birth control pills, before danocrine, before GnRH agonists, before lasers, before electrocoagulation, before laparoscopy, what was a doctor to do with a patient with pain due to endometriosis who wanted to maintain the possibility of fertility? The surgeon could perform a laparotomy and cut the disease out of the body! While this concept of removing a disease, such as endometriosis, from the body may seem strange to modern day gynecologists, it was the only treatment available for the woman of that time who hoped to become pregnant. There is much to learn from those early surgical pioneers who dared to remove the disease and leave the uterus and at least one tube and ovary behind.

Measuring the efficacy of surgical treatment of endometriosis

Measuring the response of symptoms to surgery can be confused by postoperative medical therapy, since if a patient is doing well or doing poorly, it is unclear whether this is due to medicine or surgery. Assessing endometriosis at reoperation is the most accurate way of measuring the efficacy of an operation for the disease. At reoperation, the pelvis can be surveyed to see if endometriosis is present, and if so, how much disease there is and its locations. Unfortunately, this type of report is rare in the literature. Most physicians do not keep computer tabulations of their surgical patients, so they have no systematic way to produce an ongoing comparison of the findings at initial operation with findings at subsequent reoperation. Also, assessing the extent of disease can be problematic. The revised American Fertility Society (rAFS) classification system is the most widely used classification system,[1] but it does not accurately discriminate the extent of peritoneal involvement since most of its points are directed toward adhesions and most of the endometriosis points are awarded to the ovaries. Measuring the additive diameter of the implants is cumbersome and not all lesions measured are necessarily endometriosis.[2] Pelvic mapping of involvement of separate anatomic sites involved by biopsy-proved endometriosis is the simplest and most accurate way to measure the extent of the disease.[3] For example, if a patient had six sites of involvement at her first surgery and has one site involved at reoperation, that represents a reduction of disease.

Most authors of the early 20th century presented the efficacy of conservative surgery based on pain relief or pregnancy rates. While symptoms are important, the response of symptoms does not necessarily indicate the response of the disease, since endometriosis may not have been responsible for the symptoms in the first place, and not all endometriotic lesions necessarily cause symptoms in the second place. Reoperations were mentioned by some authors mainly for their rarity of occurrence. Extent of disease was not systematically assessed during that period.

Historical evidence of efficacy of conservative laparotomy excision of endometriosis

Surgeons of the early and mid 20th century did not have available to them the concept of a randomized controlled trial (RCT). Their reports of the efficacy of conservative laparotomy were usually published as longitudinal observational studies of the outcomes observed after application of excisional surgical therapy of endometriosis at laparotomy for the treatment of pain or infertility. As today, office visits, questionnaires and phone calls served as the basis for follow-up, although the methods of measuring pain were not always clear. Similar to today, some patients were lost to follow-up. Statistical analyses were crude, usually presented as the percentage of the successfully followed population that became pregnant or was improved or not. Symptoms were not always stratified in detail. Conception attempts were not always corrected for male factors, tubal factors or ovulation disorders, as these clinical concepts which seem so obvious to us now were developed over time and were foreign to early practitioners. Before dismissing such reports, one should be cautious of becoming an 'RCT elitist',[4] who rejects any publication which is not a randomized controlled trial (RCT). It should be remembered that RCTs frequently simply confirm the findings of robust observational studies,[5] with good correlation being found of summary odds ratios between randomized and non-randomized studies.[6] The lack of an RCT does not justify discarding or ignoring data from other types of studies. With that caveat, let us examine the 'ancient' conservative selective excision laparotomy (CSEL) literature as a basis for understanding modern surgical treatment.

Smith[7] noted a clinical cure rate of symptoms of 68% in 20 patients with successful follow-up who had been treated by ovarian cystectomy or unilateral oophorectomy at CSEL or resection of peritoneal disease, while Wharton[8] in 1929 observed similar good results in 3 of 4 (75%) patients treated by CSEL.

Read and Roques in 1929 described results of CSEL among 13 patients followed between 7 months and 6 years postoperatively.[9] Nine were cured (69%) and three were improved, for a 92% improvement rate. During follow-up, two required reoperation.

Cattell and Swinton in 1936 wrote about CSEL results among 21 women, 90% of whom were considered cured of pain at an average of three years of follow-up.[10] They cited other authors studying CSEL who published clinical cure rates of between 67.5% and 95.8%.

In 1937, Pemberton reported a 70% success rate among 107 patients successfully followed out of a group of 129 undergoing CSEL.[11]

Counseller in 1938 traced 98 of 162 patients treated by CSEL. Of 13 who also received a presacral neurectomy, 3 (23%) were partially improved and 6 (46%) were greatly improved.[12] In 85 patients treated by CSEL alone, 16 (19%) were partially improved and 48 (56%) were greatly improved. One surgical death occurred.

In 1940, Payne described a group of 73 patients undergoing CSEL, 25 of whom had obliteration of the cul de sac.[13] In the 48 without obliteration of the cul de sac, complete pain relief was achieved by 67% and partial relief by 26%. Obliteration of the cul de sac was not treated in the other 2, yet complete relief was claimed for 72% and partial relief for 20%.

In 1941, Dannreuther observed an 89% improvement among 18 women treated by CSEL during follow-up lasting up to 24 months.[14]

In 1942, Holmes noted complete relief of symptoms in 7 (29%) and partial relief of symptoms in 13 (54%) of 24 patients treated by CSEL.[15] Among 35 women undergoing hysterectomy with conservation of one ovary and incomplete removal of endometriosis, the rates of complete and partial relief of symptoms were 71% and 26%, respectively.

Schmitz and Towne followed a group of 47 women for one to four years after CSEL. Ovarian cystectomy or unilateral salpingo-oophorectomy was performed, along with resection or cauterization of peritoneal disease.[16] They found complete relief of symptoms in 25 (53%) and partial relief in 12 (26%).

Bacon in 1949 reported a clinical symptomatic cure rate of 49% and a partial cure rate of 21% among 138 patients treated by CSEL.[17] Greater success (64%) was noted in patients with unilateral ovarian endometriomas who had ovarian cystectomy combined with resection of other pelvic endometriosis. Greater failure (46%) was noted in patients with bilateral ovarian endometriomas treated by cystectomy without any other obvious pelvic endometriosis. Twenty patients were reoperated and underwent hysterectomy, with endometriosis found in nine of these. The surgically documented cure rate following conservative excision of endometriosis was therefore 55%.

Counseller and Crenshaw noted a rate of improvement of 72% was noted after CSEL, rising to 91% with the addition of a presacral neurectomy.[18] Reoperation was eventually required in 9%.

From the studies reviewed above, one can draw the impression that CSEL for endometriosis was more effective than not, with cures or successful treatment of painful symptoms outnumbering failures. So strong was the thought that CSEL was effective treatment of endometriosis that Meigs in 1953 wrote that: '... recurrence is not frequent, and cure of the lesion by conservative surgery is usual'.[19] He went on to state that the cure rate among 215 cases in his own hands was 93%. When the optimism expressed in those days is compared to the pessimism prevalent today ('... endometriosis is a mysterious, enigmatic, incurable, highly recurrent disease for which surgery is futile ...'), the question is begged: Has the disease changed that much over time, or have our therapies changed? The answer is obvious: The disease has not changed, but our treatment has. Management of endometriosis in the 21st century employs medicines that treat symptoms but not the disease, as well as surgical modalities which either have never been adequately described in sufficient detail to be replicated (electrocoagulation) or whose ability to eradicate endometriosis has never been validated by a sufficient number of reoperations with biopsy control (laser vaporization). No one can answer the question: 'What happens to endometriosis after thermal ablation?' because the question is not considered important. While it is theoretically possible that endometriosis might be eradicated by either thermal ablative method, there is also the possibility that neither may burn deeply enough to eradicate all disease. Additionally, the surgeon employing thermal ablative techniques rightfully is worried about damaging underlying vital structures. Since our understanding of endometriosis is thought to be limited, it was a leap of faith to discard treatment as apparently efficacious as CSEL and embark on treating a misunderstood disease with new and incompletely understood therapies. Medical equipment manufacturers seek to produce variations on thermal ablative techniques including the argon beam coagulator or coagulation with the harmonic scalpel. Pharmaceutical companies seek to produce variations of drugs that do not treat the disease, and are bent toward an ideal world where all women with pelvic pain are placed on medical therapy without a surgical diagnosis and maintained on that therapy indefinitely. This all seems illogical and likely to be a prescription for failure. Many patients with endometriosis would agree with this and would always select excisional surgery if proper informed consent was obtained.

Modern conservative excision of endometriosis at laparotomy

Patient preparation

Candidates for conservative surgery could include any patient with endometriosis, including those with minimal disease, because if a surgeon believes that excision of endometriosis is the best treatment but cannot perform excision by laparoscopy, then laparotomy would by default be the method of choice. Since simple laparoscopic excision is increasingly performed by general gynecologists, many surgeons will use laparotomy for cases that are too difficult to handle laparoscopically. Such cases might include those with obliteration of the cul de sac (Fig. 16.1), large uterosacral ligament nodules obstructing adjacent ureters, or intestinal involvement. Preoperative imaging tests are usually not helpful. In obese patients, ultrasound might be helpful in excluding other pathologies, such as uterine fibroids, which might change the overall surgical strategy, since myomectomy or hysterectomy might be added to the procedure. When the ovaries cannot be palpated easily, ultrasound can reveal possible endometriotic cysts, which may help in selecting patients for a bowel prep, since ovarian disease is a marker for an increased risk of intestinal involvement. In patients with known or suspected bowel involvement or significant nodularity on examination, a mechanical bowel prep is helpful.

Endometriosis is a pelvic disease for the most part, and it can be approached with a pelvic incision with the patient in Trendelenburg position. A low transverse incision will be adequate for most cases, including most cases of intestinal endometriosis. A muscle-cutting incision is never necessary. Presacral neurectomy will be slightly more difficult when performed through a low transverse incision.

A self-retaining retractor is applied to the wound and the bowel is packed into the upper abdomen with moistened lap sponges. A cell-saver for recycling recovered erythrocytes is recommended. The cul de sac and rectovaginal septum of the female pelvis is the deepest possible hole in which a surgeon can operate in the human body, so long instruments will be

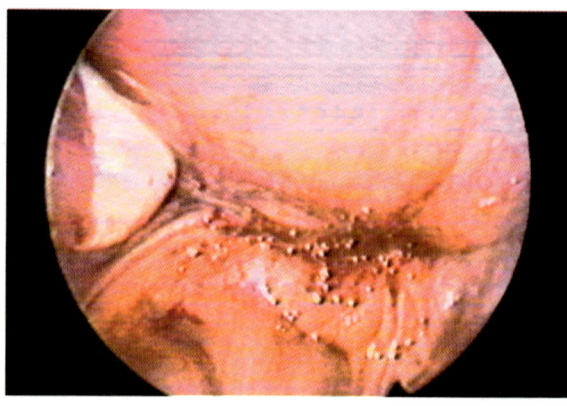

Figure 16.1

Complete obliteration of the cul de sac associated with invasive endometriosis of the uterosacral ligaments, posterior cervix, cul de sac and anterior rectal wall. The left ovary and tube are seen on the left edge of the frame. This surgical morphology may be described as 'dense adhesions behind the cervix' or 'dense adhesions between the rectum and cervix'. Such descriptions in terms of adhesions belie the endometriotic nature of this finding and the surgeon may not realize what is really going on

CONSERVATIVE EXCISION OF ENDOMETRIOSIS AT LAPAROTOMY

necessary, frequently even in thin patients. The four most useful instruments for excision of endometriosis at laparotomy are: long tonsil clamps, long Allis clamps, long right-angle clamps, and a long extension on the hand-held electrosurgical pencil. The tonsil clamps are used to grasp and elevate normal peritoneum adjacent to an area to be excised. Two tonsil clamps provide thin grasping surfaces, allowing the surgeon to 'walk' the tissue into a desired position. The Allis clamps are useful for grasping nodules of the uterosacral ligaments or nodules of the anterior rectal wall, although occasionally, a long Kocher clamp or single-toothed tenaculum will be the only instruments that can grasp nodules without tearing. The right-angle clamp is used to perform ureterolysis or angiolysis, assisted by electrosurgical cutting using the extension tip on the electrosurgical pencil. The electrosurgical pencil can also be used for cutting through parenchymous structures, such as the uterosacral ligaments or posterior cervix, when dealing with invasive disease in those areas. When using electrosurgery, it is important to remember that sufficient power should be used to get the desired effect efficiently. The exact watt setting may vary depending on the size of the active electrode, the area of the electrode in contact with the tissue, and the surgeon's technique. For a typical flat spatula electrode, pure cutting set initially at 50 watts and coagulation also set at 50 watts would be reasonable starting points. If the power is set too low, then the current density delivered to the tissue will be low and the desired effect may be blunted or absent. An expectation of a quick, clean cut may be replaced by messy coagulation with insufficient power. This is inefficient and potentially dangerous. As at laparoscopy, sufficiently high power is required for proper electrosurgery. It may be more dangerous to use inefficient low power settings than efficient higher power settings.

A traction suture of 0 Vicryl or similar is placed low on the posterior uterine fundus (Fig. 16.2). The ends of this suture are tagged with a hemostat and the thread can be pulled and attached to the self-retaining retractor or pulled by an assistant, thus elevating the uterus and exposing the posterior pelvis.

Ovarian endometriosis

If ovarian endometriotic cysts are present, they will need to be drained and excised first so other areas of involvement can be seen and treated. Attempting to bluntly dissect the ovary from its adherent attachments to the pelvic sidewall will invariably result in rupture of the ovary and spillage of the chocolate cyst contents since: '[it] is the destiny of the chocolate cyst to perforate . . .'.[20] Spillage of the contents of a chocolate cyst is not a matter of great concern, since no case of postoperative chemical peritonitis has been reported, and Sampson's original concern of spread of endometriosis from ovarian endometriomas was discarded soon after he proposed it. Ovarian chocolate cysts can usually be

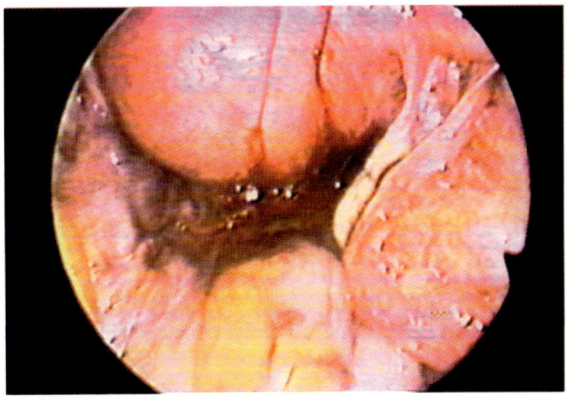

Figure 16.2

A traction suture is placed low on the posterior uterus to help draw the uterus, with the attached rectum, anteriorly in the pelvis. This strong anterior traction greatly assists the pelvic dissection

drained sufficiently through a single puncture site adjacent to the mid-portion of the Fallopian tube. The ovary, which is involved by an endometrioma cyst, is commonly adherent to the bottom of the pelvis, including adherence to a uterosacral ligament which is commonly foreshortened as well as to the lateral edge of the uterus. After the cyst is drained, the perimeter of the ovarian adherence can be seen more easily. Normal pelvic sidewall peritoneum adjacent to the adherent ovary can be incised and retroperitoneal dissection allows the ovary to be freed from the pelvic sidewall with abnormal peritoneum from the ovarian fossa still attached to it. This will ensure complete removal of all pelvic sidewall disease. The cyst wall itself can be extracted by blunt and sharp dissection. Simple drainage of a cyst, or drainage and coagulation of its epithelial lining is not very effective for permanent eradication.[21,22]

If an endometrioma cyst is densely adherent to the ipsilateral uterosacral ligament, it may be helpful to leave a portion of the ovary temporarily adherent to the uterosacral ligament, to be removed later when the ligament is resected. This technique is illustrated in Chapter 10. Ovarian endometriomas frequently obscure underlying pelvic anatomy, and it should be remembered that when endometriomas are present, there is an increased likelihood of more extensive pelvic and intestinal disease.[23] Therefore, surgical treatment which is directed solely toward ovarian endometriomas will guarantee that endometriosis will be left behind in almost 100% of patients, which is not a desirable surgical outcome. Allis clamps or tonsil clamps can be used to grasp the edges of either the cyst wall or normal ovarian cortex. A small cotton 'peanut' sponge can be helpful in bluntly stripping the cyst wall from the ovarian stroma. Occasionally, it may be more efficient to perform a wedge resection of the ovary if multiple cysts are present or if a cyst wall cannot be stripped out easily. After ovarian cystectomy or wedge resection, the ovaries can be suspended with absorbable suture from the ipsilateral round ligaments in order to keep them out of the way during subsequent pelvic dissection and to reduce the likelihood that they will become densely and confluently readherent to the pelvic sidewalls. After ovarian cystectomy, if ovarian function is suboptimal for some reason, ovarian stimulation can be expected to result in normal function.[24]

Ovarian endometriosis is often accompanied by retroperitoneal invasion by endometriosis, or the fibrosis resulting from it. Because of this, retroperitoneal structures, such as the ureter, blood vessels, or nerves, may need to be surgically freed. Surgery for invasive endometriosis is best guided by the line of demarcation between soft normal tissue and nodular fibrotic tissue which is the hallmark of invasive endometriosis. Palpation either with the fingers or with surgical instruments is frequently necessary to discriminate invasive disease from normal tissue.

Obliteration of the cul de sac

The cul de sac and uterosacral ligaments are frequently involved by endometriosis.[25] Obliteration of the cul de sac obscures direct visualization of these sites and is more than just an adhesive process binding the rectum to the posterior cervix. Identification of this impressive morphologic feature of endometriosis indicates the presence of invasive disease of the uterosacral ligaments, posterior cervix, cul de sac, and usually the anterior rectal wall. If psychic recognition of this fact by the surgeon is absent, surgery will be aimless, incomplete and seem far more difficult than it already will be. Surgery must remove disease in all these areas. This is best accomplished by an en bloc resection, which is also illustrated in Chapter 12.

Normal peritoneum lateral to the uterosacral ligaments can be put on stretch with Allis clamps then incised with scissors (Fig. 16.3) or electrosurgery. Blunt dissection lateral and posterior to the uterosacral ligaments will allow the lateral margins of the rectovaginal septum to be approached.

Retroperitoneal fibrosis can extend laterally from the invasive nodular disease of the uterosacral ligaments and encircle the ureters and uterine vessels, requiring ureterolysis (Figs 16.4, 16.5) or angiolysis. This is best done with long right-angle and tonsil clamps and electrosurgery. Two long tonsil clamps are frequently used together to stabilize the peritoneum during excision, or to grasp other tissue for traction or cutting (Fig. 16.4). The tips of the right-angle clamps are inserted alongside the ureter underneath the fibrosis encircling the ureter. By opening and closing the tips, they can be used to probe along the ureter to develop a dissection space. Once a sufficient length of the tips has been inserted alongside the ureter, the tips can be spread (Fig. 16.5), and the tissue between the

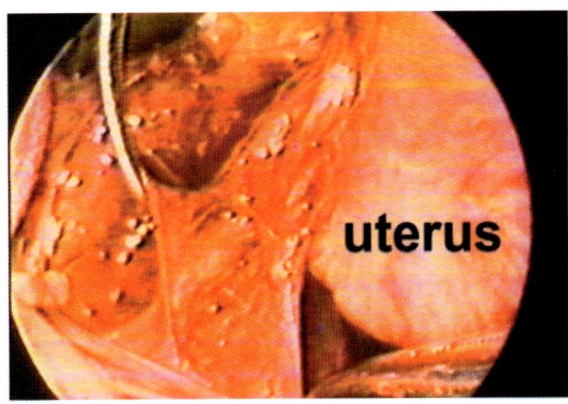

Figure 16.4

Areolar tissue surrounding the left ureter is grasped with a tonsil clamp to provide countertraction during ureterolysis

spread tips can be carefully severed with electrosurgery. By alternating the steps of blunt dissection, spreading, and cutting with electrosurgery (Fig. 16.6), the ureter can be freed from its investing fibrosis. Ureterolysis is usually necessary down to the uterine artery until the ureteral tunnel underneath the artery is found to be clear of fibrosis. In cases of exceptional fibrosis, the

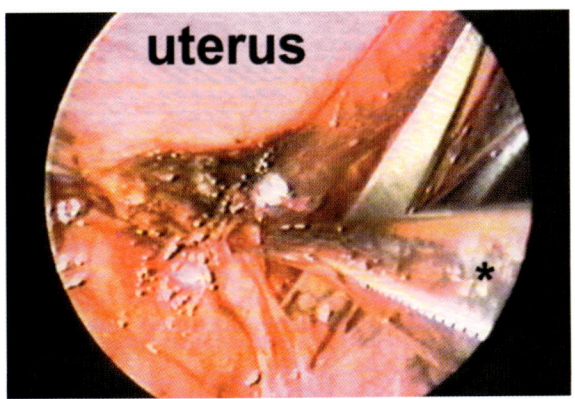

Figure 16.3

The right uterosacral ligament has been partially transected. The edge of an endometriotic nodule is being grasped with a tonsil clamp (*). Scissors behind the tonsil clamp are used to incise the normal peritoneum of the adjacent broad ligament along the peritoneal length of the uterosacral ligament

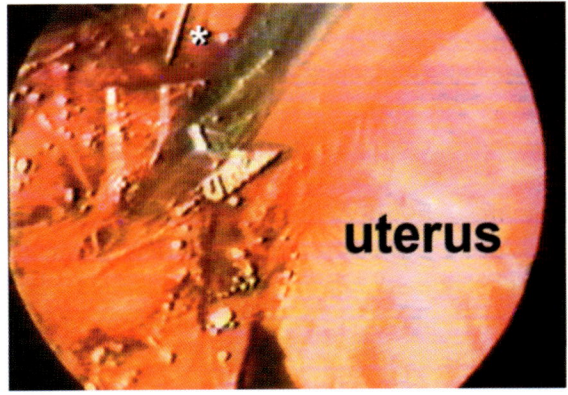

Figure 16.5

Retroperitoneal fibrotic and areolar tissue surrounding the left ureter is undermined with a right-angle clamp. The jaws of the clamp can then be spread, exposing the tissue between the jaws for cutting, either with an electrosurgical pencil tip (*) or scissors

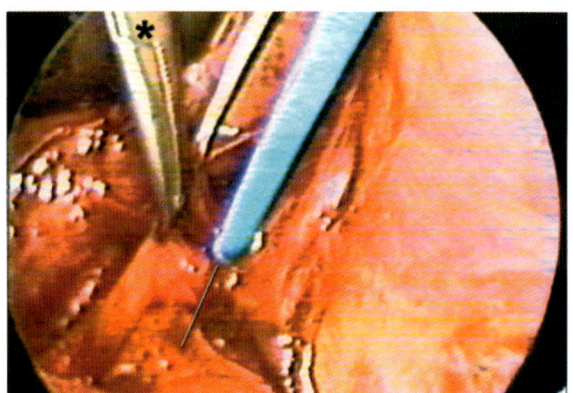

Figure 16.6

A tonsil clamp (✱) is grasping the surface of the left ureter and elevating it. This exposes the tendrils of fibrotic tissue posterior to the ureter which can be severed with the electrosurgical pencil tip

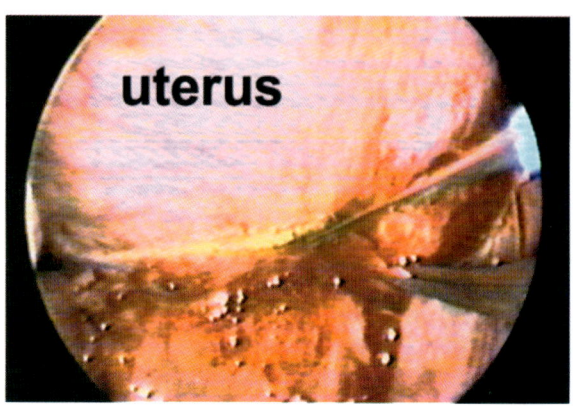

Figure 16.7

A transverse incision is created across the posterior cervix or uterus. This incision is made above the line of adherence of the bowel. The cul de sac remains obliterated

uterine artery must be ligated lateral to the fibrosis emanating from the uterosacral ligament and the dissection carried caudally alongside the uterus until the edge of the bladder is encountered. In the most severe cases, an invasive nodule of endometriosis of the uterosacral ligament may invade the ureter or even the base of the bladder, in which case segmental resection of the ureter or partial cystectomy of the urinary bladder may be necessary.

Once the ureters are seen to be well away from the uterosacral ligaments, a transverse incision is created across the posterior cervix above the line of adherence of the bowel (Fig. 16.7). This incision is created to a depth of only 1 mm or 2 mm. The transverse incision is extended bilaterally to amputate the uterosacral ligaments from the posterior cervix (Fig. 16.8). An intrafascial dissection is carried down the posterior cervix, shaving approximately 2 mm of cervical tissue until the rectovaginal septum is approached. The posterior cervix can be invaded virtually to the endocervical canal by endometriosis. If a surgeon aggressively pursues deeper lying micropockets of chocolate-colored material found within the cervical parenchyma in an effort to remove all invasive disease of the posterior cervix, mucus from the endocervical glands will eventually be encountered. Repair of the posterior cervix will be difficult because of its inherently stiff tissue. Given this possibility, shaving only about 2 mm off the back of the

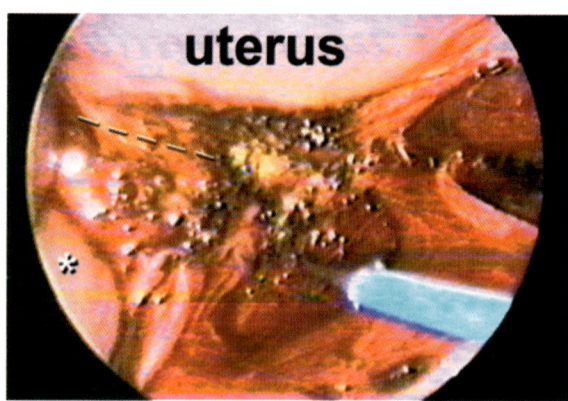

Figure 16.8

The transverse incision across the posterior cervix (– – –) is extended across the insertion of the right uterosacral ligament into the posterior cervix using electrosurgery. The normal rectal wall (✱) is seen adjacent to the obliterated cul de sac nodule which is beginning to drop away from the cervix

CONSERVATIVE EXCISION OF ENDOMETRIOSIS AT LAPAROTOMY

cervix seems to be a reasonable compromise between removal of a margin of tissue around the disease and causing too much surgical damage.

As the intrafascial dissection proceeds posteriorly down the cervix, a reddish layer of tissue will be encountered which is separate from the cervical parenchyma (Fig. 16.9). The true rectovaginal septum lies just beyond this reddish layer. Incision of this layer will expose the yellowish fatty tissue of the rectovaginal septum (Fig. 16.10), which can then be bluntly dissected by the surgeon's finger (Fig. 16.11). If finger dissection is begun prematurely against the reddish fascial layer, excessive bleeding will result as the dissection will be in the incorrect surgical plane.

The remainder of the surgery is performed as described in Chapter 13. The uterosacral ligaments are progressively dissected off the posterior cervix and the nodular mass will fall away from the cervix still attached to the anterior rectal wall. The cul de sac remains obliterated but has become simply an unimportant part of this mass. Severing the fatty lateral attachments of the rectum to the pelvic sidewall will expose the normal distal rectum as well as the lateral margins of the rectal nodule and lateral normal bowel wall. The rectum is progressively freed up from its fibrotic attachments to the sacrum and sidewalls using electrosurgery or scissors, guided in large part by finger palpation. The dissection should proceed immediately adjacent to the nodule, particularly when it is large and impinging on the sacrum, since this will help avoid damage to the nerves of the pelvic plexus which are illustrated in Chapter 17. Even unilateral damage to the pelvic plexus puts the patient at risk for permanent bladder atony. When the last posterolateral tendrils of fibrotic tissue attaching the lateral rectosigmoid colon to the pelvic sidewalls are severed, the rectum can suddenly be drawn up easily toward the incision.

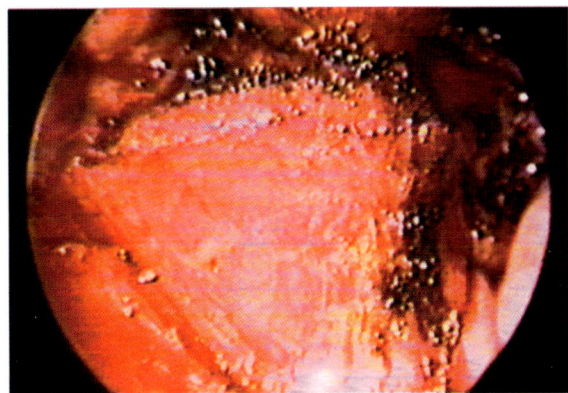

Figure 16.9

The intrafascial dissection down the posterior cervix has gone just past the level of the junction of the cervix with the posterior vagina, which area is seen at the top center of the frame. The surgeon will encounter a softer reddish layer of tissue which is the fascia of the posterior vaginal fornix. The rectovaginal septum lies just beyond this tissue

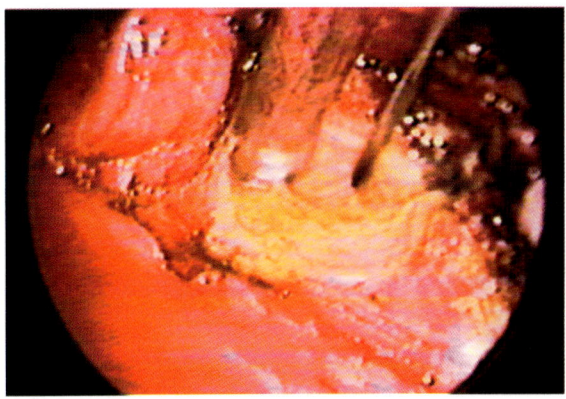

Figure 16.10

The tip of a plastic suction device is used to put the reddish fascial layer on stretch. It is then cut with the electrosurgical spatula, revealing the yellowish fatty tissue of the rectovaginal septum

Bowel resection for endometriosis

Endometriosis may be removed from the bowel by superficial, partial thickness, full thickness, or segmental bowel resection. Most patients will not require segmental bowel resection, bringing

SURGICAL MANAGEMENT OF ENDOMETRIOSIS

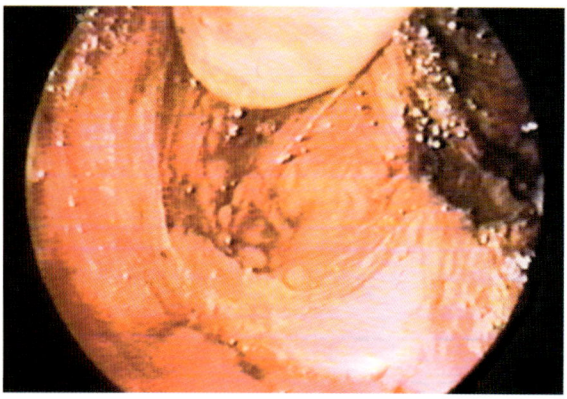

Figure 16.11

The surgeon's finger can be used to bluntly dissect down the rectovaginal septum, completing the separation of the rectal nodule from the posterior cervix and vagina

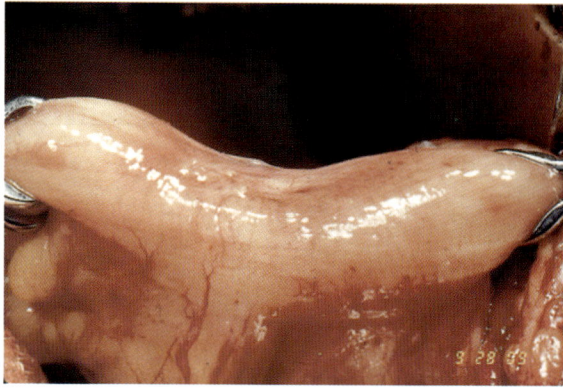

Figure 16.12

A segment of sigmoid colon is suspended between clamps. Notice the whitish nodule with surrounding erythema on the anterior antimesenteric surface. There is associated neovascularity extending to the mesentery

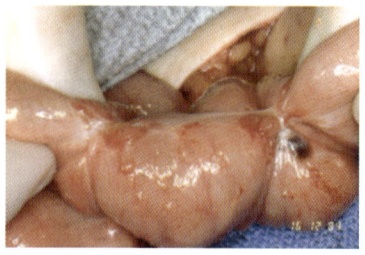

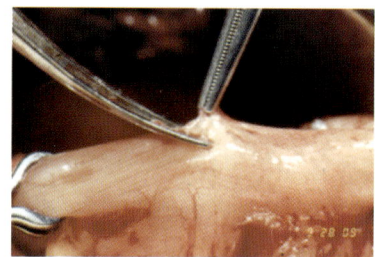

Figure 16.13

Endometriosis of the ileum is displayed between the surgeon's hands. Notice that the lesions occur primarily on the antimesenteric side of the bowel, with interlesional scarring resulting

Figure 16.14

The small superficial nodule of endometriosis of the sigmoid seen in Figure 16.12 is being removed. The nodule has been grasped and elevated while scissors are used to begin to incise normal bowel wall adjacent to the nodule

much bowel surgery for endometriosis into the province of the gynecologist. If full thickness or segmental bowel resection is anticipated, prophylactic antibiotics should be considered.

Endometriosis of the bowel, like pelvic disease, does not have a random distribution, but follows recurring patterns. Most intestinal endometriosis occurs on the antimesenteric sur- face of the bowel. Thus, the anterior surface of the rectum and sigmoid and the antimesenteric surface of the ileum (Figs 16.12, 16.13; 35 mm slides) are especially common patterns of sites of intestinal involvement.

Endometriosis of the bowel begins on the serosal surface with varying degrees of penetration into the muscularis. The mucosa is rarely

CONSERVATIVE EXCISION OF ENDOMETRIOSIS AT LAPAROTOMY

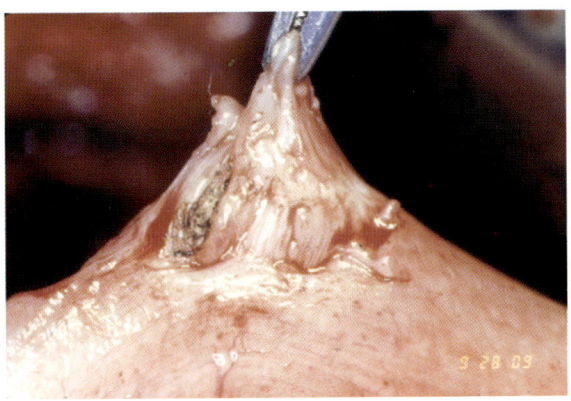

Figure 16.15
The sigmoid nodule has been partially escised. Notics the striations of the muscularis of the bowel wall. It often is possible to remove small nodules by partial thickness bowel resection carried down to the mucosa

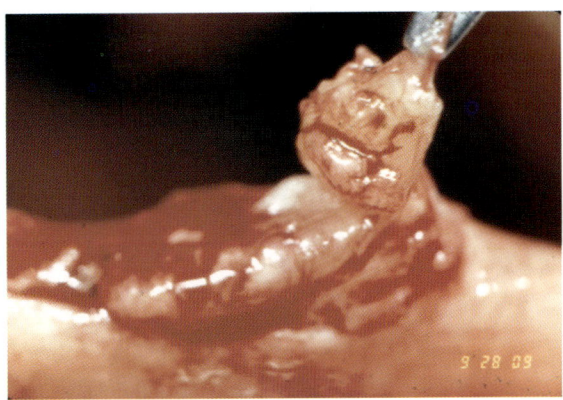

Figure 16.16
The sigmoid nodule has been almost completely removed. Notice that the defect left in the bowel wall is three to four times the diameter of the nodule which has been removed

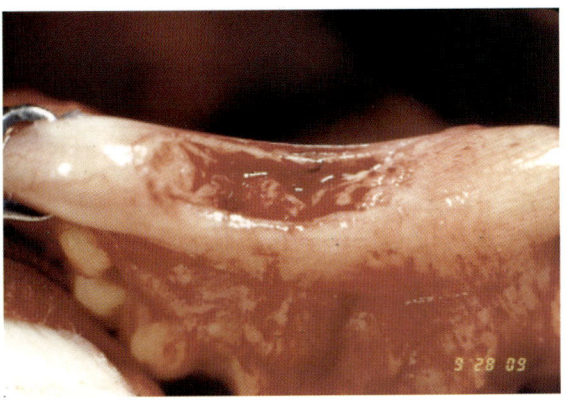

Figure 16.17
The sigmoid nodule has been completely removed. The mucosa is intact and the seromuscular layer of the bowel will be closed with interrupted 2–0 silk

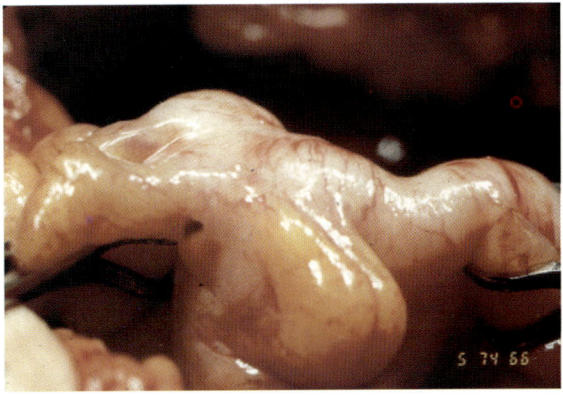

Figure 16.18
A large partially obstructing nodule of endometriosis of the sigmoid

involved. The layers of the bowel wall can frequently be peeled apart for removal of lesions without penetration into the bowel lumen.

When lesions are superficial, (Figs 16.14–16.17; 35 mm slides) they may be removed by simply picking them up with small tissue forceps and snipping underneath them with scissors. More invasive nodules will require deeper resections into the muscularis down to the mucosa and suture repair of the defect.

When a nodule is large, (Fig. 16.18; 35 mm slide) the submucosa can be involved by fibrosis related to endometriosis. In such a case, full thickness penetration of the bowel wall may be inevitable, even if the mucosa itself is uninvolved. (Fig. 16.19; 35 mm slide) The affected

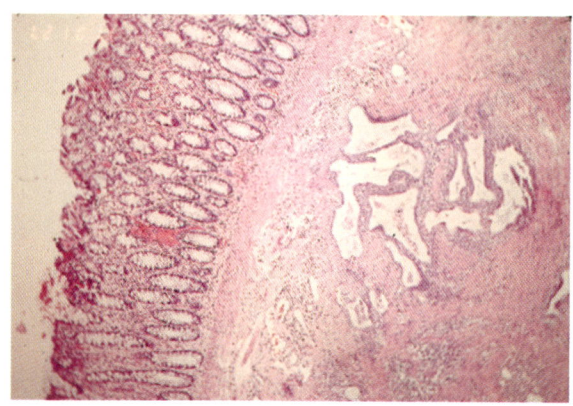

Figure 16.19
Histology of colonic endometriosis. The mucosa is seen to the left. The glands and stroma of endometriosis rarely penetrate through the mucosa. This lesion extends to the lamina propria. It is difficult to imagine how such lesions can be treated adequately or safely by thermal ablation techniques such as laser vaporization or electrocoagulation

area can be removed by disc resection and closed in two layers as illustrated in Chapter 12.

One of the interesting features of intestinal endometriosis is that the linear length of the defect left in the bowel wall after removal of a nodule will be from two to four times the diameter of the nodule. This is due to the gathering of the anterior bowel wall around the nodule. Defects up to 8 cm in length can be repaired without affecting bowel function. Double layer repair of larger defects is possible without affecting bowel function, but larger defects become increasingly tedious to repair. Segmental bowel resection will be preferable for extremely large nodules, since the huge anterior disc resection will leave only a small ribbon of posterior bowel wall which will be difficult to repair. Segmental resection will also be preferable when two or more sizeable nodules are adjacent along a length of bowel, since the repair of one defect can impede the repair of another. Segmental bowel resections will usually be done by general surgeons using techniques of their choosing. It is to be emphasized that the most difficult part of intestinal surgery for endometriosis is the pelvic dissection by the gynecologist to free up the lower rectosigmoid colon when obliteration of the cul de sac is present.

Endometriosis of the urinary tract

Invasive endometriosis of the ureter is rare. It will be apparent only when the ureter has been completely freed from all fibrosis and will be manifest as granularity of the wall of the ureter associated with obvious constriction of the ureter at that point. Segmental resection of the ureter with primary anastomosis is technically a very easy procedure. A ureteral stent will be necessary to ensure postoperative ureteral patency, since both the sutures used to repair the ureter as well as postoperative edema at the point of repair may cause temporary ureteral obstruction. This stent can be easily removed as an office procedure at six weeks. Some patients may have an impressive postoperative stent syndrome manifesting as debilitating ipsilateral renal colic during micturition which may necessitate early removal of the stent.

Endometriosis of the bladder is most frequently found on the serosal surface of the anterior cul de sac. Most endometriosis in this region is superficial and can be identified by traction on the peritoneum which will reveal the absence of a nodule in the bladder wall. Such disease can be removed by peritoneal resection. Invasive disease of the bladder muscularis will be identified when traction on the lesion reveals an underlying nodule which may not be apparent on initial visualization, while occasionally retractive fibrosis of the peritoneal surface may give evidence of invasive bladder disease. Excision of invasive bladder endometriosis will frequently require full-thickness resection even though the mucosa is rarely involved. All fibrotic tissue must be resected until only soft normal tissue remains behind. The bladder can then be repaired in one or two layers using absorbable suture. Although it is customary for urologists to recommend that a retention catheter be left in place for a week or two, this is not necessary if a watertight closure has been achieved and if the patient is able to void after removal of the catheter on the first or second postoperative day. Considering that general surgeons cannot stent the bowel after full-thickness or segmental bowel resections and anastomotic leaks of the bowel suture line rarely occur, the frequent urological recommendation to have a retention catheter in place for one to two weeks after full-thickness bladder repair seems unnecessary if a patient can void normally when the catheter is removed at the normal time.

Invasive endometriosis of the base of the bladder can result from extension of endometriosis from a uterosacral ligament nodule involving the ureter. Non-pliable fibrotic tissue will demarcate the extent of endometriosis in the wall of the bladder, and a partial cystectomy of the urinary bladder will be necessary, occasionally associated with repositioning of the ureter. Techniques for surgical treatment of endometriosis of the urinary tract are discussed in Chapter 13.

Postoperative care

Laparotomy for excision of endometriosis is usually associated with a three day stay in the hospital and recovery will be similar to any other laparotomy. If full-thickness or segmental bowel resection have been performed, the main difference will be in the timing of resumption of oral intake. For smaller full thickness resections, it may be advisable to delay beginning clear liquids until about 24 hours after completion of surgery and when bowel tones are present. If segmental bowel resection has been performed, it is advisable to delay oral intake until the passage of flatus. The diet can be graduated every two days thereafter, beginning with clear liquids, then full liquids including custard or pudding, then carbohydrates, then white meat, then diet as tolerated. The hospital stay following segmental bowel resection may range from four to seven days.

References

1. The American Fertility Society. Revised American Fertility Society classification of endometriosis. Fertil Steril 1985;43:351–4.
2. Doberl A, Bergqvist A, Jeppson S, Koskimies AI, Ronnberg L, Segerbrand E, Starup J. Regression of endometriosis following shorter treatment with, or lower dose of danazol. Acta Obstet Gynecol Scand 1984;123(Suppl):51–8.
3. Redwine DB. The distribution of endometriosis in the pelvis by age groups and fertility. Fertil Steril 1987;47:173–5.
4. Redwine DB, Wright JW, Mann C. RCT elitism. BMJ 2000;321:1077–8.
5. Benson K, Hartz. A comparison of observational studies and randomized, controlled trials. N Engl J Med 2000;342:1878–86.
6. Ioannidis JPA, Haidich A-B, Pappa M, Pantazis N, Kokori SI, Tektonidou MG et al. Comparison of evidence of treatment effects in randomized and nonrandomized studies. JAMA 2001;286:821–30.
7. Smith GVS. Endometrioma. A clinical and pathologic study of 159 cases treated at the clinic of the free hospital for women, Brookline, Massachusetts. Am J Obstet Gynecol 1929;17:806–14.
8. Wharton LR. Conservative surgical treatment of pelvic endometriosis. South Med J 1929;22:267–71.
9. Read CD, Roques F. After-results of the operative treatment of endometriomata – A study of forty-one cases. Proc Roy Soc Med 1929;22:1441–51.
10. Cattell RB, Swinton NW. Endometriosis. With particular reference to conservative treatment. N Engl J Med 1936;214:341–6.
11. Pemberton FA. Endometrioma of the female genital organs. New Engl J Med 1937;217:1–5.
12. Counseller VS. Endometriosis. A clinical and surgical review. Am J Obstet Gynecol 1938;365:877–88.
13. Payne FL. The clinical aspects of pelvic endometriosis. Am J Obstet Gynecol 1940;39:373–82.
14. Dannreuther WT. The treatment of pelvic endometriosis. Am J Obstet Gynecol 1941;41:461–74.
15. Holmes WR. Endometriosis. Am J Obstet Gynecol 1942;43:255–66.
16. Schmitz HE, Towne JE. The treatment of pelvic endometriosis. Am J Obstet Gynecol 1948;583–8.
17. Bacon WB. Results in 138 cases of endometriosis treated by conservative surgery. Am J Obstet Gynecol 1949;57:953–8.
18. Counseller VS, Crenshaw JL. A clinical and surgical review of endometriosis. Am J Obstet Gynecol 1951;62:930–9.
19. Meigs JV. Endometriosis. Etiologic role of marriage age and parity; conservative treatment. Obstet Gynecol 1953;2:46–53.
20. Fallon J, Brosnan JT, Manning JJ, Moran WG, Meyers J, Fletcher ME. Endometriosis: A report of 400 cases. Rhode Island Med J 1950;33:15–23.
21. Fayez JA, Vogel MF. Comparison of different treatment methods of endometriomas by laparoscopy. Obstet Gynecol 1991;78:660–5.
22. Beretta P, Franchi M, Ghezzi F, Busacca M, Zupi E, Bolis P. Randomized clinical trial of two laparoscopic treatments of endometriomas: cystectomy versus drainage and coagulation. Fertil Steril 1998;70:1175–80.
23. Redwine DB. Ovarian endometriosis: A marker for more severe pelvic and intestinal disease. Fertil Steril 1999;73:310–15.
24. Marconi G, Vilela M, Quintana R, Sueldo C. Laparoscopic ovarian cystectomy of endometriomas does not affect the ovarian response to gonadotropin stimulation. Fertil Steril 2002;78:876–8.
25. Redwine DB. The distribution of endometriosis in the pelvis by age groups and fertility. Fertil Steril 1987;47:173–5.

17

Endometriosis in distant sites
David B Redwine

Musculoskeletal endometriosis

Most cases of musculoskeletal endometriosis exist without evidence of pelvic disease. The symptoms and signs of disease follow a somewhat predictable course dictated by the anatomic site of involvement. Surgical treatment is most often successful.

Two cases of the posterior left thigh have been reported,[1,2] as well as two cases of the right thigh, one anteriorly,[3] and one laterally.[4] One case report of endometriosis of the right gluteus maximus exists.[5] The patients ranged in age from 24 to 36 and had noticed progressive pain or localized swelling over the course of months to years. Symptoms were typically worse during menses in most cases. Physical examination would typically show a hard, rubbery, often tender mass, in most cases, although computed tomography (CT) scan was required to diagnose a deeper lesion.[5] Local aggressive surgical excision was curative without the need for postoperative medical therapy in all but one case.[3] Cutaneous implantation of endometriosis in the surgical scar is possible.[5]

A 5 cm × 7 cm painful soft tissue mass posterior to the right fibular head which appeared over the course of seven months in a 32-year-old black woman was not associated with neuropathy or vascular involvement.[6] The pain and swelling increased during menses. Surgical exploration found the mass extended from the posterior head of the fibula under the lateral head of the gastrocnemius and completely surrounded the peroneal nerve. A biopsy showed endometriosis. The pain and swelling decreased quickly during danocrine therapy but recurred within two weeks of stopping treatment, but decreased again when treatment was resumed.

A 45-year-old nulliparous woman with right foot drop for six years developed a painful 8 cm × 15 cm swelling of the right lateral thigh.[7] CT scan showed that this connected through the obturator foramen with a pelvic soft tissue tumor. The thigh tumor was partially removed in two operations and gonadotropin-releasing hormone (GnRH) agonist therapy given for six months. This was associated with an increase in the size of the lateral thigh swelling as well as the size of the pelvic tumor by magnetic resonance imaging (MRI) scan. The serum CA–125 level was 1990 IU/ml. At reoperation, the right trochanter major was found to be invaded by the tumor, with extension into the marrow. The thigh tumor was almost completely removed, but the pelvic tumor was not. The ovaries were removed and were normal. Bleeding into the pelvic tumor several months later was associated with anemia and a CA–125 level of 10 232. She died two months later of suspected pulmonary embolus.

A 27-year-old nullipara noticed a small slightly painful lump of the left side of her neck which had been growing for about a year.[8] A 2 cm ovoid rubbery, mobile mass was removed and microscopy showed endometriosis in the secretory phase. Pelvic and pulmonary examinations were negative.

Inguinal canal endometriosis

Cullen, 1896, gave the first English-language report of endometriosis of the inguinal canal.[9] This entity usually represents nodular endometriosis (or 'adenomyoma') arising from the round ligament or from the fascial structures surrounding the external inguinal ring with surrounding fibromuscular metaplasia presenting as a painful tumor. Cullen mentions a similar case reported by von Recklinghuasen in the same year. Cullen's microscopic plates clearly indicate what would today be considered endometriosis. Because of the catamenial pain and the resemblance to eutopic endometrium, he postulated that the tumor rose from Müllerian rests.

Sampson later reported three cases of symptomatic inguinal endometriosis, the patients complaining of painful lumps of the groin which steadily grew in size with increased pain during menses. The preoperative diagnosis was inguinal hernia in two cases. Two were on the right side, and all were treated by local excision with good symptomatic relief. In one case, endometriosis was densely adherent to the femoral vein.[10] In only one of his cases was the adenomyoma attached to the round ligament and significant pelvic endometrosis was present in two of the women but none in the third. Because none of his cases had any direct contact with the peritoneal cavity or seemed to spring directly from the round ligament, he postulated vascular or lymphatic spread as the mode of origin.

A literature review of 30 cases,[11] and a series report of six cases,[12] indicate that 90% of inguinal endometriosis is right-sided, and 91% of patients have coexistent pelvic endometriosis.

A nodule can sometimes be misdiagnosed as an indirect inguinal hernia when it is present near the external inguinal ring. Occasionally, such nodules may be attached to the pubic tubercle,[13] and radiate pain toward the hip.

Endometriosis has also been reported in an inguinal lymph node,[14] as well as involving a superficial branch of the femoral vein,[15] both cases without coexisting inguinal endometriosis.

In virtually all cases of endometriosis of the groin region, the pathology has been recognized by physical examination alone. Treatment by local excision allows histologic diagnosis and produces symptomatic relief in virtually all cases, with recurrence being rare.

Central nervous system endometriosis

A 26-year-old woman had a five year history of generalized lower extremity muscle and pains with moderate lumbosacral pain radiating to the left leg for two years. Pain increased monthly about five days before menses. Headache, nausea, vomiting, stiffness of the neck and back and a fever caused hospital admission for suspected meningitis. Lumbar puncture showed normal pressure and red blood cells. A myelogram showed a mass at the level of L-1 and L-2. Laminectomy found a round tumor inside the dural sac on the left, measuring up to 1.5 cm in diameter. It was adherent to the roots of the cauda equina and two nerve roots were sacrificed for its removal. Photomicrographs illustrating the lesion show clear evidence of endometriosis. The pain was relieved although skin anesthesia in dermatomes L-1 and L-2 on the left side remained. Pain and myelogram evidence of recurrence of the tumor recurred within three months and the patient was treated with progesterone for symptomatic relief.[16]

A 27-year-old female peasant had progressively worsening lower extremity and lumbar pain for ten years. Weakness and dysuria eventually appeared and the patient eventually could not stand. MRI showed a tumor at the L-4 level of the spinal canal and at surgery the tumor was fused to the cauda equina so that complete removal was impossible. Microscopy confirmed endometriosis. Permanent danocrine therapy was begun and the patient was asymptomatic at two years follow-up.[17]

A 28-year-old woman had a two years history of cyclic low back and groin pain. MRI showed a mass 2.6 cm × 1.3 cm × 1.4 cm in dimension beneath the dura of the lumbar spinal canal. It was incompletely removed. Laparoscopy showed pelvic and intestinal endometriosis and gonadotropin-releasing hormone (GnRH) agonist therapy was administered for 12 months, with decreased pain resulting. Two years later a second operation was done for recurrent symptoms and a tumor 5 cm × 1.7 cm × 1.9 cm was found with involvement of the cauda equina. Total excision was completed and microscopy confirmed endometriosis. The uterus tubes and ovaries were removed and the patient was treated with postoperative androgen. Her cyclic pain and sphincter dysfunction resolved.[18]

A 20-year-old woman had a three year history of right sided occipital headaches unrelated to menses culminating in a severe headache and generalized seizure. An electroencephalogram showed generalized moderate slowing over the right temporal area. CT showed a well-circumscribed lesion of the right parietal area. Angiography showed the mass to be avascular. At craniotomy, a greenish-brown cystic lesion was seen on the surface of the parietal lobe, filled with thick chocolate-colored fluid. The entire lesion was excised and danocrine was given for six months. She appeared cured at one year after surgery.[19]

Peripheral nervous system endometriosis

Endometriosis on or near the sciatic nerve is the most common site of involvement of the peripheral nervous system by endometriosis. Approximately 90% of cases are right-sided. Patients may complain of pain in a sciatic distribution occurring just before and during menstruation, sometimes with motor dysfunction of the affected extremity.[20–24] The sciatic pain may become chronic in some. Endometriosis usually involves the pelvic portion of the roots of the sciatic nerve without actual invasion of the nerve, although cases of endometriosis within the sheath of the sciatic nerve after it exited the pelvis has been reported, with treatment through a skin incision over the right buttock.[20,25]

While three cases of successful medical treatment of sciatic endometriosis have been reported, one with danocrine,[26] another with GnRH agonist,[27] and the third with progestins[28] most cases have been treated surgically. At surgery, a pocket sign may be present (Fig. 17.1).[29] At the bottom of the pocket will be found a small fibrotic mass which will be adherent to the internal iliac vein near the bifurcation of the common iliac vein or to the roots of the sciatic nerve lateral to the vein, or to both (Fig. 17.2). Surgery by laparoscopy or laparotomy will be very difficult, and it is necessary to be acquainted with the anatomy of the deep pelvic sidewall and pelvic floor (Figs 17.3–17.7). The bottom of the pocket will not evert as will pockets of the cul de sac, because the nodule at the bottom of the pocket is firmly fused to underlying structures. In approaching the bottom of such a pocket laparoscopically, it is more efficient to make an incision posterior to the ureter and approach the bottom of the pocket from a medial direction (Fig. 17.3). Ligation of the internal iliac artery or vein may be necessary for

SURGICAL MANAGEMENT OF ENDOMETRIOSIS

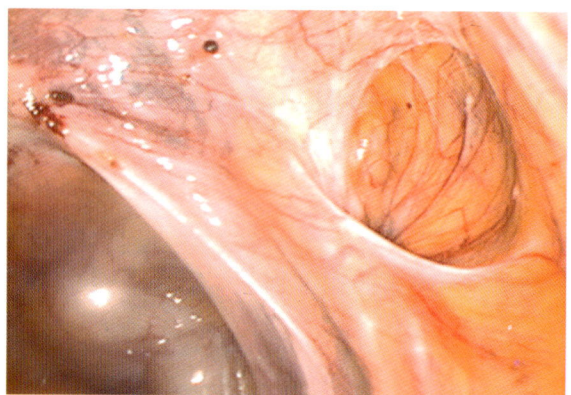

Figure 17.1
A pocket sign of the right broad ligament. The ureter forms the medial margin of the edge of the pocket opening. Small superficial hemorrhagic lesions of endometriosis are seen on the medial right broad ligament as well as on the right uterosacral ligament near its insertion into the posterior cervix

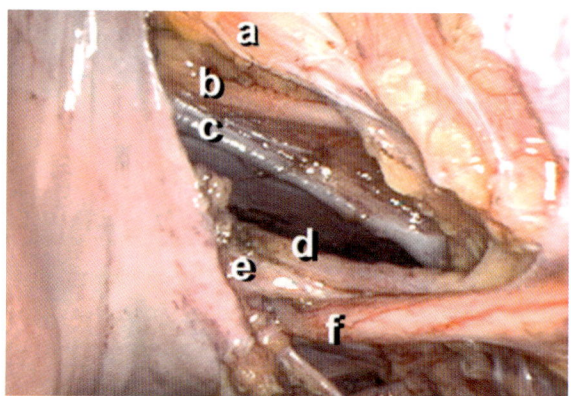

Figure 17.3
Normal anatomy of the right pelvic sidewall. The peritoneum has been opened: (a) areolar tissue which surrounds the right external iliac vein; (b) obturator nerve; (c) obturator vein; (d) hypogastric vein which is invested in some residual areolar tissue; (e) uterine artery; (f) ureter

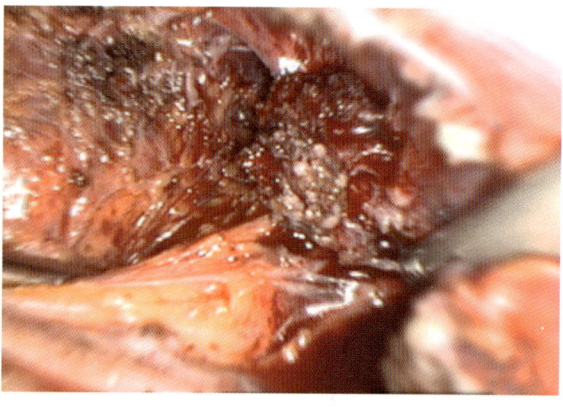

Figure 17.2
The tip of the suction-irrigator is at the posterior edge of a 1.5 cm nodular mass attached by dense fibrosis to the internal iliac vein, which is not clearly seen. The inferior roots of the sciatic nerve are hidden behind the nodule and the vein

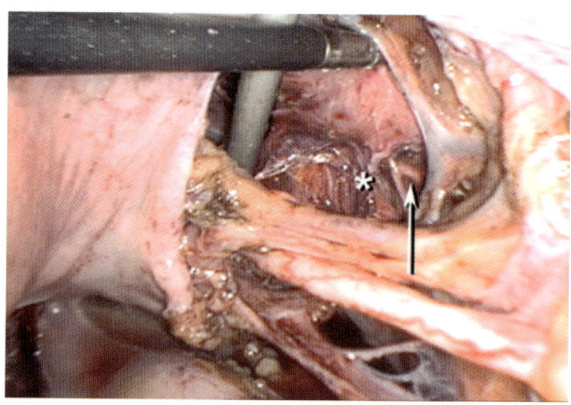

Figure 17.4
Same patient as in Fig. 17.3. The grasper is elevating the right obturator vein and the tip of the grasper is against the region of obturator internus. Note the obturator vein joining another more posterior vein to form a larger vein. The right ischial spine is hidden beneath tissue (*). The pudendal nerve (arrow) is seen traversing behind the ischial spine through the greater sciatic foramen. The roots of the sciatic nerve cannot be seen

proper exposure (Fig. 17.8). The fibrosis involving vascular structures can be intense and use of a cell-saver during surgery is recommended. The surgeon should be comfortable with repair of large arterial or venous structures with vascular suture material.

One case of endometriosis of the right obturator nerve treated by laparotomy has been reported (Fig. 17.9),[30] and another has since been encountered and treated laparoscopically.

ENDOMETRIOSIS IN DISTANT SITES

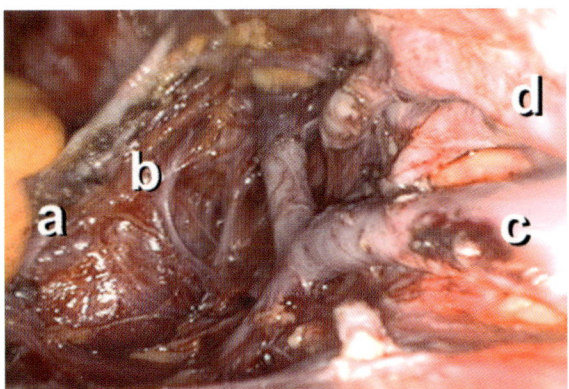

Figure 17.5
Deep view of the right posterior pelvis. (a) cut edge of peritoneum adjacent to right side of the rectum; (b) pelvic plexus; (c) right internal iliac vein; (d) right internal iliac artery. Anatomic variations are possible in this area

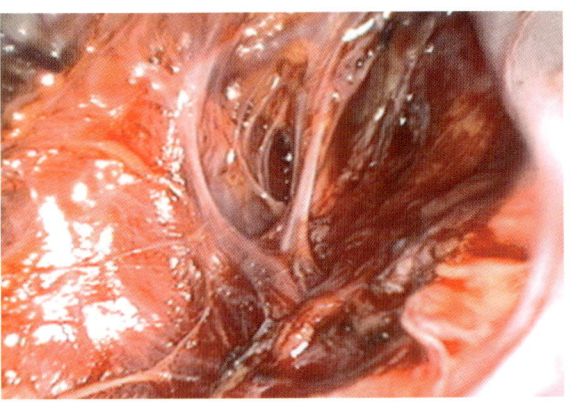

Figure 17.6
Close-up view of the right pelvic plexus. This neurological area is important for bladder and bowel function. Unilateral damage during dissection of endometriosis invading this area can result in permanent bladder atony

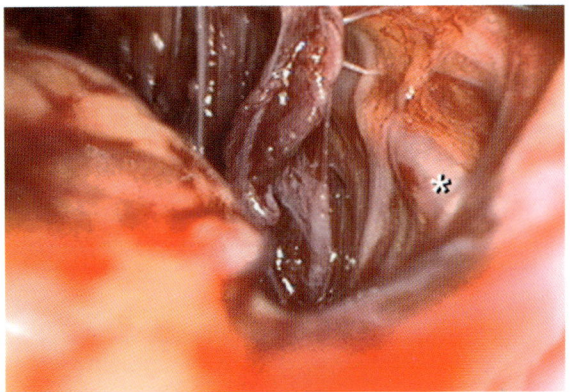

Figure 17.7
The right superior gluteal artery (✳) is seen leaving the pelvis through the greater sciatic foramen

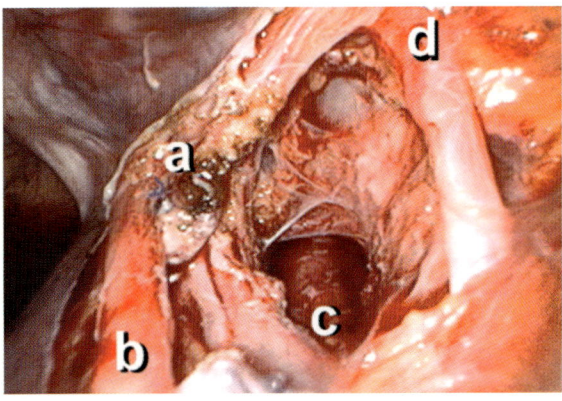

Figure 17.8
The anterior branch of the internal iliac artery, commonly called the hypogastric artery, has been ligated with blue Vicryl sutures (a), and divided to better investigate the posterior pelvic sidewall. The ureter is seen medially (b). A deep branch of the internal iliac vein (c), and the right obturator nerve (d), are also seen

In both cases, the nerve was encircled by endometriosis and fibrosis without invasion. Since the obturator nerve is shallower in the pelvis, it is easier to reach compared to the sciatic nerve. Fibrosis can be intense, but large vascular structures are rarely involved so the dissection for neurolysis is easier.

Liver endometriosis

Two cases of endometriosis of the liver have been reported in women aged 21 and 37 years.[31,32] Both patients presented with epigastric pain and the younger had episodic pain and

SURGICAL MANAGEMENT OF ENDOMETRIOSIS

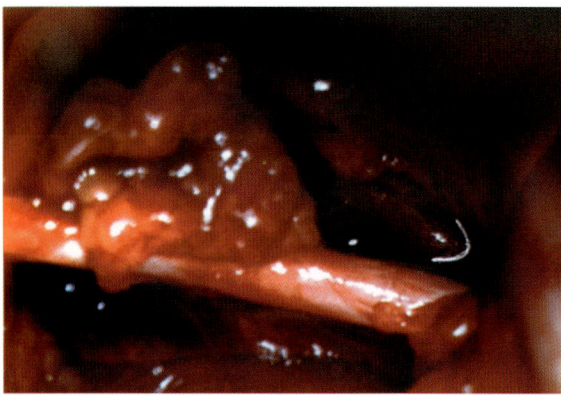

Figure 17.9
The right obturator nerve is seen as a white cord-like structure traversing the frame from left to lower right. The dissection of the nerve is almost complete. A fibrotic stricture around the nerve has already been released. Sitting atop the nerve is the fatty tissue infiltrated by endometriosis which has surrounded the nerve

nausea and vomiting. Examinations of the liver by CT and ultrasound scans were abnormal in both cases. Laparotomy was used to remove the cystic process from the left liver lobe in one patient, and from the right lobe in the other. Danocrine therapy was given postoperatively in both cases. The older patient also had a left ovarian endometrioma cyst and pelvic peritoneal endometriosis. The posterior edge of the right lobe of the liver as it joins the diaphragm can sometimes be superficially involved by endometriosis spreading from disease of the adjacent diaphragm.

One case of endometriosis of the pancreas has been reported.[33]

Cutaneous endometriosis

Most cases of cutaneous endometriosis present as tender nodules in surgical scars following surgery on the uterus, especially Cesarean section. The diagnosis is suggested by cyclic pain and tenderness during menses, with slow growth of the nodule in some patients over the course of months or years.[34–36] The lesions typically involve the rectus fascia on one side or another of low transverse incisions and may occasionally tract down toward the bladder. Actual connection with the uterus is rare. Treatment is by local excision, which will usually include a portion of rectus fascia. In cases of scar endometriosis following supracervical hysterectomy by laparotomy, a cervicocutaneous fistula of endometriosis surrounded by dense fibrosis may result, with symptoms of bleeding or discharge at the skin opening.[37] Treatment is by excision of the fistulous tract.

Endometriosis has been diagnosed in a needle tract 18 months following amniocentesis for midtrimester abortion in a woman taking oral contraceptives. She noted a midline lower abdominal wall mass which became tender during menses. She discontinued the pill after seven years but the size and character of the mass did not change. A biopsy confirmed endometriosis but the patient was lost to follow-up before complete excision could be arranged.[38] Transplantation of endometrium to the umbilicus occurred in 2 of 10 women who underwent laparoscopic hysterectomy with removal of strips of endometrium and myometrium through the unprotected umbilicus. Symptoms began two years after laparoscopic hysterectomy and included umbilical pain and cyclic swelling of the umbilicus. Diagnosis was obvious by a combination of physical examination, ultrasound, MRI and thin-needle aspiration. One of these women had undergone hysterectomy in the late luteal phase of the hormonal cycle, the other during menstruation. Local excision was performed in both cases.[39] Vulvar endometriosis has been reported in a nulligravida,[40] as well as in episiotomy scars.[41,42] Treatment is by local excision.

Thoracic endometriosis

Endometriosis in the thorax can involve either the parietal pleural surface or the parenchyma of the lung itself. Endometriosis of the pleural surface of the thorax occurs on the right in over 90% of cases and can be associated with chest pain associated with menses and shortness of breath.[43] Pneumothorax will occasionally occur. Some cases reported as thoracic endometriosis could actually be considered as diaphragmatic endometriosis. Almost 50% of patients in one retrospective review had coexisting pelvic endometriosis.[43] Treatment has usually been surgical, ranging from chest tube treatment of pneumothorax to thoracotomy with pleurectomy. Danocrine therapy was successful in one case.

Involvement of the lung parenchyma by endometriosis is uncommon and can cause painless or painful catamenial hemoptysis.[43–45] Bronchoscopy during an episode of hemoptysis helped isolate the responsible lung segment in one case with a presumptive diagnosis,[43] but was rather inconclusive in another.[44] One patient's symptoms worsened during estrogen therapy but improved somewhat with androgen therapy.[44] Simple chest x-rays have allowed diagnosis in two cases,[44,45] resulting in treatment by thoracotomy and segmental pulmonary resection.

Endometriosis in males

In older males with metastatic prostate cancer treated by orchiectomy and high dose estrogen therapy with chlorotrianisene, embryonic rests of Müllerian cells can be stimulated to bleed, sometimes heavily. Cystoscopy revealed ulcerated lesions of the bladder surrounding and obstructing the left ureter in one case in which transurethral resection was incomplete.[46] Hematuria did not respond to birth control pill therapy but eventually ceased when all hormonal therapy was stopped. Repeat cystoscopy showed a smaller mass beneath an intact mucosa. In another case where hematuria was investigated with cystoscopy, an ulceration near the right bladder dome was found and treated by segmental resection of the affected area of the bladder.[47]

One case of endometriosis of the prostate causing hematuria was diagnosed by transurethral resection in a 78-year-old man treated with chlorotrianisene after a diagnosis of prostatic cancer based on an abnormal prostate exam.[48] Adenocarcinoma of the prostate was not confirmed histologically and the patient died of a stroke at the age of 91.

Vicarious menstruation

Vicarious menstruation is the bleeding occurring during menses in an area remote from the uterus, such as the eye,[49,50] or nasal membranes. When disease processes, such as ulcerations, inflammation, or foreign bodies, have been ruled out, it is thought that vicarious menstruation may simply be due to the response of abnormally fragile capillary beds responding to the vasodilating effects of estrogen.[51]

References

1. Schlicke CP. Ectopic endometrial tissue in the thigh. JAMA 1946;132:445–6.
2. Giangarra C, Gallo G, Newman R, Dorfman H. Endometriosis in the biceps femoris. J Bone Joint Surg 1987;69:290–2.
3. Gitelis S, Petasnick JP, Turner DA, Ghiselli RW, Miller III AW. Endometriosis simulating a soft tissue tumor of the thigh: CT and MR evaluation. J Comput Assist Tomogr 1985;9:573–6.
4. Nunn LL. Endometrioma of the thigh. Northwest Med 1949;48:474–5.
5. Botha AJ, Halliday AEG, Flanagan JP. Endometriosis in gluteus muscle with surgical implantation. A case report. Act Orthop Scan 1991;62:497–9.
6. Patel VC, Samuels H, Abeles E, Hirjibiehedin PF. Endometriosis at the knee. A case report. Clin Orthop Rel Res 1982;171:140–4.
7. Oei SG, Peters AAW, Welvaart K, Bode PJ, Fleuren G-J. Aggressive endometriosis in bone. Lancet 1992;339:1477–8 (Letter).
8. Gennari L, Luciani L. Un caso di endometriosi del muscolo trapezio. Tumori 1964;51:361–5.
9. Cullen TS. Adeno-myoma of the round ligament. Johns Hopkins Hosp Bull 1896;7:112–14 (plus plates).
10. Sampson JA. Inguinal endometriosis. Often reported as endometrial tissue in the groin, adenomyoma in the groin, and adenomyoma of the round ligament. Am J Obstet Gynecol 1925;10:462–503.
11. Clausen I, Neilsen KI. Endometriosis in the groin. Int J Gynaecol Obstet 1987;25:469–71.
12. Candiani GB, Vercellini P, Fedele L, Vendola N, Carinelli S, Scaglione V. Inguinal endometriosis: Pathogenetic and clinical implications. Obstet Gynecol 1991;78:191–4.
13. Pellegrini VD, Pasternak HS, Macaulay WP. Endometrioma of the pubis: A differential diagnosis of hip pain. J Bone Joint Surg 1981;63:1333–4.
14. Mitchell AO, Hoffman AP. An unusual occurrence of endometriosis in the right groin: A case report and review of the literature. Mil Med 1991;156:633–4.
15. Recalde AL, Majmudar B. Endometriosis involving the femoral vein. South Med J 1997;70:69–74.
16. Lombardo L, Mateos JH, Barroeta FF. Subarachnoid hemorrhage due to endometriosis of the spinal canal. Neurology 1968;18:423–6.
17. Sun Z, Wang Y, Zhao L, Ma L. Intraspinal endometriosis: A case report. Chin Med J 2002;115:622–3.
18. Erbayraktar S, Acar B, Saygili U, Kargi A, Acar U. Management of intramedullary endometriosis of the conus medullaris. A case report. J Reprod Med 2002;47:955–8.
19. Thibodeau LL, Prioleau GR, Manuelidis EE, Merino MJ, Heafner MD. Cerebral endometriosis. Case report. J Neurosurg 1987;66:609–10.
20. Denton RO, Sherrill JD. Sciatic syndrome due to endometriosis of sciatic nerve. South Med J 1955;48:1027–31.
21. Hibbard J, Schreiber JR. Footdrop due to sciatic nerve endometriosis. Am J Obstet Gynecol 1984;149:800–1.
22. Salazar-Grueso E, Roos R. Sciatic endometriosis: A treatable sensorimotor mononeuropathy. Neurology 1986;36:1360–3.
23. Torkelson SJ, Lee RA, Hildahl DB. Endometriosis of the sciatic nerve: A report of two cases and a review of the literature. Obstet Gynecol 1988;71:473–7.
24. Liberman JS, Trelford J, Taylor R, Garrett V. Neurological deficits, back pain tied to endometriosis. JAMA 1983;249:686.
25. Baker GS, Parsons WR, Welch JS. Endometriosis within the sheath of the sciatic nerve. J Neurosurg 1966;25:652–5.
26. Richards BJ, Gillett WR, Pollock M. Reversal of foot drop in sciatic nerve endometriosis. J Neurol Neurosurg Psychiatr 1991;54:935–6.
27. DeCesare SL, Yeko TR. Sciatic nerve endometriosis treated with a gonadotropin releasing hormone agonist. A case report. J Reprod Med 1995;40:226–8.

28. Bjornsson OG. Cyclic sciatica of endometriosis. Case report. Acta Chir Scand 1976;142:4156.
29. Head HB, Welch JS, Mussey E, Espinosa RE. Cyclic sciatica. Report of a case with introduction of a new surgical sign. JAMA 1962;180:123–6.
30. Redwine DB, Sharpe DR. Endometriosis of the obturator nerve. J Reprod Med 1990;35:434–5.
31. Finkel L, Marchevsky A, Cohen B. Endometrial cyst of the liver. Am J Gastroenterol 1986;81:576–8.
32. Rovati V, Faleschini E, Vercellini P, Nervetti G, Tagliabue G, Benzi G. Endometrioma of the liver. Am J Obstet Gynecol 1990;163:1490–2.
33. Marchevsky AM, Zimmerman MJ, Aufes AH Jr. Endometrial cyst of the pancreas. Gastroenterology 1985;86:1589–91.
34. Kale S, Shuster M, Shangold J. Endometrioma in a cesarean scar: Case report and review of the literature. Am J Obstet Gynecol 1971;111:596–7.
35. Taff L, Jones S. Cesarean scar endometriosis. A report of two cases. J Reprod Med 2002;47:50–2.
36. Steck WD, Helwig EB. Cutaneous endometriosis. JAMA 1965;191:101–4.
37. Post op fistula: Hertzler AE. Surgical pathology of the female generative organs. Philadelphia: JB Lippincott, 1932; 225–51.
38. Kaunitz A, DiSant'Agnese PA. Needle tract endometriosis: An unusual complication of amniocentesis. Obstet Gynecol 1979;54:753–5.
39. Koninckx PR, Donders G, Vandercruys H. Umbilical endometriosis after unprotected removal of uterine pieces through the umbilicus. J Am Assoc Gynecol Laparosc 2000;7:227–32.
40. Healy JJ. Bilateral endometriosis of the vulva. Am J Obstet Gynecol 1956;72:1361–3.
41. Beischer NO. Endometriosis of an episiotomy scar cured by pregnancy. Obstet Gynecol 1966;28:15–21.
42. Hambrick E, Abcarian H, Smith B. Perineal endometrioma in episiotomy incision: Clinical features and management. Dis Colon Rectum 1979;22:550–2.
43. Foster DC, Stern JL, Buscema J, Rock JA, Woodruff JD. Pleural and parenchymal pulmonary endometriosis. Obstet Gynecol 1981;58:552–6.
44. Lattes R, Shepard F, Tovell H, Wylie R. A clinical and pathologic study of endometriosis of the lung. Surg Gynecol Obstet 1956;103:552–8.
45. Assor D. Endometriosis of the lung: Report of a case. Am J Clin Path 1972;57:311–15.
46. Pinkert TC, Catlow CE, Straus R. Endometriosis of the urinary bladder in a man with prostatic carcinoma. Cancer 1979;43:1562–7.
47. Oliker AJ, Harris AE. Endometriosis of the bladder in a male patient. J Urol 1971;106:858–9.
48. Beckman EN, Pintado SO, Leonard GL, Sternberg WH. Endometriosis of the prostate. Am J Surg Pathol 1985;9:374–9.
49. Abboud IA, Hanna LS. Bleeding from the conjunctiva. Br J Ophthal 1971;55:487–91.
50. Anderson RL. Bloody tears. JAMA 1987;257:1108.
51. Israel SL. Vicarious menstruation as an abnormal manifestation of the menstrual cycle. In: Israel SL (ed) Diagnosis and treatment of menstrual disorders and sterility. New York: Harper and Row 1963:213–16.

Subject index

Note. Page references in *italics* indicate figures/tables

A

'active electrode,' 62, 63
'add back therapy,' 28, 35, *36*
adenomyoma, 101, 226
adhesion barriers, 132
Allis clamps, 215, 216
American Fertility Society (AFS) classification system, 13, 211
anastrazole, 29
angiogenesis inhibitors, 30
appendiceal disease, 159, 160–161, *161*
    appendectomy, 167–168, *168*
    harmonic scalpel excision, 141, 144–145
'apple core' stricture, 72, *72*
arcus taurinus procedure, 102
argon beam coagulator (ABC), 103–104
argon lasers, 89–90
aromatase inhibitors, 29

B

barium enemas, 72, *72*
Berkson's fallacy, 4, 13–24, x
    menopause effects, 17–20
        pseudomenopausal treatment, 19–20, 133
    pregnancy effects, 13–17
        pseudopregnancy treatment, 15–17, 27
'Bicap' bipolar endocoagulator, 96
BiCoag dissecting forceps, 129
biopsies, 16
bipolar electrosurgery, 102–103
    monopolar *vs.*, 67–68
bladder endometriosis, 191–195
    coagulation/vaporization, CO_2 laser, 100–101
    diagnosis, 191–192
    excision, *192*, 192–195, *193*, *194*, *195*
        carbon dioxide laser, 121–122, *122*
        conservative, 222–223
        harmonic scalpel, 144, *146*, 146–147
        injury risk, 54–55
        laparotomy, 192, 222–223

physical examination, 50
symptoms, 191
blood tests, 50
blooming effect, 88, 110
blue-domed lesions, 76
bowel
    endometriosis of *see* intestinal endometriosis
    perforation risk, 91–92, 100, 160, 170
    pre-surgical preparation, 51, *51*, 73, 100, 141, 177
broad ligament, *228*
'burned out' disease, 57

C

cannulae, laser, 91
capacitive coupling, 65–67
carbon deposits, 56–57, *58*
carbon dioxide (CO_2) lasers, 87–88, 110
    advantages/disadvantages, 69, 71, 88, 95, 110
    beam distortion, 88
    coagulation/vaporization, 90–95, *91*, 129, 209
        deep infiltrating disease, 99–102
        early clinical results, 92
        initial experience, 90–92
        prospective trial, 93–95
        retrospective results, 93
    excision, 109–125
        cul de sac nodules, *121*, 121–122, *122*
        deep excision, no distortion, 115–117, *116*, *117*
        deep excision, with distortion, 117–123, *118*, *119*, *120*, *121*, *122*, *123*
        equipment, 111, *112*
        fiber, 129
        intestinal disease, 122–123, *123*
        ovarian endometriomas, *118*, 118–120, *119*, *120*
        room/patient set-up, 111, *112*
        simple excision, 113–115, *114*, *115*
        vaginal disease, *120*, 120–121, *121*
    historical perspective, 87, 109–110
    power density, 95, 110
    super-pulse/ultra-pulse systems, 88

carbon dioxide (CO_2) lasers (*cont.*)
   tissue effects, 90, 92, 110
   wavelength, 95
   see also individual anatomic structures
carcinoid tumor, 141
cecum, endometriosis, 158–159, 161, *161*
central nervous system, endometriosis, 226–227
Cesarean section scars, endometriosis, 230
chocolate cysts *see* ovarian endometrioma cysts
circuits, monopolar electrosurgery, 62
clinical trials
    laser laparoscopy, 93–95
    medical treatment, 31, *31*
Clostridium difficile, 51
coagulating shears, 138–139
   hook blade, *138*
coagulation
    coaptive, 137
    electrosurgical *see* electrosurgery
    harmonic scalpel, 137, 142
    laser *see* laser surgery
coagulation (modulated) current, 64, *64*
coaptive coagulation, 137
coelomic metaplasia theory of origin, 3
cold plasma coagulator, 104
colorectal endometriosis, 81–82, *82*, 166–167
computed tomography (CT), 72, 160, 170, 176
conservative excisional surgery, 211–224
Contact neodymium-yttrium-aluminium garnet laser *see* Nd: YAG laser
contraceptives, oral, 27
Crohn's disease, 162, *162*
cul de sac obliteration, 2, 163, *178*, *179*
   anatomic distribution, 76
   diagnosis, 160, *164*
   dyspareunia associated, 48
   excision
     carbon dioxide laser, *120*, *121*, 121–122
     conservative laparotomy, 216–219, *217*, *218*, *219*
     en bloc procedure, 179–181, *180*, *181*, *182*, *217*, *218*, *219*
     harmonic scalpel, 146
   histology, *179*
   physical examination, 50
   uterine manipulation, 51–52

cutaneous endometriosis, 230
cutting (unmodulated) current, 64, *64*
cytoscopy, 191–195

D

danazol, 19, 25–26, 32, 33–34
   infertility, 35
   post-surgery, 37, 38
deep infiltrating endometriosis, 99–102
   etiological factors, 99
diagnosis, 50
   bladder, 191–192
   cul de sac, obliteration, *164*
   diaphragm, *205*, 205–206, *206*
   differential, 49
   endometriomas, *149*, *164*
   intestinal, 160–164
   laboratory tests, 50–51
   rectovaginal, 177–178
   see also imaging scans; physical examination
diaphragmatic endometriosis, 205–210
   diagnosis, *205*, 205–206, *206*
   excision, *207*, *208*, *209*
     harmonic scalpel, 147, *147*
     laparotomy incisions, 55
   laser vaporization, 209
   symptoms, 48, 205
differential diagnosis, 49
'digital embossing,' 116, *116*
dioxin, 99
drug treatment *see* medical treatment
dwell time, 65
dyspareunia, 48

E

electrocoagulation *see* electrosurgery
electroexcision *see* electrosurgery
electrosurgery
   bipolar, 102–103
     monopolar *vs.*, 67–68
   electrocoagulation, 102–104
     argon beam coagulator (ABC), 103–104
     bipolar, 103
     cold-plasma coagulator, 104
     helica thermal coagulator, 104
     limitations, 68, 102–103

INDEX

excision, 71–86, 127
    disease distribution and, 74–77
    equipment, *74*
    laparoscopic entry technique, 73–74
    modality selection, 71–72
    monopolar, 68–69, *69*
    preoperative preparation, 73
    radical *see* radical laparoscopic endometrial excision (RLEE)
  monopolar *see* monopolar electrosurgery
  see also laser surgery; *specific techniques/instruments*
electrosurgical pencil, 215
electrosurgical scissors, 71–72
  hook scissors, 62–63, *63, 65*
en bloc excision, 77, 77–79, *78, 79*
endometrioma cysts *see* ovarian endometrioma cysts
endometriosis
  Berkson's fallacy and *see* Berkson's fallacy
  deep infiltrating disease, 99–102
  diagnosis *see* diagnosis
  differential diagnosis, 49
  disease distribution
    distant sites, 223–232
    pretreatment identification, 74–77
    see also specific regions affected
  etiological factors, 99, 177
  fertility and, 14–15
    see also infertility; pregnancy
  medical treatment *see* medical treatment
  menopause and, 17–18, 27
  origins, 7–8
    Sampson's theory *see* reflux menstruation
    transplantation theory, 30
  pregnancy and, 13–17, 21
  superficial disease, 114, 115–116, *116*
    electrocoagulation, 102–104
    intestinal, 165, *165*
  symptoms, 47–49
  visual identification, 56, *56*–58, *57*
epigastric vessels, *53, 54*
episiotomy scars, 230
estrogen–progestogen combinations, 27
estrogens, 27
ethylnorgestrienone (R2323), 28, 33, 35
etiological factors, 99, 177

Sampson's theory *see* reflux menstruation
European Quality of Life Questionnaire (EuroQoL), 82, *83*
Everest bipolar dissector, 144
examination *see* physical examination

F
fiber laser excision, 127–135
  equipment, 128–129
    see also Nd:YAG laser
  technique, 129–132, *130, 131*
    trocar placement, 129, *129*
'fibretom,' 89
forceps, BiCoag dissecting, 129

G
Gestrinone, 33, 35
gestrinone, 28
gluteal artery, 229
gonadotrophin-releasing hormone (GnRH)
  agonists, 19–20, 27–28, 33, *33*, 133
    pain relief, 34, *34*–35, *36*
    post-surgery, 37–38, *38*
    side-effects, 28
  antagonists, 29
Griffith's work, intestinal endometriosis, 158
groin, endometriosis, 226
Guilford double-blind trial of laser laparoscopy, 93–95

H
harmonic scalpel, 137–148
  blades, 137–140, *138, 139*
  coagulation, 137, 142
  excision, 142–147
    adherent ovary, 144
    appendix, 144–145
    bladder disease, *146*, 146–147
    cul de sac obliteration, 146
    diaphragmatic, 147, *147*
    external iliac, 144
    intestinal disease, 145, *145, 146*
    periureteral fibrosis, 144, *144*
    pneumodissection, 141, 142–143
    suturing, 143
    ureteral endometriosis, 142, 144, *144*

harmonic scalpel (cont.)
   foot pedal, 138
   generator, 138
   handpiece, 138
   patient inspection/documentation, 141–142
   safety considerations, 140–141
Hasson technique, 129–130
helica thermocoagulator, 104
helium-neon laser, 87
hemoptysis, 231
hemostasis, argon beam coagulator, 103–104
hepatic endometriosis, 229–230
hook scissors, 62–63, *63*, 65
Hudson technique, 129
hydrodissection, 113
hydronephrosis, 76, *76*, 195
hydroureteronephrosis, 48
hypogastric artery, *229*
hysterectomies, 99

I
ileal endometriosis, 159, *162*
   excision, 166, *166*, *167*, 220
     harmonic scalpel, 144
   laparotomy incisions, 55, *56*
imaging scans, 50–51, 72, *72*, 160, 170, 176
   see also specific modalities
immune system, problems, 5–6
incision placement, laparotomy, 55, *56*
infertility, 13–15, 20, 21
   medical treatment, 32, 35–37, *36*, *37*
inguinal canal, endometriosis, 226
insulation breaks, safety issues, 66–67
intestinal endometriosis, 157–173
   capacitive coupling risk, 66
   coagulation/vaporization, 100–101
   diagnosis, 160–164
   excision, 164–168, 219–222, *220*, *221*
     appendectomy, 167–168, *168*
     carbon dioxide laser, 122–123, *123*
     colon resection, 166–167
     complications, 169–171
     harmonic scalpel, 145
     ileal resection, 166, *166*, 167
     laparotomy, conservative, 219–222, *220*, *221*
     laparotomy, conversion to, 168–169, *169*
     mucosal skinning, 165–166, *166*
     postoperative care, 169
     preparation, 51, *51*, 73, 141, 177
     superficial lesions, 165
   histology, *222*
   historical case reports, 157–159
   perforations and, 91–92, 100, 160, 170
   sites of involvement, 159, *159*
     appendix *see* appendiceal disease
     cecum, 158–159, 161, *161*
     colorectal, 81–82, *82*, 166–167
     cul de sac *see* cul de sac obliteration
     ileum *see* ileal endometriosis
     sigmoid *see* sigmoid colon endometriosis
   symptoms, 48, 159–160
   see also rectovaginal endometriosis
intracorporeal knot tying, *165*
intravenous pyelogram (IVP), 72, 76

K
kidney, endometriosis, 201–202
Kocher clamp, 215
KTP lasers, 89–90, 96, *96*, 97

L
laboratory tests, 50–51
laparoscopy
   advantages, 127
   bladder surgery, 192–195
   conversion to laparotomy, 168–169, *169*
   deep infiltrating disease, 99–102, *101*
   electrosurgery and *see* electrosurgery
   entry technique, 73–74
   laser therapy and *see* laser surgery
   operative laporoscope, *91*
   radical excision *see* radical laparoscopic endometrial excision (RLEE)
   retrovaginal disease diagnosis, 177–178, *178*
   safety, 104–105
   suturing, 143
laparosonic coagulating shears, 138, *139*, 139–140, *143*
laparotomy
   conservative, 211–224
     bladder disease, 192, 222–223
     cul de sac obliteration, 216–219
     efficacy, 211–214

INDEX

intestinal resection, 219–222, *220, 221*
ovarian endometriosis, 215–216
patient preparation, *214,* 214–215, *215*
ureteral disease, 222
conversion to from laparoscopy, 168–169, *169*
incision placement, *55, 56*
postoperative care, 223
laser cannulae, 91
laser scalpels, 89, 128–129, *129*
laser surgery
adhesion formation, 98
coagulation/vaporization, 87–108, 137
deep infiltrating disease, 99–102, *101*
diaphragmatic endometriosis, 209
ovarian endometriomas, 95–98
coaptive, 137
excision, 69, 109–125, 127
fiber laser *see* fiber laser excision
history, 87, 109
lasers used, 87–90
see also specific lasers/techniques
levonorgestrel, 26, 32
add back therapy, 28
post-surgery, 38
liver, endometriosis, 229–230
Lockyer, Cuthbert, 157
Lumenis, Ultrapulse 'L' laser, 110, 111, *111*
lynestrenol, 26

M

magnetic resonance imaging (MRI), 50, 72, 160, 192
males, endometriosis, 231
matrix metalloproteinase inhibitors, 30
medical treatment, 25–45
clinical evidence, 31, *31*
efficacy, 31–33, 137
established treatments, 25–28
experimental treatments, 28–31
following surgery, 37–38
infertility, 32, 35–37, *36, 37*
pain relief, 32, 33–35, *36, 38, 39*
post-surgery, 37–38
pseudomenopausal regimen, 19–20, 133
pseudopregnancy regimen, 15–17, 27
see also individual drugs
medicolegal action, 171

medroxyprogesterone acetate (MPA), 26, 32–33
pain relief, 34
post-surgery, 37
side-effects, 26
menopause, 17–20, *21*
pseudomenopausal treatment, 19–20, 133
menstruation
reflux *see* reflux menstruation
vicarious, 231
mesoappendix, harmonic scalpel excision, 144–145
mestranol, 27
meta-analysis, 31
mifepristone, 28–29
modulated (coagulation) current, 64, *64*
monopolar electrosurgery, 61–70
circuits, 62
excision, 68–69, *69*
instrumentation, 62–63
power density, 61, 63–64, *64,* 68
safety, 65–68
bipolar *vs.*, 67–68
capacitance coupling, 65–67
dwell time, 65, 68
insulation breaks, 66–67
power settings, 65
waveforms, *64,* 64–65
'mucosal skinning,' 165–166, *166,* 183, 183–184, *184*
Müllerian epithelium, 2
musculoskeletal endometriosis, 225–226

N

nafarelin, 19, 202
natural killer cells, 6
Nd:YAG laser, 88–89
contact laser scalpels, 89, 128–129, *129*
fiber laser excision, 128–129
technique, 129–132, *130*
necrobiosis, 16
negligence, 171
neodinium-yttrium-aluminium-garnet laser *see* Nd:YAG laser
nervous system, endometriosis, 226–229
nodular *see* adenomyoma
nodules, isolated pelvic, 81, *81, 82*
norethindrone acetate, 26, *33*

norethynodrel, 27
Novak's coelomic metaplasia theory, 3, 7

O
obese patients, 214
obturator nerve, endometriosis, 228–229, 230
ONO-4817, 30
oophorectomy, 17–18
oral contraceptives (combination estrogen-progestogen), 27, 34, 38
ovarian endometrioma cysts, 2, 48, 149–156, 151
   coagulation/vaporization, 95–98, 96
      harmonic scalpel, 142
      results, 97–98
   diagnosis, 149, 164
   excision, 150, 150–154, 151, 152, 153, 154
      carbon dioxide laser, 118, 118–120, 119, 120
      conservative laparotomy, 215–216
      fiber laser, 131
      harmonic scalpel, 144
      radical laparoscopic, 80–81
   isolated nodules, 81, 82
   oophorectomy, 17–18
   ovarian remnant syndrome, 154–155, 155
   pathogenesis, 95
   symptoms, 149
ovarian remnant syndrome, 154–155, 155
ovaries
   adherent to pelvic sidewall, 144
   endometriosis see ovarian endometrioma cysts
   structure, 2

P
pain, 47–49, 97–98
   differential diagnoses, 49
   mapping, 127–128, 141–142
   'memory,' 94
   pelvic pain score, 36
   relief, 32, 33–35, 36, 38, 39
patient preparation, 47–59, 73
   bowel preparation, 51, 51, 73, 100, 141, 177
   laboratory tests and imaging scans, 50–51
      see also specific techniques
   physical examination see physical examination
   surgical considerations, 51–58
      laparotomy incision placement, 55

   patient positioning, 52
   trocar placement see trocar placement
   uterine manipulation, 51–52, 74
   visual identification, 56, 56–58, 57
patient support, 170–171
pelvic plexus, 219, 229
pelvis
   endometriosis symptoms, 47–48
   examination, 49–50
   pain score, 36
pentoxifylline, 30–31, 37
peripheral nervous system, endometriosis, 227–229, 228, 229, 230
peritoneum, 56, 56–57, 57
periuretal fibrosis, 144, 144, 197
'peri-visceritis,' 188
physical examination, 49–50, 72
   bladder, 50
   cul de sac, 50
   pre-harmonic scalpel surgery, 141–142
   rectovaginal, 50, 176, 176–177
   umbilicus, 49, 49
   uterosacral ligament, 50, 72, 74, 74
   uterus, 50, 51–52
   vaginal, 49, 49–50
pleural surface, endometriosis, 231
plume, abdominal, 112–113
pneumodissection, 141, 142–143
pneumothorax, 231
pocket sign, 227, 228
polychlorinated biphenyls, 99
postoperative care, laparotomy, 223
potassium titanyl phosphate (KTP) lasers, 89–90, 96, 96, 97
pouch of Douglas, 74, 176
'powder burn' lesion, 114
power density
   carbon dioxide lasers, 95, 110
   monopolar electrosurgery, 63–64, 64, 68
   calculation, 61
pregnancy, 13–17, 21
   endometriosis and fertility, 14–15
   endometriosis prophylaxis, 13–14
   endometriosis 'treatment,' 14, 15
preparation of patient see patient preparation
progesterone receptor modulators, 28–29, 38

progestogens, 26–27, 32
  see also specific drugs
prostrate cancer, male endometriosis, 231
pseudocyst, ovarian, 153–154
pseudomenopausal endometriosis, 17–18
pseudomenopause treatment, 19–20, 133
pseudopregnancy, 15–17, 27

R
radical laparoscopic endometrial excision (RLEE), 77–84, *83*
  colorectal endometriosis, 81–82
  en bloc excision, 77, *77–79*, *78*, *79*
  isolated nodules, 81, *81*, *82*
  ovarian endometriomata, 80–81
  results and reoperation, 82–84, *84*, *85*
  variations, 79–80, *80*
raloxifene, post-surgery, 38
randomized clinical trials (RCTs), 31
  Guildford study, laser laparoscopy, 93–95
rectal manipulator, 122–123
rectosigmoid colon endometriosis, 160, 184–186, *185*, *186*, *187*
  harmonic scalpel excision, 145, *145*, *146*
  see also cul de sac obliteration
rectovaginal endometriosis, 75, 128, 175–190
  coagulation/vaporization, 101
  cul de sac obliteration see cul de sac obliteration
  diagnosis, laparoscopic, 177–178, *178*
  etiology and pathogenesis, 177
  excision, 179–188
    carbon dioxide laser, *116*, 116–117, *117*, *123*, 188
  physical examination, 50, *176*, 176–177
  presentation, 175–176
  see also intestinal endometriosis; vaginal endometriosis
rectum see colorectal endometriosis; rectovaginal endometriosis
reflux menstruation, 1–11, ix–x
  dangers of theory, 6–7
  immune system arm, 5–6
  peritoneal circulation, 4–5
renal endometriosis, 201–202
retroperitoneal fibrosis, 132, *154*, 196–197, *198*
RLEE see radical laparoscopic endometrial excision (RLEE)

RU486, 28–29
Runge/Hughesdon/Brosens pseudocyst, 153–154

S
safety, electrosurgery, 65–68
Sampson's theory of reflux menstruation see reflux menstruation
scalpels
  harmonic see harmonic scalpel
  Nd:YAG laser, 89, 128–129, *129*
  power application, 61
scar tissue, endometriosis, 230
sciatic nerve, 227–228, *228*, *229*, 230
scissors see electrosurgical scissors
selective progesterone receptor modulators (SPRMs), 28–29, 38
Sexual Activity Questionnaire (SAQ), 82, *83*
sigmoid colon endometriosis, 162–163, *163*
  excision, 81–82, *220*, *221*
  see also rectosigmoid endometriosis
skin, endometriosis, 230
spinal cord, endometriosis, 226–227
Spraygel, 132
subcutaneous emphysema, 52, *52*
super-pulse/ultra-pulse systems, 88
support, patient, 170–171
surgical techniques, 127
  electrosurgery see electrosurgery
  laser surgery see laser surgery
  see also specific techniques
Swiftlase carbon dioxide laser, 88

T
tampons, dioxin pollution and, 99
'thermal blooming,' 88, 110
thoracic endometriosis, 231
T lymphocytes, dioxin pollution and, 99
tonsil clamps, 215, *216*, *217*, *218*
traction, 113–114, *114*
traction suture, 215, *215*
transabdominal ultrasound, 72
transplantation theory, 30
transrectal ultrasound, 50, 72
trocar placement, 52–55, *53*, *54*, *55*
  fiber excision sites, *129*, 129–132
tumor necrosis factor-α (TNFα) inhibitors, 30

U

Ultrapulse 'L' laser, 110, 111, *111*
ultrasound
    diagnostic scans, 50, 72
    excision *see* harmonic scalpel
umbilical endometriosis
    physical examination, 49, *49*
    post-surgical, 230
    symptoms, 48–49
    trocar insertion, 52–55, *53*
unmodulated (cutting) current, 64, *64*
ureteral endometriosis, 48, 76, *76*, 77, 195–201
    excision, *196*, *197*, *198*, *199*, *200*, *201*, *202*
        conservative laparotomy, 222
        harmonic scalpel, 142, 144, *144*
    superficial, *131*
urinary tract endometriosis, 191–203, 222–223
    bladder *see* bladder endometriosis
    incidence, 128
    kidney (renal), 201–202
    laparotomy, 192, 222–223
    ureter *see* ureteral endometriosis
uterosacral ligament
    endometriosis involvement, *131*, 151
        excision, 78, *78*, 100, *199*, 216
        nodules, 100
    physical examination, 50, 72, 74, *74*
uterus
    manipulation, 51–52, 74, *74*, 129
    physical examination, 50, 51–52

V

vaginal endometriosis, 74–76, 128, 180–183, *183*
    carbon dioxide laser therapy
        coagulation/vaporization, *101*, 101–102
        excision, *120*, 120–121, *121*
    diagnosis, 160
    posterior fornix, 74–75, *75*, 80, *80*, 176
        physical examination, *49*, 49–50
    see also rectovaginal endometriosis
Valchev uterine manipulator, 74, *74*
vaporization, laser *see* laser surgery
vascular endothelial growth factor (VEGF), 30
Veress needle technique, 73–74
vicarious menstruation, 231
visual identification of disease, 56, 56–58, *57*
vulvar endometriosis, 230

W

waveforms, electrosurgical, 64–65
    modulated (coagulation) current, 64, *64*
    unmodulated (cutting) current, 64, *64*